Antidotes

Robert J Flanagan PhD FRCPath
Consultant Biochemist

Alison L Jones MD FRCP(E)
Consultant Physician and Consultant Clinical Toxicologist

Guy's and St Thomas' Hospital Trust, London

With a section on Antidotes and Chemical Warfare by

Timothy C Marrs MD DSc FATS MRCP FRCPath
Food Standards Agency

and

Robert L Maynard CBE MRCP FRCPath
Department of Health, London

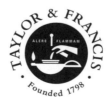

London and New York

First published 2001
by Taylor & Francis
11 New Fetter Lane, London EC4P 4EE

Simultaneously published in the USA and Canada
by Taylor & Francis Inc,
29 West 35th Street, New York, NY 10001

Taylor & Francis is an imprint of the Taylor & Francis Group

© 2001 Robert J Flanagan, Alison L Jones

Typeset in Baskerville by
Prepress Projects Ltd, Perth, Scotland
Printed and bound in Great Britain by
TJ International, Padstow, Cornwall

Every effort has been made to ensure that the advice and information
in this book is true and accurate at the time of going to press.
However, neither the publishers nor the authors can accept any legal
responsibility or liability for any errors or omissions that may be
made. In the case of drug administration, any medical procedure or
the use of technical equipment mentioned within this book, you are
strongly advised to consult the manufacturer's guidelines.

British Library Cataloguing in Publication Data
A catalogue record for this book is available from the British Library

Library of Congress Cataloging in Publication Data
A catalog record for this book has been requested.

ISBN 0–748–40965–3

[Hermes to Odysseus] Look; here is a drug of real virtue that you must take with you into Circe's palace to save yourself from disaster. But I must explain how she works her black magic. She will begin by mixing you a pottage, into which she will put her poison. But even with its help she will be unable to enchant you, for this antidote that I am going to give you and describe will rob it of its power. When Circe strikes you with her long wand, you must draw your sword from your side and rush at her as though you meant to take her life. She will shrink from you in terror and invite you to her bed. Nor must you hesitate to accept the goddess' favours, if you want her to free your men and treat you kindly. But make her swear a solemn oath by the blessed gods not to try on you any more of her tricks, or when she has you stripped she may rob you of your courage and your manhood.

Then the Giant-killer handed me a herb he had plucked from the ground, and showed me what it was like. It had a black root and milk-white flower. The gods call it Moly, and it is an awkward plant to dig up, at any rate for a mere man. But the gods, can do anything.

Homer, *The Odyssey*. Translated by EV Rieu.
London: Penguin Books, 1946, p. 163

Contents

Acknowledgements

We thank Dr Tim Marrs and Dr Bob Maynard for contributing Chapter 7 and for help with parts of Chapters 5 and 6, and Helaina Checketts (Medical Toxicology Unit Librarian), the staff of the Wellcome Library for the History of Medicine, Dr Jenny Pronczuk de Garbino (World Health Organization), Dr Paul Dargan, Dr Roy Goulding, Dee Cook (Archivist to the Society of Apothecaries), John Ramsey, Lynn Saliba and the staff of the British Library, John Trestrail, Dr Katherine Watson, Dr Paul Wax and Dr David Zuck for assistance.

Preface

The aim of this book is to provide up-to-date information on the development and clinical use of antidotes, their proposed mechanism of action, toxicity and availability and practical aspects of their clinical use. The antidotes discussed are primarily those either in current use or under consideration or development. Some other compounds of mainly historical interest are also mentioned where appropriate.

Like any other ideal drug, the ideal antidote would be selective in action, efficacious, non-toxic, easy to administer by lay personnel using a minimum of special apparatus, cheap and have a long shelf-life. Unfortunately, like most drugs, most antidotes present various problems in supply and in use, as will become evident in the ensuing pages.

The book contains information on the antidotal treatment of poisoning with substances encountered in not only Western Europe/North America/Australasia, but also developing countries. We cover doses and routes of administration, and also instances where antidote administration complicates or compromises toxicological analyses. The reader is referred to standard toxicological texts for detailed information on the diagnosis and management of poisoning.

Most antidotes differ from other drugs not only in the way they are used, but also in the way in which their efficacy and toxicity can be assessed. Antidotes used to treat acute poisoning are usually used only in life-threatening situations, and then as only a single dose or short course of treatment. For many antidotes, detailed toxicity data such as required for most drugs used chronically are not available. Indeed, many antidotes, particularly older ones, were introduced into clinical practice after minimal animal toxicity studies. Furthermore, randomized clinical trials of antidote use are rarely possible in acutely poisoned patients. Although trials in patients can be designed, these often use historical controls or patient groups treated conventionally, and therefore the results may be difficult to interpret. Consequently, the investigator is more than usually reliant on animal studies when attempting to develop new antidotes.

Despite much research, no effective treatment (antidotal or otherwise) exists for a number of common poisons. The need for antidotes effective in the later stages of paracetamol (acetaminophen) poisoning (section 4.16.1) and in paraquat poisoning (Chapter 8) is clear. Even when effective antidotes are known, the questions of clinical diagnosis and appropriate use of the antidote remain, as does the logistic problem of availability and supply of less commonly used or expensive antidotes. Against this background it is perhaps not surprising that inappropriate use of existing antidotes and use of obsolete compounds still continues. We hope that this volume will help encourage (i) proper use of existing antidotes, (ii) recognition of their potential toxicity and (iii) the development of more effective, safer compounds with a long shelf-life where needed.

Few books have been devoted to antidotes. This volume is aimed at research workers, staff of poisons information centres, drug information pharmacists, clinical toxicologists and veterinary surgeons. It should also be of interest to medical students, trainee pharmacists, emergency physicians and anaesthetists. The references have been verified from original sources as far as possible, even to 1585.

Foreword

In times past, when poisoning was probably a more common hazard than it is today and when wilful poisoning was more likely to be perpetrated, much effort was directed to fashioning antidotes and, above all, to obtaining one that was 'universal' in its action. Most of the compounds so devised, often secretly and to the accompaniment of much ceremony, were in all likelihood little more than palliatives. Yet, even to this day, it is a popular belief than recovery from poisoning rests upon antidotes.

Yet, if this concept is seldom realized in practice, there is still a place for specific antidotes in clinical toxicology, so long as they are rationally designed and are used with understanding and discrimination. That is where this book offers valuable guidance, listing as it does the recognized antidotes and setting out the indications for their use, together with their limitations.

Invaluable as this text can be educationally, it may well prove indispensable to accident and emergency departments, besides serving as a reminder to pharmacies as to the antidotes that may be needed in treating poisoned patients.

Roy Goulding BSc MD FRCP FRCPath OBE
London
February 2001

Antidote Nomenclature and Dosage

Names of drugs and poisons change with time and often differ between countries. We have tried to use current international approved names for pharmaceuticals, but so many subtle changes have been introduced in recent years (use of mesilate rather than mesylate for methanesulphonate, for example) that it has been impossible to include every new name. However, we have given Chemical Abstracts Service (CAS) Registry Numbers (RN) whenever possible (and when appropriate tried to make it clear which numbers refer to salts, hydrates, racemates, etc., another frequent cause of confusion). Similarly, when discussing dosages we have tried to be clear when referring to salts, etc. and when to free bases. However, we would still consider cross-referral to an appropriate local or national formulary mandatory before any patient treatment is initiated.

Abbreviations

AACT	American Academy of Clinical Toxicology
AAG	α_1-acid glycoprotein
ACE	angiotensin-converting enzyme
AChE	acetylcholinesterase
ACTH	adrenocorticotrophic hormone
ADH	alcohol dehydrogenase
A&E	accident and emergency department
AIDS	acquired immune deficiency syndrome
ALDH	aldehyde dehydrogenase
cAMP	3',5'-cyclic adenosine monophosphate
ANTU	1-naphthalenylthiourea
4-AP	4-aminopyridine
ARDS	adult respiratory distress syndrome
ATA	aurintricarboxylic acid
BAL	British anti-lewisite (dimercaprol)
BGDTC	N-benzyl-D-glucaminedithiocarbamate
BH-6	obidoxime dichloride (see Table 5.1)
BSO	buthionine sulphoxamine
CAS	Chemical Abstracts Service
CDTA	1,2-cyclohexanediaminetetra-acetate
CNS	central nervous system
COHb	carboxyhaemoglobin
CP20	deferiprone
CS	2-chlorobenzilidene malononitrile
CSF	cerebrospinal fluid
CSL	Commonwealth Serum Laboratories (Australia)
DAM	diacetylmonoxime
DBcAMP	dibutyryl 3',5'-cyclic adenosine monophosphate
DEDTC	diethyldithiocarbamate
DFO	deferoxamine (desferrioxamine)
DFP	di-isopropyl phosphofluoridate
DHEDTC	diethyldithiocarbamate
DMAP	4-(N,N-dimethylamino)phenol
DMHP	1,2-dimethyl-3-hydroxypyridin-4-one (deferiprone)
DMPA	N-(2,3-dimercaptopropyl)phthalamidic acid
DMPS	sodium D,L-2,3-dimercaptopropanesulphonate
DMSA	meso-2,3-dimercaptosuccinic acid
DTPA	diethylenetriaminepenta-acetate (pentetic acid)
EAPCCT	European Association of Poisons Centres and Clinical Toxicologists
ECG	electrocardiogram
EDTA	ethylenediaminetetra-acetate
EEG	electroencephalogram
EHBP	etidronic acid
EHDP	etidronic acid

EHPG	ethylene bis-2-hydroxyphenylglycine
ELISA	enzyme-linked immunosorbent assay
FDA	US Food and Drug Administration
Fio_2	proportion of oxygen in inspired air
G6PDH	glucose-6-phosphate dehydrogenase
GABA	γ-aminobutyric acid
GCS	Glasgow coma scale
GF	cyclosarin
GFR	glomerular filtration rate
GM-CSF	granulocyte–macrophage colony-stimulating factor
GSH	reduced glutathione
GSSG	oxidized glutathione
H	bis(2-chloroethyl)sulphide (sulphur mustard, 'mustard gas')
Hb	haemoglobin
HBED	N,N'-bis(2-hydroxybenzyl)ethylenediamine-N,N'-diacetic acid
HBO	hyperbaric oxygen
HD	bis(2-chloroethyl)sulphide
HI-6	asoxime dichloride (see Table 5.1)
HIV	human immunodeficiency virus
HJ-6	asoxime dichloride (see Table 5.1)
HMP	hexose monophosphate pathway
HMT	hexamethylenetetramine
5-HT	5-hydroxtryptamine
i.m.	intramuscular
INR	international normalized ratio
i.p.	intraperitoneal
IPCS	International Programme on Chemical Safety
iPTH	immunoreactive parathyroid hormone
ITU	intensive treatment unit
i.v.	intravenous
L1	deferiprone
LD_{50}	median lethal dose
LFT	liver function test
LSD	lysergic acid diethylamide
LüH-6	obidoxime dichloride (see Table 5.1)
MAOI	monoamine oxidase inhibitor
MBGDTC	N-(4-methoxybenzyl)-D-glucaminedithiocarbamate
MDA	methylenedioxyamphetamine
MDEA	methylenedioxyethylamphetamine
MDMA	methylenedioxymethylamphetamine
MESH	Medical Subject Headings
4-MP	4-methylpyrazole (fomepizole)
NAC	N-acetyl-L-cysteine
NAPA	N-acetyl-D,L-penicillamine
NAPQI	N-acetyl-4-benzoquinoneimine
NBO	normobaric oxygen
NMDA	N-methyl-D-aspartate
NPIS	National Poisons Information Service (UK)

OP	organophosphorus
OPs	organophosphorus compounds
2-PAM	pralidoxime iodide (see Table 5.1)
2-PAMCl	pralidoxime chloride (see Table 5.1)
2-PAMI	pralidoxime iodide (see Table 5.1)
2-PAMM	pralidoxime methanesulphonate (see Table 5.1)
PAPP	4-aminopropiophenone
PIH	pyridoxal isonicotinoyl hydrazone
PNU	N-3-pyridylmethyl-N'-(4-nitrophenyl)urea
p.o.	by mouth
P_2S	pralidoxime methanesulphonate (see Table 5.1)
PS-ODN	phosphorothioate oligodeoxynucleotide
RN	(CAS) Registry Number
SAH	S-adenosyl-L-homocysteine
SAIMR	South African Institute of Medical Research
SAM	S-adenosyl-L-methionine
s.c.	subcutaneous
SSRIs	selective serotonin reuptake inhibitors
TEPP	tetraethylpyrophosphate
TETA	triethylenetetramine
TECZA	triethylenetetramine
THP-12-aneN$_4$	N,N',N'',N'''-tetrakis(2-hydroxypropyl)1,4,7,10-tetraazacyclododecane
TNF-α	tumour necrosis factor α
TP	thiopronine
TCA	tricyclic antidepressant
V_D	volume of distribution
VX	O-ethyl-S-[2-(diisopropylamino)ethyl]methyl phosphonothioate
WHO	World Health Organization
w/v	weight per volume
w/w	weight for weight

General Introduction

Contents

1.1 INTRODUCTION

Most poisoned patients recover with little more than reassurance and/or supportive care. In more severe cases of poisoning, supportive measures directed particularly at the cardiovascular and respiratory systems may be required. Measures to promote the elimination of drugs or other poisons from the body are not often indicated, and antidotal therapy, if available, is rarely needed except in the treatment of paracetamol (acetaminophen) poisoning. However, the administration of an antidote can be life-saving in the appropriate circumstances and may also help reduce morbidity and also health care costs by shortening the duration of treatment. Some antidotes suggested for use in the treatment of some common types of poisoning are listed in Appendix 1.

In clinical practice, the word 'antidote' tends to be used to denote specific drug therapy for poisoning with a poison or group of poisons. Substances such as activated charcoal, which is given in the first instance to prevent absorption of poison(s), or diuretics such as frusemide (furosemide), which is given to maintain or enhance urine flow and thus aid excretion of water-soluble poisons, tend not to be termed antidotes (Tables 1.1 and 1.2). This said, it is perhaps not surprising that there is no generally accepted definition of an antidote. A World Health Organization (WHO) Working Group has proposed the definition 'a therapeutic substance used to counteract the toxic action of a specified xenobiotic' (Meredith *et al.*, 1993a; Pronczuk de Garbino *et al.*, 1997). This is a very broad definition, and encompasses nearly all of the drugs and other agents used to treat poisoning (see Meredith *et al.*, 1984), as does the Index Medicus *Medical Subject Headings* (MESH) definition: 'agents counteracting or neutralizing the action of poisons'. An alternative definition is 'a substance used to treat poisoning which has a specific effect depending on the poison'.

Definition of an antidote

- 'Medicine given to counteract the action of poison' (*Shorter Oxford Dictionary*)
- 'Therapeutic substance used to counteract the toxic action of a specified xenobiotic' (Meredith *et al.*, 1993a)
- 'Substance used to treat poisoning which has a specific action depending on the poison'

Unfortunately, it is difficult to evaluate the efficacy of antidotes and/or develop new ones in clinical practice because patient treatment has to continue notwithstanding, and thus studies in appropriate laboratory animals are important (Bateman and Marrs, 2000). Use of some antidotes, such as 4-(N,N-dimethyl)aminophenol (DMAP) and hydroxocobalamin for cyanide poisoning (Germany and France respectively) and silibinin for poisoning with *Amanita* fungi (Austria and Germany), appears to reflect national practices. Nevertheless, the evaluation of antidotes has been the subject of a major initiative undertaken by the International Programme on Chemical Safety (IPCS) in recent years (Spoerke *et al.*, 1987; Pronczuk de Garbino, 1997; Pronczuk de Garbino *et al.*, 1997; Johnson *et al.*, 2000). Three volumes of a planned series of 13 on the evaluation of antidotes and procedures used in the treatment of poisoned patients have been published thus far (Meredith *et al.*, 1993a,b, 1995). These volumes discuss naloxone, flumazenil and dantrolene; antidotes for poisoning by cyanide; and antidotes for poisoning

CHAPTER 1

TABLE 1.1
Substances given to minimize absorption and/or enterohepatic recirculation of poisons, or ameliorate external effects

Substance	Poison(s)	Rationale for use
Activated charcoal (multiple dose)	Aspirin, barbiturates, digoxin, paraquat, theophylline and others	Inactivate unabsorbed poison; interrupt enterohepatic recirculation; trap poison in the small intestine
[Apomorphine]	Many	Induce vomiting
Dimethicone	Soaps, shampoos	Anti-foaming agent
[Fuller's earth, bentonite]	Paraquat	Bind unabsorbed poison
[Ipecacuanha]	Many	Induce vomiting
Magnesium citrate, [magnesium sulphate], [lactulose], sorbitol	Many	Induce catharsis; enhance elimination of unabsorbed poison
Milk	Acids, alkalis	'Neutralize' poison
Osmotically balanced polyethylene glycol/ electrolyte solution	Iron, lead, zinc salts, packets of illicit drugs	Solution used for whole-bowel irrigation
Polyethylene glycol (Macrogol)	Phenol (carbolic acid)	Prevent skin absorption/ damage, whole bowel irrigation
Starch	Iodine	Inactivate unabsorbed poison

Note
Substances in square brackets [ ] are no longer recommended.

by paracetamol. Separate handbooks on the use of antidotes and the use of antivenins were planned as part of this series.

1.2 MECHANISM OF ACTION OF ANTIDOTES

The antidotes discussed below are thought to act in a variety of ways (Figure 1.1). Some, such as the opioid antagonist naloxone, simply compete with a poison for receptor site(s), whereas others, chelating agents for example, aim to bind the poison to form less toxic complexes that may readily be excreted. Other antidotes act either by inhibiting toxic metabolism or by aiding detoxification of reactive metabolite(s) once formed. Examples here include the use of inhibitors of alcohol dehydrogenase such as 4-methylpyrazole (4-MP, fomepizole), which may be used to treat poisoning with ethylene glycol, and the administration of sulphydryl donors such as N-acetylcysteine (NAC) or methionine to prevent or ameliorate hepatorenal damage after the ingestion of paracetamol. Yet other antidotes aim to by-pass or reverse the toxic effects of a poison. Examples here include the use of glucagon to by-pass the toxicity of β-adrenoceptor-blocking drugs such as propranolol, and the use of pralidoxime to

TABLE 1.2

Substances given to reverse or ameliorate toxic effects due to particular poisons

Effect	Substance	Examples of poison
Acidosis	Sodium bicarbonate	Ethylene glycol, iron, methanol, salicylates
Allergic reactions	Corticosteroids, promethazine	
Bronchospasm	Salbutamol, terbutaline, theophylline	β-Blockers, chlorine
Cardiac arrhythmia	[Amiodarone]	Digoxin
	Esmolol	Theophylline, methylene-dioxymethamphetamine (MDMA)
	Lignocaine	Chloral, tricyclic antidepressants
	Magnesium sulphate	Drugs causing prolongation of QT duration
	Potassium chloride	Digoxin, disopyramide
	Sodium bicarbonate	Tricyclic antidepressants
Cerebral oedema	Mannitol	
Convulsions	[Chlormethiazole], diazepam, [paraldehyde], phenytoin, thiopentone	Many
Delirium/agitation	Chlorpromazine	Amphetamines
	Diazepam	Lysergide (LSD) and others
	Haloperidol	
Eye injury	Tetracaine	
Fluid retention, left ventricular failure	Frusemide (furosemide)	
Hypersensitivity reactions	Chlorpheniramine	Hallucinogenic mushrooms, N-acetyl-L-cysteine (NAC)
Hypoglycaemia	D-Glucose (dextrose)	Insulin, oral hypoglycaemic agents, ethanol (children)
Hypokalaemia	[Potassium chloride]	Chloroquine
Hypotension	Adrenaline (epinephrine), dopamine, dobutamine, isoprenaline, noradrenaline (norepinephrine)	Barbiturates, chloroquine, digoxin, paracetamol (late presentation) and others
Hypoxia	Oxygen	
	– Normobaric	Many
	– Hyperbaric	Hydrogen peroxide gas embolism (Mullins and Beltran, 1998)
		Carbon monoxide, cyanide, etc.
		Quinine (Wolff et al., 1997)
		Rattlesnake venom-induced tissue necrosis (Kelly et al., 1991)

TABLE 1.2 *(continued)*

Effect	Substance	Examples of poison
Muscular rigidity (e.g. during mechanical ventilation)	Pancuronium bromide	
Nausea/vomiting	Metoclopramide, ondansetron	Paracetamol
Respiratory tract injury	Sodium bicarbonate (nebulized)	Chlorine
Stress ulceration	Cimetidine, ranitidine	Many

Note
Substances in square brackets [ ] are no longer recommended.

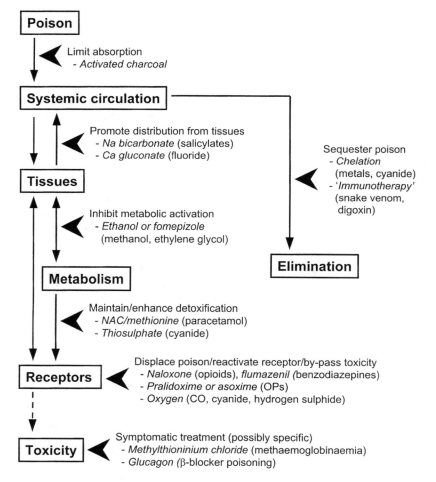

Figure 1.1: Simplified summary of the sites/mechanism of action of some antidotes (adapted from Saviuc and Danel, 1993)

reactivate acetylcholinesterase after poisoning with organophosphorus (OP) insecticides or chemical warfare (nerve) agents (Lapostolle *et al.*, 1999a,b).

Only antidotes with clinical value are discussed here in any depth. For many of these compounds, adequate toxicity and pharmacokinetic data in man are lacking, particularly in relation to the doses used in the treatment of acute poisoning (Vale and Meredith, 1986; Pronczuk de Garbino, 1997). Thus, with the possible exception of use of relatively non-toxic compounds such as D-glucose (dextrose) (Hoffman and Goldfrank, 1995) and naloxone, which may be administered in part as diagnostic tests (Table 1.3), antidotal therapy should be commenced only after thorough clinical examination of the patient, due consideration of the evidence that exposure has occurred and evaluation of the results of appropriate laboratory tests. Some antidotes, such as dicobalt edetate, may cause serious dose-related adverse effects or hypersensitivity reactions, and the balance between risk and potential benefit must be clear before the antidote is given. Teratogenicity and fetotoxicity are concerns when antidotes are given in pregnancy, although usually treatment of the mother takes precedence and is critical to the survival of the fetus. Antidotes, such as naloxone, that simply antagonize pharmacological effects do not alter the pharmacokinetics of the poison and, thus, once the antidote has been given, the patient must be observed until the risk of recurrence of toxicity has diminished. This is particularly important where the elimination half-life of the antidote is short and that of the poison is long. A classic example is the use of naloxone (plasma half-life 30–80 min) to treat poisoning with dextropropoxyphene (half-life 8–24 h).

As noted above, a few antidotes are given before analytical confirmation of the diagnosis can be obtained. Lack of response to a particular antidote does not necessarily indicate the absence of a particular poison or group of poisons. Naloxone, for example, will usually rapidly and completely reverse coma due to opioids such as morphine and codeine. However, the absence of response may merely mean that insufficient antidote has been administered, an agent with partial opioid agonist/antagonist activity has been taken (for example buprenorphine) or that consciousness is depressed for other reasons such as head injury, hypoxic brain damage, hypoglycaemia or the presence of other non-opioid drugs.

Some antidotes react with poisons or their toxic metabolite(s) to form new compounds or complexes. Examples include the chelating agents used to treat poisoning with metal

CHAPTER 1

TABLE 1.3
Antidotes which have been administered as diagnostic agents

Agent	Poison/condition
Calcium disodium edetate	Lead (chronic)
Deferoxamine (DFO)	[Iron], aluminium (chronic)
Flumazenil	Benzodiazepines
D-Glucose (dextrose)	Hypoglycaemia
Naloxone	Opioid agonists (e.g. morphine, dextropropoxyphene)
Sodium dimercaptopropane- sulphonate (DMPS)	Mercury (chronic)

Notes
Deferoxamine challenge is no longer used as a test for iron overload.
Administration of flumazenil is contraindicated if multiple drug ingestion has occurred (see section 5.13).

ions and antidigoxin F_{ab} antibody fragments. Here, not only the toxicity, pharmacokinetics, etc. of the poison and of the antidote, but also the toxicity and pharmacokinetics of the antidote–poison complex or complexes, must be considered when making the decision to give the antidote. The possibility of precipitating an acute withdrawal reaction or of exacerbating the toxicity of co-ingested poison(s) must be borne in mind in other cases. Examples include the use of naloxone to reverse coma and respiratory depression in opioid-dependent subjects and the use of flumazenil to reverse the central effects of a benzodiazepine if a tricyclic antidepressant is also present.

There are concerns regarding the possible adverse effects of some antidotes used for long periods of time. An example is the use of chronic chelation therapy to help remove excess iron in people requiring repeated blood transfusion (section 2.3.1). In addition, there are concerns that some antidotes, such as pyridostigmine used prophylactically, may exert adverse effects, as has been suggested in the case of the so-called Gulf War syndrome (Pennisi, 1996; see section 7.3.5).

Any discussion of antidotes is complicated by the need to compare and contrast the mode of action, efficacy and toxicity of certain antidotes, for example chelating agents used to treat poisoning with metal ions, while simply listing other compounds whose use appears relatively straightforward. In addition, some antidotes, most notably those used to treat cyanide poisoning, are usually used in combination and are thus best discussed together.

The ideal antidote

- Efficacious
- Non-toxic
- Simple to administer either alone or with other antidotes
- Readily available (long shelf-life)
- Cheap

1.3 ANTIDOTE AVAILABILITY

In Western Europe, Australasia, Scandinavia and the USA, the antidotes (excluding normobaric oxygen) most commonly used in treating acute poisoning are NAC and naloxone, which were used, respectively, in 10,586 (0.48 % of all human poison exposures reported) and 7,044 (0.32 %) cases reported to the Toxic Exposure Surveillance System of the American Association of Poison Control Centers in 1997 (Litovitz *et al.*, 1998). Other antidotes used included flumazenil (0.10 % of cases), antivenins (0.039 %), atropine (0.035 %), ethanol (0.033 %), hyperbaric oxygen (0.024 %), phytomenadione (0.015 %), pyridoxine (0.013 %) and deferoxamine (desferrioxamine) (0.013 %). Overall, 17 compounds account for all antidote use in the USA, excluding antivenins (Bowden and Krenzelok, 1997). Note that these data refer to reports of acute poisoning incidents only, most (74.9 %) of which are managed at home/on-site. Thus, the use of, for example, deferoxamine in treating iron and aluminium overload does not feature.

A list of antidotes that should be considered for holding at acute hospitals and at regional/national centres is given in Table 1.4. Further details, including suggested dosage regimens, are given in Appendix 2. The UK National Poisons Information Service

TABLE 1.4

Antidotes that should be held at acute hospitals/regional centres

Antidote	Principal indication(s)
Acute hospitals	
N-Acetylcysteine (or D,L-methionine)	Paracetamol poisoning
Amyl nitrite	Cyanide poisoning
Atropine	Poisoning with cholinesterase inhibitors
Benzatropine	Drug-induced dystonic reactions
Calcium disodium edetate	Lead poisoning
Calcium gluconate	
Gel, topical	Hydrofluoric acid burns
10 % (w/v), i.v.	Poisoning with calcium channel blockers
Dantrolene	Drug-induced malignant hyperthermia
Deferoxamine	Aluminium poisoning, iron overload
Dicobalt edetate	Cyanide poisoning
Dimercaprol	Poisoning with arsenic, lead, mercury
Ethanol	Poisoning with ethylene glycol, methanol
Flumazenil	Benzodiazepine toxicity
Glucagon	Poisoning with β-adrenoceptor blockers
Isoprenaline	Poisoning with β-adrenoceptor or calcium channel blockers
Leucovorin	Exposure to folate reductase inhibitors
Methylthioninium chloride (methylene blue)	Methaemoglobinaemia
Naloxone	Poisoning with opioid agonists or partial agonists
D-Penicillamine	Wilson's disease (copper poisoning)
Phytomenadione (vitamin K$_1$)	Poisoning with anticoagulants
Procyclidine	Drug-induced dystonic reactions
Pyridoxine (vitamin B$_6$)	Poisoning with isoniazid
Sodium nitrite	Cyanide poisoning
Sodium thiosulphate	Cyanide poisoning
Regional/national centres	
Antidigoxin antibody fragments	Poisoning with cardiac glycosides
Antivenins	Snake bite etc.
Fomepizole	Poisoning with ethylene glycol, methanol
Pralidoxime mesilate	Poisoning with OP insecticides or nerve agents
Prussian Blue	Thallium poisoning
Sodium 2,3-dimercaptopropanesulphonate (DMPS)	Poisoning with arsenic, bismuth, copper, mercury
meso-2,3-Dimercaptosuccinic acid (DMSA)	Lead poisoning

CHAPTER 1

(NPIS) on-line database TOXBASE (http://www.spib.axl.co.uk/) has details of antidote availability in the UK and information on the calculation of antidote doses etc. The antidotes cited reflect clinical experience in Western Europe/North America, and these same antidotes are likely to be needed sooner or later in other parts of the world. The list does not differ greatly from that suggested to be held in the event of a 'chemical incident', i.e. a chemical spillage or other accident involving release of toxic chemical(s) into the workplace or into the environment (Pronczuck de Garbino, 1998) (Table 1.5).

Estimating requirements to hold local/regional/national stocks of effective, but expensive or rarely needed, antidotes is difficult, especially in countries where there are many other pressures on health care resources. Special factors may include antidote suitability to treat poisoning encountered locally and training staff to administer the antidote appropriately. Identification of a reliable manufacturer or importer, the cost of production or purchase (many antidotes are used so rarely that production costs must be subsidized by the state or an equivalent body), the minimum quantity of

TABLE 1.5
Selected antidotes and other drugs that may be needed in the event of a chemical spillage or other accident (adapted from Pronczuk de Garbino, 1998)

Substance	Poison (other indication)
Adrenaline (epinephrine)	(Anaphylaxis, cardiac arrest, myocardial depression)
Amyl nitrite	Cyanides
Atropine	OP insecticides and nerve agents, carbamate pesticides
Corticosteroids	(Bronchospasm, laryngeal oedema, mucosal oedema)
Calcium disodium edetate	Lead
Calcium gluconate	Hydrofluoric acid, fluoride, oxalate
Diazepam	OP insecticides and nerve agents (convulsions, excitation, anxiety, hypotonia)
Dicobalt edetate	Cyanides
Dimercaprol	Arsenic, gold, mercury (inorganic)
1,4-Dimethylaminophenol (DMAP)	Cyanides
Sodium dimercaptopropanesulphonate (DMPS)	Cobalt, gold, lead, mercury (inorganic), nickel
Dimercaptosuccinic acid (DMSA)	Arsenic, mercury (organic, inorganic), lead, bismuth
Hydroxocobalamin	Cyanides
Methylthioninium chloride (methylene blue)	(Methaemoglobinaemia)
Naloxone	Opioids
Noradrenaline (norepinephrine)	(Myocardial depression, vasodilatation)
Obidoxime	OP insecticides and nerve agents
Oxygen	Carbon monoxide, cyanides, hydrogen sulphide (hypoxia)
Polyethylene glycol (Macrogol 400)	Phenol (skin contamination)
Pralidoxime	OP insecticides and nerve agents
Salbutamol	(Bronchoconstriction)
Sodium nitrite	Cyanides
Sodium thiosulphate	Cyanides
Terbutaline sulphate	(Bronchospasm)
Tetracaine hydrochloride (eyedrops)	(Eye irrigation)

antidote that has to be purchased, the optimum storage conditions and the most appropriate location(s) of storage/distribution centre(s), and the shelf-life of the preparation under different storage conditions, are further considerations. Lall *et al.* (1996) have produced a guide to the use of antidotes specifically aimed at India.

Where antidote use has at best a marginal effect on outcome, as with the use of flumazenil in benzodiazepine self-poisoning, economic as well as clinical considerations determine that it is rarely used in such patients. On the other hand, where a cheap, ubiquitous and effective antidote is available, such as ethanol in treating methanol or ethylene glycol poisoning, economic considerations dictate that it will continue to be used in this role in many places despite the introduction of fomepizole, which has the advantages of longer duration of action and fewer adverse effects (section 4.2.2). Similarly, oral methionine is safe and effective in treating paracetamol poisoning if the patient presents within 12 h of the ingestion. D,L-Methionine tablets are cheap, have a long shelf-life and do not require special precautions in storage. In addition, administration is much simpler than giving intravenous (i.v.) or oral NAC provided the patient does not vomit and has not been given oral activated charcoal (section 4.16.1). Methionine thus presents a simple treatment option for paracetamol poisoning if NAC administration is not practicable.

1.4 HISTORY OF ANTIDOTE DEVELOPMENT

The word antidote comes from the Greek *antidotos* (*anti* = against, *didonai* = to give), hence the dictionary definition of an antidote ('any agent administered to prevent or counteract the action of a poison'). Through the ages the natural human fascination with, and fear of, poisons has been paralleled by an interest in antidotes. Stones of both natural (talismans, amulets, 'snake stones') and animal origin, parts of plants and animals and mixtures of the same together with various minerals, incantations and other devices have at various times been endowed with protective power against poisons, and indeed against disease in general (Tichy, 1977; Trestrail, 1988; Wax, 1998).

The Chinese Emperor Shen Nung (*c.* 2000 BC) is said to have experimented with poisons and antidotes. One of the earliest references to possible use of a pharmacological antidote occurs in Homer's *Odyssey* (approximately ninth century BC), in which Odysseus is advised to protect himself against Circe's poison by taking 'moly'. It has been suggested that 'moly' could have been *Galanthus nivalis* (snowdrop), which contains an orally active cholinesterase inhibitor, galanthamine (section 5.8), and which may have been used as an antidote against poisonous plants containing anticholinergic agents such as *Datura stramonium* (thorn apple) (Plaitakis and Duvoisin, 1983). Galanthamine is also found in Caucasian snowdrop (Voronov's snowdrop, *G. woronowii*).

1.4.1 Theriacs and the mithridatium

The widespread study and use of poisons in ancient Greece and in Rome (self-poisoning was the form of state execution practised in classical Athens, for example) was accompanied by an intensive search for a universal antidote, the *alexipharmica* or *theriac*. In time, the term alexipharmica was used to refer to a mode of treatment, such as the induction of emesis by using a feather. Theriac (which had originally been used to refer to poisonous reptiles or wild beasts) was used as the term for the actual antidote. Ingestion of the early theriacs (*c.* 200 BC) was said to make people 'poison-proof' against bites of all venomous animals except the asp. Their ingredients included wild thyme, apoponax, aniseed, fennel, parsley, meru and anmi, and were documented in the works of Nicander of Colophon (204–135 BC). As simple antidotes, compounds that excite vomiting – lukewarm oil, warm water, mallow, linseed tea – were recommended.

A well-known universal antidote was that developed by the work of King Mithridates VI of Pontus (132–63 BC), a survivor of seemingly repeated poisoning attempts. In perfecting his antidote he performed acute toxicity experiments on criminals and slaves. His product, the *mithridatium*, contained at least 36 ingredients and was said to protect against spiders, scorpions, vipers, aconite, sea slugs and all other poisons. Mithridates took his mixture every day. Ironically, as an old man, Mithridates is said to have attempted suicide by poison, but reputedly was unsuccessful because he had become poison-proof (he may indeed have become tolerant to opium). Galen (*c.* 129–201 AD) described Mithridates' experiences in a series of three books: *De Antidotis I, De Antidotis II* and *De Theriaca ad Pisonem* (Anonymous, 1585; Corner, 1915; Coturri, 1959; Watson, 1966; Jarcho, 1972).

The theriac of Andromachus, also known as 'Venice treacle' or 'galene', is probably the most famous theriac. Andromachus the elder (Archiater) (37–68 AD), physician to the Roman emperor Nero, added to the mithridatium ingredients such as the flesh of vipers, squill and generous amounts of opium, and removed others. Altogether, 73 ingredients were described. It was claimed to counteract 'all poisons and bites of venomous animals' as well as being of value in a host of other medical problems such as colic, jaundice and dropsy. It was used both therapeutically and prophylactically. As evidence of its efficacy, Galen reportedly demonstrated that fowl receiving poison followed by theriac had a higher survival rate than fowl receiving poison alone.

By mediaeval times the theriac of Andromachus contained over 100 ingredients. Its initial production period was followed by a process of maturation lasting several years. The final product was often more solid than liquid in consistency. Other theriacs were named after famous physicians (Damocrates, Nicolaus, Amando, Arnauld and Abano) who contributed additional ingredients. Over the centuries, certain localities were celebrated for their own brand of theriac, notable centres of production including Cairo, Venice, Florence, Genoa, Bologna and Istanbul (see front cover).

Whether these preparations had any value is doubtful. It has been suggested that the theriac may have had an antiseptic effect on the gastrointestinal tract, while others have stated that theriac's sole benefit derived from its formulation with opium (Bierman, 1994; Hopkins and Lehmann, 1995). The efficacy of theriacs was finally questioned by William Heberden (1710–1801) in Cambridge in his essay 'Antitheriaka: An essay on mithridatium and theriaca' (Heberden, 1745; Paulshock, 1982; Swann, 1985). Both mithridatium and theriac were removed from the Edinburgh Pharmacopoeia in 1756; London followed suit in 1788 (Cowan, 1985). The last ceremonial production of theriac in Paris took place in 1790. Nevertheless, pharmacopoeias in France, Spain and Germany continued to list these agents until the late 1870s (Bernhard, 1893). Theriac was still available in the early twentieth century in France, Italy and Turkey. Even in 1984 'Teriaca secondo la formula di Andromacho' was still available in Rome, although lacking the exotic ingredients of former years and recommended not as an antidote, but for 'insomnia, nerves, and digestive disorders' (Bierman, 1994).

1.4.2 Sealed earth and other remedies

Terra sigillata (= 'sealed earth') dates from the time of Herodotus (fifth century BC). A red clay, which came originally from a hill on the island of Lemnos, was mixed with goat's blood, and stamped or sealed with a representation of the goddess Diana. It was said to be an antidote to all poisons: poisoned liquids drunk from a cup made from the clay were said to be rendered harmless. At one time, it was included as part of the theriac of Andromachus. Demand for *terra sigillata* continued into the fifteenth century. Similar 'antidotal clays' were found in Italy, Malta, Silesia and England.

In mediaeval times stones such as serpentine (said to protect against the bites of serpents and the stings of other animals), turquoise (Turkish or lucky stone – reputed to provide protection from poisons and venomous reptile bites) and bloodstone (haematite, which when powdered was said to cure snake bite) were valued, as were bezoars (calcareous and other growths found inside animals). The word bezoar comes from the Persian *pad-zahr* = 'an expeller of poisons', cited by the Arab physician Avenzoar *c*. 1140, and known to the Hebrews as *Bel Zaard* = 'Master' or 'every cure for poisons'. Over the years regional variations of bezoar stones were popularized, including varieties from Persian wild goat, Peruvian llama and Swiss chamois. Historical antidotes to snake bite included songs, prayer, ritual dances, onions, garlic, herbs, gunpowder, opium, vinegar, tobacco, paraffin and alcohol (ethanol). The Neapolitan dance tarantella was long thought a remedy for tarantism, epidemic dancing mania, thought to be caused by a bite from the south European wolf spider tarantula (*Lycosa tarantula*).

In part 1 of his *Treatise on Poisons and Their Antidotes* (1198), Moses Maimonides (1135–1204) discussed the bites of snakes and mad dogs, and the stings of bees, wasps, spiders, and scorpions. He also described the use of cupping glasses for bites (a forerunner of modern suction devices), and was one of the first to differentiate the haemolytic (hot) from the neurotoxic (cold) effects of poison (Rosner, 1968). In part 2, he discussed mineral and vegetable poisons, and their antidotes. He suggested that emesis should be induced by hot water, *Anethum*, and much oil, followed by fresh milk, butter and honey, all of which should be vomited. Although rejecting some contemporary treatments, he advocated the use of the great theriac and the mithridatium as first- and second-line agents in the treatment of snake bite (Rosner, 1968).

Toadstones and unicorn horn were also promoted as universal antidotes. Toadstones (from the heads of old toads) were reputed to have the ability to extract poison from the site of a venomous bite or sting. Ctesias (390 BC) was the first to chronicle the wonders of the 'unicorn' horn, claiming that drinking water or wine from the 'horn of the unicorn' would protect against poison. The horn was usually narwhal tusk or rhinoceros horn, and was greatly valued (Lucanie, 1992). In mediaeval times it was said that the unicorn horn was worth ten times its weight in gold. To give further credence to its use, a 1593 study on arsenic-poisoned dogs reportedly showed that the horn was protective. Ambroise Paré (1510–90) argued against the use of bezoars and unicorn horn and related the tale of a cook who, being condemned to death for theft, agreed to take corrosive sublimate (mercuric chloride) together with a bezoar so that the king, Charles IX, should have evidence of the efficacy of the bezoar. The cook died in agony some seven hours later (Orfila, 1821).

William Piso (1611–78) is said to have been among the first to recognize the emetic properties of ipecacuanha (ipecac), the ground-up roots of *Uragoga ipecacuanha*.

CHAPTER 1

1.4.3 Antidotal treatment in the nineteenth century

In the early nineteenth century the scientific study of toxicology was pioneered by Matthieu Joseph Bonaventure Orfila (1787–1853) in Paris, his pupil Sir Robert Christison (1797–1872) in Edinburgh and Alfred Swaine Taylor (1806–80) at Guy's Hospital in London. Among other things, rationalization of the use of antidotes, the 'counter-poisons' (contre-poisons) of Orfila, was attempted. Contemporary developments in resuscitation techniques such as laryngeal intubation prior to artificial ventilation (dating from the 1770s), and in other emergency procedures such as the stomach pump or its variants, must, however, be borne in mind. A further technique, i.v. injection, was also developed in the nineteenth century and became in time a major advance in drug treatment, including antidotal treatment.

The use of the stomach pump {the 'gum-elastic probe or tube fitted with a syringe of Boerhaave [Herman Boerhaave (1668–1738) of Leiden], as refined by Dupuytren [Baron Guillaume Dupuytren (1777–1835) of Paris], and Renault (Casimir Renault of Paris)'} to wash out the stomach and remove any remaining poison when an emetic could not be swallowed was suggested by Renault (1801) for use in arsenic poisoning on the basis of experiments in animals. Christison (1835) states that the first successful use of the device in a patient (a child) poisoned with opium was by Philip Syng Physick (1768–1837) in Philadelphia (1812). In Great Britain the stomach pump patented by John Read (1760–1847) in 1820, and publicized by Sir Astley Paston Cooper (1768–1841) of Guy's Hospital for the treatment of poisoning in 1823, enjoyed popularity for a number of additional applications, including the administration of enemata (Owen, 1995).

Orfila (1821) classed poisons broadly as '*Irritants, Narcotics, Narcotico-acrids*, and *Septics* or *Putrefiants*'. Christison (1835) was among the first to remark upon 'compound poisoning', i.e. poisoning with mixtures of compounds not necessarily having the same effects as each other. This being said, the sentiments expressed in the introduction to *A Popular Treatise on the Remedies to be Employed in Cases of Poisoning and Apparent Death* (Orfila, 1818) ring true today, even acetic acid in the form of vinegar and sodium chloride still finding a place in treating poisoned patients (see sections 4.1 and 4.16), although not for the purposes (usually gastrointestinal decontamination) envisaged by Orfila:

> Before speaking of the treatment of poisoned persons, we shall examine, under the title of *Counter-poisons*, those substances which have been regarded as such by several physicians: we shall reject such as are useless or dangerous, and recommend only those the efficacy of which has been demonstrated by reiterated experiments. These are the *white of eggs, milk, common salt, vinegar, lemon juice, soap, gall-nuts*, and some other substances which may be procured with the greatest facility.

His definition of the ideal antidote too (Orfila, 1821) has hardly aged, even though his animal experiments seem cruel by today's standards:

1 It ought to be such as may be taken in a large dose without any danger.
2 It ought to act upon the poison, whether it be in a fluid or solid state, at a temperature equal, or inferior to that of the human body.
3 Its action ought to be prompt.
4 It ought to be capable of combining with the poisons, in the midst of the gastric liquors, mucous, bilious, and other fluids, which may be contained in the stomach.

5 Lastly, in acting upon the poison, it ought to deprive it of all its deleterious properties.

At this time, chemical analysis was in its infancy, and many of the antidotal treatments recommended were based on reactions observed *in vitro*, such as the neutralization of acids by alkali and vice versa or the precipitation of barium sulphate by adding sodium sulphate to a solution of a soluble barium salt. Associated effects such as the evolution of heat or carbon dioxide were deemed of secondary importance. Induction of vomiting remained an almost universal aim, even if poisoning originated from a mercurial substance applied topically. The method used to treat colic arising from occupational lead poisoning (painters' colic) at l'Hôpital de la Charité in Paris is one of the few examples of contemporary treatment of chronic poisoning, yet even here induction of vomiting featured prominently (Table 1.6). Christison (1835) noted that the British method of treating lead colic (a dose of a laxative followed 1 h later by a dose of opium) was usually effective and was much less traumatic than the French treatment. This latter purgative regime, with the addition of oral dosage with a mixture of arsenic trioxide, potassium carbonate, peppermint water, laudanum (tincture of opium) and lemon juice, was also advocated for snake bite, but only after cauterization of the bite site with a white-hot iron, concentrated sulphuric acid, boiling oil or some other caustic agent (Orfila, 1818)!

Orfila's suggested treatment regime for a patient who had swallowed a concentrated acid (Table 1.7) aimed not only to induce vomiting, but also to neutralize the poison, and is notable for its list of contraindicated ('irritant') substances. Subsequent treatment aimed to reduce inflammation by topical administration of compresses or leeches, rehydrate the patient by administration of oral fluids such as sweetened mallow tea and bring about pain relief by giving diethyl ether, laudanum, boiled poppy heads or other mild analgesic preparation, again in sweetened tea. This same regimen was also recommended for the later stages of poisoning with many other agents. Wine was always to be avoided until recovery was effected.

Tartar emetic (a highly toxic potassium antimony tartrate) was widely prescribed in Victorian times (Table 1.7), but proved exceedingly unreliable in inducing emesis when given orally. Indeed, it was often used as a homicidal poison! Even such apparently innocuous substances as common salt (sodium chloride) or Epsom salts (magnesium sulphate), when given in aqueous solution to induce vomiting for example, have been responsible for many deaths, especially in children, when the patient (victim) failed to vomit and absorbed a fatal dose of the erstwhile emetic (Taylor, 1859). Deaths from salt poisoning in children when given as an intended emetic continued even into the latter part of the twentieth century in Western countries.

1.4.3.1 The 'black bottle'

Although violently dismissed by Orfila (1818, 1821) on the basis of his own experiments in dogs, in which he, as usual, tied off the oesophagus after administration of the poison and putative antidote to prevent vomiting, the first suggestion that orally administered wood charcoal might have an antidotal role in poisoning came from experiments reported by the French physician Michel Bertrand (1774–1857). These experiments were performed in dogs from 2 February 1811, and were reported in November and December 1813. On 6 February 1813, Bertrand himself claimed to have taken 4 grains

TABLE 1.6

Treatment of the colic of painters (Orfila, 1818) (dr = drachm, gr = grain, oz = ounce)

Day	Treatment	Preparation
1	Purgative clyster (enema) – morning	Boil (10 min) 4 oz senna leaves in $^1/_2$ pint water, and add when strained $^1/_2$ oz sodium sulphate and 4 oz antimonial wine
	Purgative drink	Boil (15 min) 2 oz broken-up cassia fistula; add 1 oz magnesium sulphate and 3 gr potassium antimony tartrate in 1 pint water 'If the disease be very powerful, an ounce of the syrup of buckthorn, and 2 dr of the confection of Hamech are to be mixed with this drink'
	Anodyne clyster – evening	Mix 6 oz sweet oil and 12 oz red wine. Give $1^1/_2$ dr treacle and (optional) $1^1/_2$ gr opium internally
2	Emetic	Dissolve 6 gr potassium antimony tartrate in a large glass of water and give in divided doses 1 h apart. To facilitate vomiting, give freely warm water sweetened with honey
	Sudorific potion	Boil (1 h) 1 oz each of guaiacum, china root and saraspirilla in $3^1/_2$ pints water. Add 1 oz sassafras and $^1/_2$ oz liquorice, boil for a few minutes and strain
	Anodyne clyster – evening	Mix 6 oz sweet oil and 12 oz red wine. Give $1^1/_2$ dr treacle and (optional) 1 gr opium internally
3[a]	Gently purgative potion	Boil 1 oz senna leaves in 1 pint sudorific potion (day 2) and strain. Give in four doses 45 minutes apart
4[a]	Purgative drink	Boil 1 oz senna leaves in $1^1/_2$ glasses water until reduced to a glass. Strain, and add $^1/_2$ oz sodium sulphate, 1 dr powdered jalap and 1 oz syrup of buckthorn
5[a]	Gently purgative potion	Boil 1 oz senna leaves in 1 pint sudorific potion (day 2) and strain. Give in four doses 45 minutes apart
6[a,b]	Purgative drink	Boil 1 oz senna leaves in $1^1/_2$ glasses water until reduced to a glass. Strain, and add $^1/_2$ oz sodium sulphate, 1 dr powdered jalap (bryony) and 1 oz syrup of buckthorn

Notes

a   On days 3, 4, 5 and 6 the sudorific potion and the anodyne clyster of day 2 were given, except that the sudorific potion was omitted on day 5.

b   'If notwithstanding all these means, the patient does not evacuate', the following mixture was given orally in 12 bolus doses 2 h apart: 10 gr scammony, 10 gr jalap, 12 gr gamboge, and $1^1/_2$ dr confection of Hamech mixed with a 'sufficient quantity' of syrup of buckthorn; in between doses the patient was made to drink of the sudorific potion (see day 2).

TABLE 1.7
Treatment to be administered after ingestion of concentrated acids (Orfila, 1818)

1	Magnesia in water (1 ounce per pint), one glass every 2 min in order to procure vomiting; whilst obtaining magnesia give several glasses of water, of a decoction of linseed, or of any other emollient drink
2	If magnesia is unavailable, give half an ounce of soap dissolved in a pint of water
3	If neither magnesia nor soap is available, give Spanish white or chalk, pulverized coral, crabs eyes, prepared pearls, or burnt hartshorn diffused in water
4	Clysters (enemas) prepared with the same substances should also be given
5	Do not give potashes, soda, treacle, tartar emetic, syrup of ipecacuanha; do not tickle the throat with a finger, feather, etc.

of mercuric chloride mixed with powdered wood charcoal with only minor discomfort, while on 16 February he is said to have taken 5 grains of arsenic trioxide mixed with charcoal and sugar, again experiencing minimal discomfort (Orfila, 1821). In 1831, before the French Academy of Medicine, the pharmacist Pierre Touéry is said to have survived the ingestion of 10 times the lethal dose of strychnine mixed with 15 g of charcoal (Andersen, 1946).

One of the first reports of charcoal used in a poisoned patient was by William P. Hort in North Carolina in 1829. A 40-year-old male patient had accidentally ingested mercuric chloride. Intense pain in the upper gastrointestinal tract ensued, and a large quantity of magnesium sulphate was given at 3 h. The patient's condition having deteriorated considerably at 20 h, some 3 pints of blood was removed by venesection, and beaten egg white mixed with sugar prescribed. By 44 h his condition had worsened, with stomach pain, diarrhoea and hypotension. Finely pulverized charcoal, one teaspoonful hourly in gruel, was prescribed and recovery began shortly after the first dose. Charcoal was continued for several days, the interval between doses being increased slowly. The patient eventually made a full recovery (Hort, 1834).

Meanwhile, the absorptive properties of charcoal of animal origin were being exploited as a chemical reagent (Rand, 1848). Graham and Hofman (1853) in London, for example, used ivory-black or animal charcoal as a means of extracting strychnine from beer. However, [Sir] Alfred Baring Garrod (1819–1907), working at Aldersgate Medical School in London, performed the first controlled studies of purified animal charcoal in the treatment of poisoning (Garrod, 1846). The charcoal used ('carbo animalis purificatus') was prepared by digesting bone or ivory-black in dilute hydrochloric acid, washing and drying, and heating to redness in a covered crucible. Using frogs, dogs, cats, guinea pigs and rabbits, he demonstrated the potential benefits of charcoal in the management of strychnine poisoning. He also emphasized the importance of early utilization of charcoal and the use of the proper ratio of charcoal to poison. Other toxic substances, such as aconite, morphine, mercuric chloride and hemlock, were also studied. Subsequently, Benjamin Howard Rand (1827–1883) of Philadelphia reported a number of animal charcoal efficacy studies in a human subject, presumably himself. Morphia, extract of belladonna, digitalis, hydrocyanic acid and strychnine were among the poisons co-ingested with charcoal, minimal toxicity being reported (Rand, 1848).

By 1855, powdered animal charcoal suspended in sugared water was being used in London to treat poisoning with atropine, strychnine and other alkaloids (Garrod, 1857; Taylor, 1859).

CHAPTER 1

1.4.3.2 Snake antivenins

Interest in the treatment of snake bite was fuelled by rapid colonial expansion during the second half of the nineteenth century (Figure 1.2). In 1886–7, Henry Sewall (1855–1936) working in Michigan had shown that pigeons dosed subcutaneously (s.c.) with increasing doses of crotalid venom acquired a degree of tolerance or immunity against the venom. Léon Charles Albert Calmette (1863–1933), working at the Pasteur Institute in Saigon in 1892 and then in Paris, thought that snake antivenin might be manufactured by injecting animals with increasing doses of heated venom (Calmette, 1894a,b, 1895, 1896). Calmette and his co-workers used cobra venom, whereas Césaire-Auguste Phisalix (1852–1906) and Gabriel Bertrand (1867–1962), who in 1884 had discovered that heat inactivated snake venom while working at the Paris Natural History Museum, used viper venom (Phisalix and Bertrand, 1894a–d; Phisalix, 1922).

At the Pasteur Institute, horses and donkeys were injected with increasing doses of cobra venom until they could withstand some 200 times the fatal dose of active venom in a naive animal without showing signs of toxicity. Serum obtained from such animals was tested in rabbits that were also given snake venom and, if efficacy was proved, the serum was preserved with antiseptic precautions in 10-mL tubes. The antiserum so prepared had a shelf-life of at least 2 years. Low-temperature drying was also introduced, the product being marketed as dry, light-yellow scales for reconstitution in purified water before use (Calmette, 1907). At the time it was hoped that a single antivenin prepared in this way might give protection against bites from a variety of snakes, but this has not proved to be the case (section 3.1).

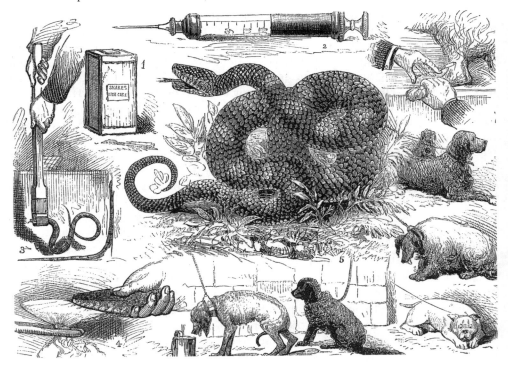

Figure 1.2: 'Australian Experiments in Snake Poisoning' (*Illustrated Sporting and Dramatic News*, 6 October 1877, p. 60)

1.4.4 Antidotes since 1900

Some milestones in the development of modern antidotes are given in Table 1.8. Some compounds, such as flumazenil and physostigmine, appear to be able to cause serious toxicity in some patients while playing a useful role in others. Many other 'antidotes' have been shown to be ineffective, whereas others are positively dangerous especially when given to poisoned patients. Some indication of the heroic nature of the emergency treatment of poisoning even up to the 1960s is given by consideration of the contents of physicians' 'antidote kits' (Tables 1.9 and 1.10) – many of the remedies applied and procedures instituted would have been familiar to Orfila at the beginning of the nineteenth century. Zuck (1987) has noted that some of the suggested treatments, for example keeping an opiate-poisoned patient awake by encouraging walking while infusing strong black coffee per rectum, were mutually incompatible aims. It is noteworthy that the teaching of poisons treatment was long the province of forensic pathologists/toxicologists, who increasingly had little practical experience of patient management (Christison, 1835; Taylor, 1859; Blyth and Blyth, 1906; Witthaus, 1911; Kaye, 1961). This is perhaps one reason why some outmoded remedies continued to be advocated for so long despite the lack of objective evidence of efficacy.

1.4.4.1 *Gastrointestinal decontamination – the role of activated charcoal*

In 1900 the Russian Ostrejko demonstrated that heating ('activating') charcoal under carbon dioxide markedly enhanced its adsorbing power. Leopold Lichtwitz (1908) again called attention to the potential value of oral activated charcoal in treating acute poisoning, as did a number of other workers in papers that appeared mainly in the German literature prior to 1939. After World War II, A. Harrestrup Andersen (1946) in Copenhagen began to publish a series of quantitative experimental studies on the absorptive properties of activated charcoal towards a number of compounds at various times and pH values (Holt and Holz, 1963). However, despite this considerable body of knowledge, oral activated charcoal was used only rarely in treating acute poisoning until L. Emmett Holt and Peter Holz (1963) drew renewed attention to its potential value in limiting the absorption of a wide range of compounds (Corby *et al.*, 1970; Picchioni, 1970; Greensher *et al.*, 1987; AACT/EAPCCT, 1997a). Crome *et al.* (1977) showed that use of multiple doses as opposed to a single dose of activated charcoal reduced the absorption of nortriptyline in volunteers and thus was more likely to be effective in limiting drug absorption after overdosage.

More recently the valuable role of multiple-dose oral activated charcoal in treating acute poisoning with carbamazepine, dapsone, phenobarbitone, quinine and theophylline has become clear. Leaving a dose of charcoal in the stomach after gastric lavage may reduce the absorption of residual poison but, more importantly, repeating the dose every 4 h or so serves to interrupt enterohepatic recirculation should this occur, and may enhance excretion by adsorbing poison that diffuses into the small intestine (Neuvonen and Elonen, 1980; Neuvonen *et al.*, 1980; Berg *et al.*, 1982; Lee and Roberts, 1991; AACT/EAPCCT, 1999). Activated charcoal is cheap and safe when given by mouth, except for the risk of aspiration into the airway if the patient vomits. Hence appropriate airway protection must be ensured if charcoal is given to a patient with a Glasgow coma scale (GCS) score of 8 or less. Vomiting should be treated (for example with an antiemetic drug) since it may reduce the efficacy of charcoal treatment.

TABLE 1.8

Some milestones in the development of modern antidotes (note that years cited refer to the date of publication, not necessarily to the date of introduction)

Year	Milestone
1813	First use of oral charcoal to limit absorption of poison
1818	Description of intubation and artificial ventilation in treating poisoning with carbon monoxide and other asphyxiant gases
1829	Use of oral charcoal to treat mercuric chloride poisoning
1846	First controlled trials of purified animal charcoal in limiting absorption of poisons
1868	Supplemental oxygen used to treat carbon monoxide poisoning
1884	Use of supplemental oxygen suggested in cyanide poisoning
1888	Use of amyl nitrite to treat cyanide poisoning
1894	First reports of the preparation of snake antivenin
1894	Cobalt salts suggested for treating cyanide poisoning
1895	Sodium thiosulphate suggested for treating cyanide poisoning
1900	Activation of charcoal perfected
1911	Use of supplemental oxygen to treat barbiturate poisoning
1933	Sodium nitrite plus sodium thiosulphate recommended for use in cyanide poisoning
1933	Use of methylthioninium chloride (methylene blue) to treat chemically induced methaemoglobinaemia
1941	Synthesis of opioid antagonist nalorphine reported
1942	Hyperbaric oxygen used to treat carbon monoxide poisoning
1945	Dimercaprol (British anti-lewisite, BAL) introduced to treat arsenic poisoning
1948	Discovery that disodium edetate (disodium EDTA) is a strong heavy metal chelator
1949	*meso*-2,3-Dimercaptosuccinic acid (*meso*-DMSA) synthesized
1951	Reactivation of acetylcholinesterase by nucleophilic reagents reported
1952	Use of hydroxocobalamin in cyanide poisoning suggested
1953	Clinical use of calcium disodium edetate to treat lead poisoning
1955	Introduction of cholinesterase reactivator pralidoxime
1956	Introduction of sodium dimercaptopropanesulphonate (DMPS)
1956	Use of D-penicillamine to treat Wilson's disease
1960	Use of dicobalt edetate suggested in cyanide poisoning
1963	Use of oral activated charcoal re-advocated
1964	Introduction of cholinesterase reactivator obidoxime
1965	Use of DMSA in treating occupational lead poisoning
1969	Use of 4-dimethylaminophenol (DMAP) suggested in cyanide poisoning
1970	H (Hagedorn) series oximes introduced for use in soman and sarin poisoning
1971	Use of oral Prussian Blue to treat thallium poisoning
1973	Opioid antagonist naloxone introduced to clinical use
1974	Cysteamine and methionine introduced for treating paracetamol poisoning
1976	F_{ab} antidigoxin antibody fragments made available for clinical use
1977	Use of repeat (multiple) dose oral activated charcoal suggested after overdosage
1978	Introduction of muscle relaxant dantrolene
1979	*N*-Acetylcysteine (NAC) introduced for treating paracetamol poisoning
1981	Benzodiazepine antagonist flumazenil introduced
1986	Hydroxocobalamin for treating cyanide poisoning becomes practical proposition
1988	Oral DMSA advocated to treat lead poisoning in children
1997	Crotalid venom F_{ab} antivenin fraction used clinically

TABLE 1.9

Suggested composition of a physician's antidote kit (Blyth and Blyth, 1906)

Instruments

Stomach pump or tube	Bistoury, forceps and tubes (for performing
Lancet	tracheostomy)
Hypodermic syringe	Glass syringe with cannula (for transfusions)
	Battery (interrupted current)

Emetics

Apomorphine (2 % solution for	Mustard
s.c. injection)	Zinc sulphate (30-grain powders, or solid)
Ipecacuanha	

Antidotes

Acetic acid (to neutralize poison)	Magnesia (calcined) (to neutralize poison)
Aromatic spirits of ammonia	Morphine meconate (10 %)
Atropine sulphate (0.8 % for	Muscarine (5 %)
s.c. injection)	Pilocarpine nitrate (5 %)
Brandy	Potassium permanganate (crystals)
Chloral	Potassium tri-iodide (to precipitate alkaloids)
Chloroform	Strychnine nitrate (2 % solution for s.c. injection)
Chloric ether (i.e. ethyl chloride)	Tannin (to precipitate alkaloids)
Coffee extract	Wyeth's dialysed iron (for arsenic poisoning)
French oil of turpentine	

TABLE 1.10

Suggested composition of a physician's antidote kit (Brookes and Alyea, 1946)

'The kit is suggested for use by the physician with each container having the dose carefully written on the label.'

Amyl nitrite pearls	Magnesia (calcined)
Apomorphine tablets	Morphine sulfate tablets (10 mg)
Atropine tablets	Olive oil
Caffeine-sodium benzoate	Potassium permanganate (1 % aq. Sol.) (to be
Powdered animal charcoal	diluted 20 times)
Chloroform	Sodium sulphate
Aromatic spirits of ammonia	Strychnine sulfate tablets (2 mg)
Cocaine hydrochloride	Whiskey
tablets (0.03 g)	Hypodermic syringe
Epinephrine tablets (1 mg)	Stomach tube
Tincture iodine (7 %)	Funnel
Cupric sulfate (powdered)	
Limewater	

'The following can be secured at the site where the poisoning occurred: boiled water; hot, strong, black coffee; eggs; heat applications such as water bottles, etc.; milk; mustard; salt; soap; starch; tea; vinegar.'

Mention must be made of 'Multiple Antidote' (Blyth and Blyth, 1906). This consisted of a saturated solution of ferrous sulphate (100 parts), water (800 parts), magnesia (88 parts), and animal charcoal (44 parts). It was recommended that the charcoal and magnesia were kept mixed together in the dry state in a well-corked bottle. When needed, the ferrous sulphate solution was mixed with eight times its bulk of water and the charcoal/magnesia mixture added with constant stirring. This concoction was to be administered in wineglass-full doses in cases of poisoning with arsenic, zinc, opium, digitalis, mercury or strychnine. It was said to be useless in poisoning with antimony, caustic alkalis or phosphorus, but efficacy against other poisons seems unlikely.

A similar preparation, the so-called 'universal antidote', originated in the USA in the 1940s and was said to adsorb/neutralize ingested poisons. It consisted of burnt toast (two parts), strong tea (one part) and milk of magnesia (one part). The toast was supposed to adsorb toxic agents in the same way as activated charcoal, the tannic acid was supposed to precipitate heavy metal ions and some alkaloids, thereby preventing absorption, and the milk of magnesia was supposed to neutralize acids. However, much of this was wishful thinking – burnt toast has no adsorptive properties, tannic acid is a hepatotoxin and neutralization of ingested acids generates heat, thereby exacerbating the problem. A more modern version marketed in the USA as Unidote and Res-Q contained activated charcoal (two parts), tannic acid (one part) and magnesium oxide (one part), but was probably equally useless.

The use of syrup of ipecac to induce emesis after the ingestion of poisons was advocated widely for many years, even for use outside hospital (Cashman and Shirkey, 1970). The principal emetic constituents of ipecac are the alkaloids cephaeline and emetine (methylcephaeline; Figure 1.3). However, current thinking is that this mixture should not be used routinely as there is no evidence that ipecac administration improves outcome. Ipecac may delay the administration or reduce the effectiveness of oral activated charcoal, oral antidotes and whole-bowel irrigation, and should not be administered to a patient with impaired consciousness or in whom impaired consciousness may develop, or one who has taken a corrosive substance or hydrocarbon, the ingestion of which is prone to cause aspiration (AACT/EAPCCT, 1997b).

The administration of osmotic cathartics such as sorbitol, magnesium citrate or magnesium sulphate, either alone or in combination with activated charcoal, has been said to minimize toxicity arising from oral ingestion of poison(s) and was once routine treatment (Kaye, 1961). However, there is no evidence that administration of cathartics reduces the bioavailability of ingested poisons or improves outcome in poisoned patients, hence the routine use of cathartics has not been endorsed. If a cathartic is used, it should be limited to a single dose in order to minimize the risk of adverse effects (AACT/EAPCCT, 1997c). Similarly, there is as yet no evidence that whole-bowel irrigation via the enteral administration of large amounts of an osmotically balanced polyethylene glycol electrolyte solution (whole-bowel irrigation) improves outcome in patients poisoned with sustained- or modified-release (enteric-coated) preparations. However, it may be considered in such patients, and substantial quantities of tablets may be recovered this way. This mode of treatment may also have value in treating patients who have ingested iron, lead or zinc salts, or packets of illicit drugs (AACT/EAPCCT, 1997d).

Fuller's earth (*terre à Foulon*, Lloyd's reagent), a diatomaceous clay used in mediaeval and later times for fulling (washing) wool, has been advocated for oral administration with the aim of adsorbing ingested poisons and is still recommended by some for use in

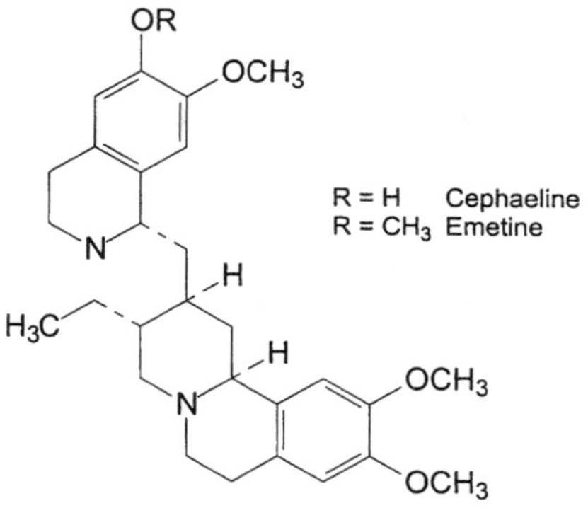

Figure 1.3: Structural formulae of cephaeline and emetine

paraquat poisoning (see Chapter 8), although activated charcoal is thought to be equally effective.

1.4.4.2 *The Scandinavian experience*

A major advance in the treatment of poisoned patients came with the realization that some antidotes given in hospital often killed rather than cured. Central stimulants (analeptics) such as methylphenidate, nikethamide and picrotoxin were commonly used to treat poisoning with sedative drugs such as barbiturates even into the 1960s (Thienes and Haley, 1964; Loennecken, 1967) despite increasing concern that effects such as hyperthermia, arrhythmias, convulsions, psychosis and death were due to the treatment rather than the primary poison (Clemmesen and Nilsson, 1961; Kaye, 1961). Nowadays, of course, the emphasis on supportive care, pioneered in Denmark from the 1940s onwards (Clemmesen and Nilsson, 1961), has done away with these practices and reduced the in-patient mortality from barbiturate overdose from up to 25 % [or even up to 45 % in moderate to severe poisoning (Heinrich, 1939)] to no more than 1–2 % in most countries (Locket and Angus, 1952). More recently the administration of sodium bicarbonate together with large volumes of fluid (so-called forced alkaline diuresis), sometimes combined with administration of diuretics such as frusemide, to treat barbiturate poisoning has been discontinued, although sodium bicarbonate alone is still sometimes used to treat poisoning with relatively water-soluble barbiturates such as barbitone and phenobarbitone (section 4.16).

Even though the Fell–O'Dwyer apparatus for the treatment of morphine poisoning by intubation and ventilation had been introduced in the USA in the 1880s (Zuck, 1987), opiate poisoning too used to be treated by giving analeptics such as caffeine orally or rectally, or nikethamide. The effects of these compounds were transient at best (Figure 1.4). However, the situation was altered dramatically in the early 1950s with the introduction of the partial opioid antagonists levallorphan and nalorphine (Bodman, 1953, 2000; Figure 1.5). Nowadays the pure opioid antagonist naloxone is used in treating patients acutely poisoned with opioids and related compounds such as pentazocine. A further opioid antagonist, diprenorphine, is used widely in veterinary medicine because it has a longer half-life than naloxone in many animal species. Even naloxone administration can cause problems however, as an acute withdrawal syndrome

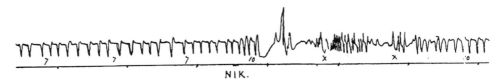

Figure 1.4: Effect of nikethamide (NIK) on respiration depressed by pethidine in a patient lightly anaesthetized with thiopentone and cyclopropane (Bodman, 1953)

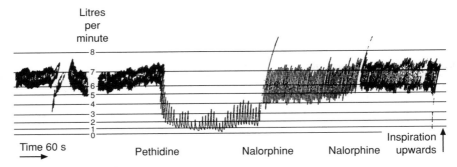

Figure 1.5: Nalorphine 3 mg reversing respiratory depression caused by 50 mg pethidine in a patient lightly anaesthetized with cyclopropane. Gaddum's spirometer (Bodman, 1953)

can be precipitated if it is given incautiously to an opioid-dependent individual (section 5.19.2).

Benzodiazepine poisoning was also made the subject of pharmacological intervention, this time with i.v. theophylline (aminophylline). Its action in reversing benzodiazepine-induced sedation was thought to be via an effect on central nervous system (CNS) adenosine metabolism (Warren *et al.*, 1984). However, simple supportive care and the availability of the benzodiazepine antagonist flumazenil (section 5.13) have rendered theophylline treatment of benzodiazepine poisoning obsolete.

Administration of ammonium chloride, arginine or ascorbate was advocated until quite recently to promote urinary acidification to treat poisoning with basic drugs, such as amphetamines, fenfluramine, phencyclidine and quinine, that are in part excreted unchanged. The rationale for the treatment was that pharmacokinetic studies in volunteers showed that the proportion of the dose excreted unchanged within a given period was increased in acid as opposed to alkaline urine. However, urine acidification may be dangerous in the presence of myoglobinuria or rhabdomyolysis, and has never been shown to be beneficial when used to treat acute poisoning with the compounds listed above. Arginine administration has been associated with hyperkalaemia and hyperglycaemia (Spoerke *et al.*, 1986). The use of acetazolamide to promote urinary alkalinization to treat salicylate poisoning, for example, may be associated with exacerbation of metabolic acidosis, and is no longer recommended. Sodium bicarbonate (section 4.16) is the preferred method of enhancing renal elimination of salicylates.

Dimercaprol (2,3-dimercaptopropanol), the first metal-complexing agent to be used clinically, was designed by Sir Rudolph Peters (1889–1982) and his group at Oxford to treat poisoning with the arsenical vesicant war gas lewisite [dichloro(2-chlorovinyl)arsine], hence its original (American) name British anti-lewisite (BAL). Antidotes to OP pesticides and nerve agents were developed as a result of the search for antidotes to the nerve agents. Pralidoxime, the first oxime acetylcholinesterase reactivator, was introduced in 1955 (Wilson and Ginsburg, 1955). However, despite much effort there is still no effective antidotal treatment for poisoning with the two most effective chemical warfare agents developed and first used in World War I, phosgene and sulphur mustard (H, mustard gas) (see Chapter 7).

In more recent times, D-fructose (D-(−)-fructopyranose) was given i.v. to treat severe ethanol poisoning, but its use is no longer recommended because of the risk of adverse effects, including lactic acidosis and hyperuricaemia. Prenalterol (2–15 mg slowly i.v.) was advocated for use in treating poisoning with β-adrenoceptor blockers (Kulling *et al.*, 1983) but has been replaced by more specific agents such as noradrenaline, adrenaline and isoprenaline (section 5.17). A list of antidotes no longer recommended for use is given in Table 1.11. The seemingly ineffective antidotal treatment of paraquat poisoning is discussed in Chapter 8. Doubtless other compounds discussed in the following pages will in time join the ever-growing list of obsolete antidotes.

1.4.4.3 Antidotal treatment of paracetamol poisoning

It would not be appropriate to end this historical diversion without mention of paracetamol (acetaminophen) poisoning. Although hepatorenal damage and, in some cases, death from liver failure due to paracetamol overdosage are still a major concern (section 4.16.1), it seems certain that had not effective antidotal therapy for patients presenting within 10–15 h of the overdose been developed as a result of the basic studies of Jerry Mitchell, Bernard Brodie and their group (Mitchell *et al.*, 1974) working in Bethesda, Maryland, paracetamol would not today be one of the most widely used, effective and safest drugs available provided always that the recommended dose is not exceeded.

Mitchell *et al.* (1974) suggested that sulphydryl donors, in particular cysteamine, should prove effective in treating paracetamol poisoning, and indeed this proved to be the case when cysteamine was given i.v. within 10 h of the overdose (Prescott *et al.*, 1974). An important factor here in establishing efficacy was the availability of quantitative plasma paracetamol data in relation to estimated time after ingestion and outcome in untreated patients. These same data (see Figure 4.22) have reappeared many times in different guises throughout the world, often without reference to the original source.

Unfortunately, cysteamine had unacceptable side-effects (nausea, vomiting, drowsiness and cardiotoxicity) at the doses used [2 g over 10 min, with a further 1.2 g over the next 20 h – a regrettable factor here was that, owing to a miscalculation, twice the intended dose suggested on the basis of dose-ranging studies in volunteers was given to patients; most of the adverse effects were observed during the loading dose (LF Prescott, personal communication, 1998)]. Oral methionine (McLean, 1974; McLean and Day, 1975) was soon found also to be effective and free of adverse effects, although the occurrence of vomiting complicates treatment with an orally administered antidote as does prior oral dosage with charcoal. Nowadays, a further sulphydryl donor, *N*-acetylcysteine (NAC), given i.v. (Prescott *et al.*, 1979) or orally, has assumed pre-eminence among antidotes for paracetamol poisoning (section 4.16.1), and indeed is probably the most commonly administered antidote in the world today (Litovitz *et al.*, 1998).

TABLE 1.11

Some antidotes and related agents generally considered obsolete for the designated indication (adapted from Decker, 1983; Pronczuk de Garbino *et al.*, 1997; Wax, 1998)

Type of antidote	Agent(s)	Indication(s)
Analeptic (some also emetic)	Amphetamine, bemegride (Eukraton, Megimide), caffeine ('strong coffee'), camphor (also camphorated oil), cocaine, cycliton, doxapram, hexazole (cyclohexylethyltriazole, azoman), hexetone, leptazol (penta-methylenetetrazole, pentylene-tetrazole, cardiazol, metrazol), lobeline, methylamphetamine, methylphenidate (Ritalin), neospiran, nikethamide (Coramine), picrotoxin (cocculin), sodium benzoate, strychnine	Poisoning with sedative/hypnotic drugs
	Atropine, caffeine, camphor, digitalis glycosides, ethanol	Phosgene poisoning
Cathartic	Castor oil, colocynth, croton oil, jalap, magnesium hydroxide, mannitol, sodium phosphate, sodium sulphate, syrup of peach blossom, turpentine	Oral ingestion of poison(s)
Chelating agents	Aurintricarboxylic acid (ATA) Calcium disodium edetate, cysteine/cystine, diethyldithio-carbamate (DEDTC), dithizone (diphenylthiocarbazone)	Beryllium poisoning Thallium poisoning
Demulcent/oral adsorbent	Barley water, bread, butter, 'gruel', egg white (albumen), fresh meat (finely chopped), linseed meal, olive oil, rice, soup, treacle	Poisoning with corrosive substances
Emetic (usually aqueous solution or extract)	Apomorphine, castor oil, copper sulphate (blue vitriol), gall nuts/oak bark, linseed, magnesium sulphate, mallow, mustard powder, potassium antimony tartrate (tartar emetic), soap suds, sodium chloride (common salt), sugar, tincture of iodine, warm water, willow bark, zinc sulphate (white vitriol, white copperas)	Oral ingestion of poison(s); snake bite; later stages of carbon monoxide poisoning
Metabolic	Dimercaprol, cimetidine, cysteamine, D-penicillamine	Paracetamol poisoning

Type of antidote	Agent(s)	Indication(s)
Metabolic (continued)	Cysteine	1-Naphthalenylthiourea (ANTU) poisoning
	D-Fructose	Ethanol poisoning
	Guanidine precursors	Botulism
	Glyceryl monoacetate (Monoacetin)	Fluoroacetate poisoning; fluoride poisoning
	Methionine	Arsenic poisoning; poisoning with carbon tetrachloride and other chlorinated hydrocarbons
	Sulphadimidine	Poisoning with *Amanita* fungi
	Tocopherol (vitamin E)	Paraquat poisoning
	Tolonium chloride	Methaemoglobinaemia
Miscellaneous	Acetic acid (vinegar)	Carbon monoxide poisoning; hydrogen sulphide poisoning; opiate poisoning; poisoning with arsenic salts
	Acetone	Poisoning with cyanoacrylates
	Aconitine	Poisoning with digitalis glycosides
	β-Aminopropionitrile	Burns caused by caustic substances
	Ammonia	Cyanide poisoning; opiate poisoning; phosgene poisoning; snake/scorpion bites
	Ammonium acetate/ammonia	Formaldehyde poisoning
	Amyl nitrite	Poisoning with sedative/hypnotic drugs; chloroform poisoning; digitalis poisoning; iodine poisoning; poisoning with nitrates; strychnine poisoning
	Ascorbate	Lead poisoning, arsenic poisoning; poisoning with nitrates
	Atropine	Benzene, cyanides, phenol, physostigmine, morphine, nitrobenzene, opium
	Auric chloride	Snake bite
	Bibron's antidote (potassium iodide, mercurous chloride and bromine)	Snake bite
	Bromobenzene	Selenium poisoning
	Calcium salts	Lead poisoning; poisoning with chlorinated hydrocarbons
	Carbon dioxide (5 % v/v)/oxygen (95 % v/v)	Poisoning with bromides, carbon monoxide, diethyl ether
	Chlorine	Hydrogen sulphide poisoning; cyanide poisoning
	Corticosteroids	Treatment of hydrocarbon-induced pneumonitis
	Cyclophosphamide	Poisoning with gold salts; paraquat poisoning
	Curarine	Strychnine poisoning
	Diacetylmonoxime (DAM)	Physostigmine poisoning; OP pesticide poisoning

TABLE 1.11 (*continued*)

Type of antidote	Agent(s)	Indication(s)
Miscellaneous (continued)	Emetine	Phosgene poisoning
	Fantus' antidote (calcium sulphide i.v.)	Mercury poisoning
	'Guaco' juice	Snake bite
	'Gum glucose' (gum arabic + D-glucose, both 25 % w/v)	Phosgene poisoning
	Hall's antidote (potassium iodide and quinine)	Mercuric chloride poisoning
	Hydrogen peroxide	Cyanide poisoning
	Hypochlorite	Snake bite
	Magnesium sulphate	Poisoning with tetraethyl lead
	Methylene blue (methylthioninium chloride)	Carbon monoxide poisoning; cyanide poisoning
	Milk	Metal fume fever
	Muscarine	Poisoning with anticholinergics such as atropine
	Nitroglycerine	Digitalis poisoning; ergotism
	Pilocarpine	Poisoning with anticholinergics such as atropine
	Potassium ferrocyanide	Copper poisoning
	Potassium tri-iodide	Lead poisoning; mercury poisoning; poisoning with opiates and other alkaloids
	Potassium permanganate	Poisoning with alkaloids and other basic drugs, and with fluoride salts; treatment of snake bite; cyanide poisoning
	Prenalterol	Poisoning with β-blockers
	Propylene glycol	Poisoning with phenolphthalein
	Rabbit brain	Poisoning with *Amanita* fungi
	Sodium formaldehyde sulphoxylate	Poisoning with mercuric chloride
	Sodium lactate	Poisoning with procainamide and quinidine
	Sodium salicylate	Beryllium poisoning
	Sodium salts (citrate, sulphate)	Lead poisoning
	Sodium thiosulphate	Poisoning with hypochlorites; iodine poisoning
	Sulphuric acid (dilute), sulphuretted waters ('sulphur baths')	Lead poisoning
	Theophylline	Benzodiazepine poisoning
	Tincture of gentian	Strychnine poisoning
	Tincture of iodine	Oral ingestion of lead, mercury, and silver salts; quinine, strychnine, phenol poisoning
	Tobacco (boiling water extract)	Mushroom poisoning
	Turpentine (spirits, oil)	Cyanide poisoning; phosphorus poisoning
	Urease + urea	Phosgene poisoning
	Yohimbine	Tricyclic antidepressant poisoning
	Zinc phosphide	Mercury poisoning

Type of antidote	Agent(s)	Indication(s)
Neutralizing agent	Chalk, cream, flour, lime water, magnesium carbonate, magnesium hydroxide ('milk of magnesia'), potassium carbonate, sodium bicarbonate, sodium carbonate (soda), starch paste, wall plaster	Acidic poisons
	Acetic acid (vinegar), citric acid (lemon juice, lime juice, orange juice), hydrochloric acid	Alkaline poisons
Opioid antagonist	Levallorphan (Lorfan), nalorphine (Nalline)	Poisoning with opioids
Oral adsorbent	Cyanide antidote solutions 'A' and 'B'	Cyanide poisoning
	Cholestyramine	Poisoning with digitalis glycosides; chlordecone poisoning
	Ferric hydroxide/magnesium hydroxide ('antidotum arsenici'); 'hydrated sesquioxide of iron', 'dialysed iron'	Poisoning with arsenic salts
	Ferrous sulphate (copperas)	Cyanide poisoning
	Iron filings	Poisoning with copper salts and mercury salts
	Meconic acid	Poisoning with mercury salts
	Mercury	Poisoning with mercuric chloride
	Potassium sulphide	Poisoning with lead and other toxic metals
	Sodium chloride	Poisoning with silver salts
	Sodium phosphate (phospho-soda)	Poisoning with iron salts; lead poisoning
	Sugar	Poisoning with copper salts
	Sulphates (calcium, magnesium, sodium)	Poisoning with soluble barium and lead salts
	Tannins [cold tea, oak bark or galls, Cinchona bark (Peruvian bark)]	Poisoning with alkaloids and other basic drugs; poisoning with cardiac glycosides; poisoning with mercuric chloride and with potassium antimony tartrate
	'Universal antidote'	Ingested poisons
Sedative	Chloral, chloroform, diethyl ether, potassium bromide, tribromoethanol (Avertin)	Agitation/convulsions (as in poisoning with picrotoxin or strychnine)
	Digitalis alkaloids, ethanol, paraldehyde, sodium bromide (intrathecal)	Delirium tremens
Urine pH modifier	Acetazolamide, sodium lactate	Alkalinization
	Ammonium chloride, arginine, ascorbate, hydrochloric acid, phosphoric acid	Acidification

REFERENCES

AACT/EAPCCT (American Academy of Clinical Toxicology and European Association of Poisons Centres and Clinical Toxicologists). Position statement: single-dose activated charcoal. *J Toxicol Clin Toxicol* 1997a; 35: 721–41.

AACT/EAPCCT (American Academy of Clinical Toxicology and European Association of Poisons Centres and Clinical Toxicologists). Position statement: ipecac syrup. *J Toxicol Clin Toxicol* 1997b; 35: 699–709.

AACT/EAPCCT (American Academy of Clinical Toxicology and European Association of Poisons Centres and Clinical Toxicologists). Position statement: cathartics. *J Toxicol Clin Toxicol* 1997c; 35: 743–52.

AACT/EAPCCT (American Academy of Clinical Toxicology and European Association of Poisons Centres and Clinical Toxicologists). Position statement: whole bowel irrigation. *J Toxicol Clin Toxicol* 1997d; 35: 753–62.

AACT/EAPCCT (American Academy of Clinical Toxicology and European Association of Poisons Centres and Clinical Toxicologists). Position statement and practice guidelines on the use of multi-dose activated charcoal in the treatment of acute poisoning. *J Toxicol Clin Toxicol* 1999; 37: 731–51.

Andersen AH. Experimental studies on the pharmacology of activated charcoal. I. Adsorption power of charcoal in aqueous solutions. *Acta Pharmacol* 1946; 2: 69–78.

Anonymous. *A discourse of the medicine called Mithridatium, declaring the firste beginninge, the temperament, the noble vertues, and the true use of the same: compiled rather for those which are to use it, than for the learned.* London, 1585 [copy in Wellcome Library].

Bateman N, Marrs TC. Antidotal studies. In: *General and Applied Toxicology*, 2nd edn. Ballantyne B, Marrs TC, Syversen T (eds). London: Macmillan, 2000: 425–35.

Berg MJ, Berlinger WG, Goldberg MJ, Spector R, Johnson GF. Acceleration of the body clearance of phenobarbital by oral activated charcoal. *N Engl J Med* 1982; 307: 642–4.

Bernhard J. *Les Médicaments Oubliés. La Thériaque: Étude Historique et Pharmacologique.* Paris: Baillière, 1893.

Bierman AI. Medical fiction and pharmaceutical facts about theriac. *Pharmaceut Hist* 1994; 24(3): 5–8.

Blyth AW, Blyth MW. *Poisons: Their Effects and Detection*, 4th edn. London: C Griffin, 1906: 717–34.

Bodman RI. The depression of respiration by the opiates and its antagonism by nalorphine. *Proc R Soc Med* 1953; 46: 923–30.

Bodman R. Nalorphine – the first opiate antagonist. *Proc Hist Anaesth Soc* 2000; 27: 27–32.

Bowden CA, Krenzelok EP. Clinical application of commonly used contemporary antidotes: a US perspective. *Drug Safety* 1997; 16: 9–47.

Brookes VJ, Alyea HN. *Poisons: their Properties, Chemical Identification, Symptoms, and Emergency Treatments.* New York: Van Nostrand, 1946: 27.

Calmette A. Propriétés du sérum des animaux immunisés contre le venin des serpents; thérapeutique de l'envenimation. *CR Acad Sci* 1894a; 118: 720–2.

Calmette A. Contribution a l'étude du venin des serpents: immunisation des animaux et traitement de l'envenimation. *Anal de l'Inst Pasteur* 1894b; 8: 275–94.

Calmette A. Contribution a l'étude des venins, des toxines at des sérums antitoxiques. *Anal de l'Inst Pasteur* 1895; 9: 225–51.

Calmette A. Sur le serum antivenimeux. *CR Acad Sci* 1896; 122: 203–5.

Calmette A. *Les Venins, les Animaux Venimeux et la Sérothérapie Antivenimeuse.* Paris: Masson, 1907 (English translation: Austen EE. London: Bale, Sons and Danielsson, 1908).

Cashman TM, Shirkey HC. Emergency management of poisoning. *Pediatr Clin N Am* 1970; 17: 525–34.

Christison R. *A Treatise on Poisons, in Relation to Medical Jurisprudence, Physiology, and the Practice of Physic*, 3rd edn. Edinburgh: A and C Black, 1835: 524.

Clemmesen C, Nilsson E. Therapeutic trends in the treatment of barbiturate poisoning: the Scandinavian method. *Clin Pharmacol Ther* 1961; 2: 220–9.

Coby DG, Fiser RH, Decker WJ. Re-evaluation of the use of activated charcoal in the treatment of acute poisoning. *Pediatr Clin N Am* 1970; 17: 545–56.

Corner GW. Mithridatium and theriac, the most famous remedies of old medicine. *Johns Hopkins Med Bull* 1915; 26: 222–6.

Coturri E. *De Theriaca ad Pisonem*. Florence: Olschki, 1959.

Cowan DL. Expunctum est mithridatium. *Pharmaceut Hist* 1985; 15(3): 2–3.

Crome P, Dawling S, Braithwaite RA, Masters J, Walkey S. Effect of activated charcoal on absorption of nortriptyline. *Lancet* 1977; ii: 1203–5.

Decker WJ. Antidotes: some ineffective, insufficiently tested, outmoded, and potentially dangerous therapeutic agents. *Vet Hum Toxicol* 1983; 25 (Suppl 1): 10–15.

Garrod AB. Purified animal charcoal: an antidote to all vegetable and some mineral poisons. *Trans Med Soc Lond* 1846; 1 (New series): 195–204.

Garrod AB. On the influence of liquor potass and other alkalies on the therapeutic properties of henbane, belladonna and stramonium. *Med Times Gazette* 1857; 36 (New series 15): 589–90.

Graham T, Hofman AW. Report upon the alleged adulteration of pale ales by strychnine. *Q J Chem Soc* 1853; 5: 173–7.

Greensher J, Mofenson HC, Caraccio TR. Ascendency of the black bottle (activated charcoal). *Pediatrics* 1987; 80: 949–51.

Heberden W. *Antitheriaka: an essay on Mithridatium and Theriaca*. Cambridge, 1745.

Heinrich A. Zur Therapie der Schlafmittelvergiftungen. *Klin Wschr* 1939; 18: 1410–16.

Hoffman RS, Goldfrank LR. The poisoned patient with altered consciousness: controversies in the use of a 'coma cocktail'. *J Am Med Assoc* 1995; 274: 562–9.

Holt LE, Holz PH. The black bottle: a consideration of the role of charcoal in the treatment of poisoning in children. *J Pediatr* 1963; 63: 306–14.

Hopkins KD, Lehmann ED. Successful medical treatment of obesity in 10th century Spain [Letter]. *Lancet* 1995; 346: 452.

Hort WP. Case of poisoning with corrosive sublimate, in which the administration of charcoal afforded great relief. *Am J Med Sci* 1834; 6: 540–1.

Jarcho S. Medical numismatic notes. VII: Mithridates IV. *Bull NY Acad Med* 1972; 48: 1059–64.

Johnson MK, Jacobsen D, Meredith TJ, Eyer P, Heath AJ, Ligtenstein DA, Marrs TC, Szincz L, Vale JA, Haines JA. Evaluation of antidotes for poisoning by organophosphorus pesticides. *Emerg Med* 2000; 12: 22–37.

Kaye S. *Handbook of Emergency Toxicology*, 2nd edn. Springfield, IL: Charles C Thomas, 1961.

Kelly JJ, Sadeghani K, Gottlieb SF, Ownby CL, Van Meter KW, Torbati D. Reduction of rattlesnake-venom-induced myonecrosis in mice by hyperbaric oxygen therapy. *J Emerg Med* 1991; 9: 1–7.

Kulling P, Eleborg L, Persson H. β-Adrenoceptor blocker intoxication: epidemiological data. Prenalterol as an alternative in the treatment of cardiac dysfunction. *Hum Toxicol* 1983; 2: 175–81.

Lall SB, Peshin SS, Chablani V, Seth SD. *Antidotes in Poisoning*. New Delhi: National Poisons Information Centre, 1996.

Lapostolle F, Bismuth C, Baud F. Classification of antidotes based on mechanism of action. Part I. *Sem Hôp Paris* 1999a; 75: 45–52.

Lapostolle F, Bismuth C, Baud F. Classification of antidotes: practical considerations. Part II. *Sem Hôp Paris* 1999b; 75: 108–14.

Lee DC, Roberts JR. Use of oral activated charcoal in medical toxicology. In: *Contemporary Management in Critical Care*, Volume 1 (Part 3): *Critical Care Toxicology*. Hoffman RS, Goldfrank LR (eds). New York: Churchill Livingstone, 1991: 43–60.

Lichtwitz L. Die Bedeutung der Adsorption für die Therapie. *Ther Gegenwart* 1908; 49: 542–6.

Litovitz TL, Clark LR, Soloway RA. 1997 Annual report of the American Association of Poison Control Centers toxic exposure surveillance system. *Am J Emerg Med* 1998; 16: 443–97.

Locket S, Angus J. Poisoning by barbiturates: success of conservative treatment. *Lancet* 1952; i: 580–2.

Loennecken SJ. *Acute Barbiturate Poisoning: Treatment with Modern Methods of Resuscitation*. Bristol: Wright, 1967.

Lucanie R. Unicorn horn and its use as a poison antidote. *Vet Hum Toxicol* 1992; 34: 563.

McLean AEM. Prevention of paracetamol poisoning [letter]. *Lancet* 1974; i: 729.

McLean AEM, Day PA. The effect of diet on the toxicity of paracetamol and the safety of paracetamol–methionine mixtures. *Biochem Pharmacol* 1975; 24: 37–42.

Meredith T, Caisley J, Volans G. Emergency drugs: agents used in the treatment of poisoning. *Br Med J* 1984; 289: 742–8.

Meredith TJ, Jacobsen D, Haines JA, Berger J-C (eds). *Naloxone, Flumazenil and Dantrolene as Antidotes. IPCS/CEC Evaluation of Antidotes Series*, Volume 1. Cambridge: Cambridge University Press, 1993a.

Meredith TJ, Jacobsen D, Haines JA, Berger J-C, van Heijst ANP (eds). *Antidotes for Poisoning by Cyanide. IPCS/CEC Evaluation of Antidotes Series*, Volume 2. Cambridge: Cambridge University Press, 1993b.

Meredith TJ, Jacobsen D, Haines JA, Berger J-C (eds). *Antidotes for Poisoning by Paracetamol. IPCS/CEC Evaluation of Antidotes Series*, Volume 3. Cambridge: Cambridge University Press, 1995.

Mitchell JR, Thorgeirsson SS, Potter WZ, Jollow DJ, Keiser H. Acetaminophen-induced hepatic injury: protective role of glutathione in man and rationale for therapy. *Clin Pharmacol Ther* 1974; 16: 676–84.

Mullins ME, Beltran JT. Acute cerebral gas embolism from hydrogen peroxide ingestion successfully treated with hyperbaric oxygen. *Clin Toxicol* 1998; 36: 253–6.

Neuvonen PJ, Elonen E. Effect of activated charcoal on absorption and elimination of phenobarbitone, carbamazepine and phenylbutazone in man. *Eur J Clin Pharmacol* 1980; 17: 51–7.

Neuvonen PJ, Elonen E, Mattila MJ. Oral activated charcoal and dapsone elimination. *Clin Pharmacol Ther* 1980; 27: 823–7.

Orfila MP. *A Popular Treatise on the Remedies to be Employed in Cases of Poisoning and Apparent Death; including the Means of Detecting Poisons, of Distinguishing Real from Apparent Death, and of Ascertaining the Adulteration of Wine*. Trans. Price W. London: W Phillips, 1818.

Orfila MP. *A General System of Toxicology, or, A Treatise on Poisons, drawn from the Mineral, Vegetable, and Animal Kingdoms, considered as to their relations with Physiology, Pathology, and Medical Jurisprudence*, Volumes 1 and 2, 2nd edn. Trans. Waller JA. London: E Cox, 1821.

Owen B. A man named Read. *Proc Hist Anaesth Soc* 1995; 17: 86–92.

Paulshock BZ. William Heberden, M.D., and the end of theriac. *NY State J Med* 1982; 82: 1612–15.

Pennisi E. Chemicals behind the Gulf War Syndrome? *Science* 1996; 272: 479–80.

Phisalix C, Bertrand G. Atténuation du venin de vipère par la chaleur et vaccination du cobaye contre ce venin. *CR Acad Sci* 1894a; 118: 288–91.

Phisalix C, Bertrand G. Sur la propriété antitoxique du sang des animaux vaccinés contre le venin de vipère. *CR Acad Sci* 1894b; 118: 356–8.

Phisalix C, Bertrand G. Observations à propos de la Note de M. Calmette relative au venin des serpents. *CR Acad Sci* 1894c; 118: 935–6.

Phisalix C, Bertrand G. Sur la reclamation de M. Calmette à propos du sang antitoxique des animaux immunises contre le venin des serpents. *CR Acad Sci* 1894d; 118: 1071–2.

Phisalix M. *Animaux Venimeux et Venins: La Fonction Venimeuse Chez Tous les Animaux; les Appareils Venimeux, les Venins et Leurs Propriétés; les Fonctions et Usages des Venins; l'Envenimation et Son Traitement*, Volumes 1 and 2. Paris: Masson, 1922: 759–62.

Picchioni AL. Activated charcoal: a neglected antidote. *Pediatr Clin N Am* 1970; 17: 535–43.

Plaitakis A, Duvoisin RC. Homer's moly identified as *Galanthus nivalis* L.: physiologic antidote to stramonium poisoning. *Clin Neuropharmacol* 1983; 6: 1–5.

Prescott LF, Newton RW, Swainson CP, Wright N, Forrest ARW, Matthew H. Successful treatment of severe paracetamol overdosage with cysteamine. *Lancet* 1974; i: 588–92.

Prescott LF, Illingworth RN, Critchley JAJH, Stewart MJ, Adam RD, Proudfoot AT. Intravenous *N*-acetylcysteine: treatment of choice for paracetamol poisoning. *Br Med J* 1979; 2: 1097–100.

Pronczuk de Garbino J. Evolution of antidotal therapy in recent decades. *Arch Toxicol* 1997 (Suppl 19): 261–70.

Pronczuk de Garbino J. Chemical disasters. In: *International Occupational and Environmental Medicine*. Herzstein JA, Bunn WB, Fleming LE, Harrington JM, Jeyaratnam J, Gardner IR (eds). St. Louis: Mosby, 1998: 660–8.

Pronczuk de Garbino J, Haines JA, Jacobsen D, Meredith T. Evaluation of antidotes: activities of the International Programme on Chemical Safety. *J Toxicol Clin Toxicol* 1997; 35: 333–43.

Rand BH. On animal charcoal as an antidote. *Med Examiner* 1848; 4: 528–33.

Renault C. *Nouvelles Expériences sur les Contre-poisons de l'Arsenic, etc.* Paris, Fructidor an IX (1801).

Rosner F. Moses Maimonides' treatise on poisons. *J Am Med Assoc* 1968; 205: 98–100.

Saviuc P, Danel V. Les antidotes. In: *Les Intoxications Aiguës*. Danel V, Barriot P. (eds). Paris: Arnette, 1993: 109–17.

Spoerke DG, Smolinske SC, Wruck KM, Rumack BH. Infrequently used antidotes: indications and availability. *Vet Hum Toxicol* 1986; 28: 69–75.

Spoerke DG, Spoerke SE, Rumack BH. International opinion concerning indications, safety and availability of poison centre antidotes and treatment. *Hum Toxicol* 1987; 6: 361–4.

Swann JP. The universal drug: theriac through the ages. *Med Heritage* 1985; 1: 456–8.

Taylor AS. *On Poisons in Relation to Medical Jurisprudence and Medicine*, 2nd edn. London: J Churchill, 1859: 1–5.

Thienes CH, Haley TJ. *Clinical Toxicology*, 4th edn. London: Kimpton, 1964: 99.

Tichy W. *Poisons: Antidotes and Anecdotes*. New York: Sterling, 1977.

Trestrail JH. *Antidotes – Exotic, Foreign, Investigational*. Grand Rapids, MI: Spectrum Health Regional Poison Center, 1988 [unpublished syllabus].

Vale JA, Meredith TJ. Antidotal therapy: pharmacokinetic aspects. In: *New Concepts and Developments in Toxicology*. Chambers PL, Gehring P, Sakai F (eds). Amsterdam: Elsevier, 1986: 329–38.

Warren JB, O'Brien M, Dalton N, Turner CT. Aminophylline inhibition of diazepam sedation: is adenosine blockade of GABA-receptors the mechanism? *Lancet* 1984; i: 463–4.

Watson G. *Theriac and Mithridatium: A Study in Therapeutics*. London: Wellcome Historical Medical Library, 1966.

Wax PM. History. In: *Goldfrank's Toxicologic Emergencies*, 6th edn. Goldfrank LR, Flomenbaum NE, Lewin NA, Weisman RS, Howland MA, Hoffman RS (eds). Stamford, CT: Appleton & Lange, 1998: 1–18.

Wilson IB, Ginsburg S. A powerful reactivator of alkylphosphate-inhibited acetylcholinesterase. *Biochim Biophys Acta* 1955; 18: 168–70.

Witthaus RA. *Manual of Toxicology*. New York: Wood, 1911.

Wolff RS, Wirtschafter D, Adkinson C. Ocular quinine toxicity treated with hyperbaric oxygen. *Undersea Hyperbaric Med* 1997; 24: 131–4.

Zuck D. Forty years back: a case of morphine poisoning. *Today's Anaesthetist* 1987; 2: 95–6.

Agents Used to Treat Poisoning with Toxic Metals and Organometallic Compounds

Contents

2.1 INTRODUCTION

Metal ions such as lead and cadmium inhibit enzymes containing sulphydryl (thiol) moieties via mercaptide formation. Other endogenous ligands also contribute to binding in tissues. The aim of therapy is to administer relatively non-toxic compounds that bind toxic metal ions more strongly than cellular macromolecules, thus forming non-toxic complexes that may in turn be readily excreted (Aaseth, 1983; Jones, 1991; Klaassen, 1996). A range of chelating and other agents is used to treat poisoning with metal ions, in the treatment of metal storage diseases, in particular in Wilson's disease (genetic caeruloplasmin deficiency), and in haemochromatosis, and to aid the elimination of metallic radionuclides from the body. A list of chelating agents and related compounds that have been suggested for clinical use is given in Table 2.1. A further non-water-soluble compound, potassium iron(III) hexacyanoferrate(II) (Prussian Blue), is given orally to sequester thallium in the intestine prior to elimination in faeces. A second metal-complexing agent, ammonium tetrathiomolybdate, has been suggested for use in symptomatic patients with Wilson's disease, although D-penicillamine is much more widely used in practice to treat this condition.

A chelate is a coordination compound in which a central atom (usually a metal) is joined by covalent bonds to two or more other atoms of one or more other molecules or ions (ligands), so that heterocyclic rings are formed with the central (metal) atom as part of each ring. Ligands offering two groups for attachment to the metal are termed bidentate (two-toothed); three groups, tridentate; etc. The ideal chelating agent for clinical use in treating poisoning with metal ions would be (i) water-soluble, (ii) resistant to metabolism, (iii) able to reach sites where metal ions accumulate, (iv) able to displace metal ions from endogenous ligands and (v) form non-toxic, readily excretable chelates that are stable at physiological pH. In addition, the agent should have a low affinity for Ca^{2+} because this ion is readily available for chelation in plasma and should not interfere in the metabolism of other metal ions present in physiological concentrations.

The word chelate is derived from the Greek 'χηελα' = *chela*, a claw, which alludes to the way in which the metal atom is bound. The most stable chelate rings are five-membered; as the number of members increases above six so the stability of the ring decreases. The stability of metal chelates also varies with the metal ion and with the ligand. Lead and mercury have greater affinity for sulphur and for nitrogen than for oxygen in ligands. Calcium, on the other hand, has a greater affinity for oxygen than for nitrogen or sulphur. These differences in affinity serve as the basis of selectivity of action of a chelating agent in clinical use. This said, with the exception of the deferoxamine–Fe^{3+} complex (ferrioxamine), little is known of the actual form in which metal ions are excreted after administration of a chelating agent.

Chelating agents which themselves contain thiol moieties may interact with endogenous thiols, thereby increasing blood reduced glutathione (GSH), for example, and either directly or indirectly alter the distribution of metal ions in tissues. It has been postulated that GSH availability is important in moderating the toxicity of mercuric chloride (Naganuma *et al.*, 1990), and in reversing the inhibition of Δ-aminolaevulinate dehydratase by lead and in facilitating lead removal by chelation (Paredes *et al.*, 1985). Dimercaptosuccinic acid (DMSA), either alone or together with calcium disodium edetate (calcium disodium EDTA), has been found to increase blood GSH (Flora *et al.*, 1995a).

■ CHAPTER 2 ■

TABLE 2.1

Summary of chelating agents suggested for use in treating poisoning with metal ions

Chelating agent	Metal/metal complex[a]
N-Acetyl-L-cysteine (NAC)	(As, Hg)
N-Acetyl-D,L-penicillamine (NAPA)	(Hg)
Aurintricarboxylic acid (ATA)	(Be)
N-Benzyl-D-glucaminedithiocarbamate (BGDTC)	(Cd, Ni)
Calcium disodium edetate (calcium disodium EDTA)	Pb (Be) [ointment: Cr^{6+} ulcers]
Calcium trisodium diethylenetriaminepenta-acetate (DTPA)	Pu, Am (Fe)
1,2-Cyclohexanediaminetetra-acetate (CDTA)	(Ni)
Deferiprone (DMHP, L1)	Fe
Deferoxamine (desferrioxamine, DFO)	Fe, Al
Diethyldithiocarbamate (DEDTC)	(Ni)
4,5-Dihydroxy-1,3-benzenedisulphonic acid (Tiron)	(Fe)
2,3-Dihydroxybenzoic acid	(Fe)
Dihydroxyethyldithiocarbamate (DHEDTC)	(Ni)
Etidronic acid (EHDP)	(U)
N,N'-bis(2-Hydroxybenzyl)ethylenediamine-N,N'-diacetic acid (HBED)	(Fe)
Dexrazoxane	(Fe)
Dimercaprol (British anti-lewisite, BAL)	As, Hg, Au (Bi, Cu, Pb in children)
N-(2,3-Dimercaptopropyl)phthalamidic acid (DMPA)	(As, Hg)
meso-2,3-Dimercaptosuccinic acid (DMSA)	Pb (Be, Ni)
Ethylenebis-2-hydroxyphenylglycine (EHPG)	(Fe)
N-(4-Methoxybenzyl)-D-glucaminedithiocarbamate (MBGDTC)	(Cd)
D-Penicillamine	As, Pb, Cu
Pyridoxal isonicotinoyl hydrazone (PIH)	(Fe)
Rhodotorulic acid	(Fe)
Sodium 2,3-dimercaptopropanesulphonate (DMPS)	As, Bi, Cu, Hg
Thiopronine (TP)	(Bi)
N,N',N'',N'''-Tetrakis(2-hydroxypropyl)1,4,7,10-tetra-azacyclododecane (THP-12-ane N_4)	(Cd)
Triethylenetetramine (trientine, TETA)	Cu

Note

a Symbols in round brackets = treatment of largely theoretical value rather than established clinical use.

Once chelation therapy is initiated there is a tendency for any chelate to dissociate and release metal ions back into the circulation; for this reason it is important to maintain a constant excess of chelating agent. Efficacy is usually assessed by urinary/ biliary excretion of metal ion – unfortunately few studies have also looked at clinical markers of efficacy (Kosnett, 1992). Haemodialysis may be required to remove a chelate complex in patients, such as those with renal failure, in whom urine flow is inadequate despite the use of fluids and diuretics. Most agents used to treat poisoning with metal ions can chelate several different elements (Aaseth, 1983; Table 2.1). One concern when giving chronic chelation therapy is thus the risk of causing trace element depletion. A further consideration is that most chelating agents used clinically are relatively polar and, hence, water-soluble. For this reason most penetrate cell membranes poorly, and treatment is most likely to be effective if the chelating agent is given while the metal is still in the circulation or in the extracellular space.

Chelation of a metal ion tends to increase the lipid solubility of both the metal ion and the chelating agent. A fundamental concern in the use of chelation therapy is thus the risk of enhancing toxicity by increasing absorption or by favouring distribution into lipid-rich tissues such as the CNS (Kosnett, 1992). Calcium disodium edetate, for example, should not be given orally to treat lead poisoning because of the risk of enhancing lead absorption from the gastrointestinal tract. On the other hand, oral deferoxamine (DFO) or DMSA may be used to treat acute ingestion of iron or cadmium salts, respectively, as these agents effectively prevent absorption of the metal ion in question and thus reduce the potential for toxic damage. Oral DFO is of no value in treating haemochromatosis, however, as its bioavailability is negligible when given by mouth. Despite much research there is still no clinically effective chelating agent for use in chronic poisoning with not only cadmium, but also beryllium, manganese and radium (Jones and Cherian, 1990; Jones, 1991).

Chelating agents are usually used alone, but there is interest in developing combinations of agents, one of which would mobilize the metal ion from tissues into blood, while the other would favour excretion into urine and/or bile. One practical example of this has been the concomitant administration of calcium disodium edetate and dimercaprol in treating lead poisoning in children, although the value of this approach has been questioned because of the risk of dimercaprol enhancing tissue, especially brain, lead absorption. More recently, the effect of combined treatment with calcium disodium edetate and DMSA on lead excretion and other parameters of lead intoxication has been studied in rats (Flora *et al.*, 1995a).

The steps involved in the mobilization of most metal ions from tissue deposits by chelating agents are unknown. In the case of iron mobilization from tissues, the rate of mobilization may be enhanced by reducing agents such as ascorbic acid (vitamin C) or low-formula-mass chelators such as nitrilotriacetate or phosphonates. Ascorbate or xanthine may be required to mobilize Fe^{3+} from ferritin (Funk *et al.*, 1985; Topham *et al.*, 1989), while the small chelators may act to transfer iron to larger chelators such as DFO (Harris, 1984; Harris *et al.*, 1987). Ascorbate or B vitamins can also enhance lead excretion when given with a chelating agent such as edetate in experimental animals, although the underlying mechanism(s) are unknown (Jones, 1991). There seems no reason to suppose that such examples of synergy cannot occur with other metal ion/ chelating agent combinations.

Chelation therapy may be indicated in pregnancy, and thus the developmental toxicology of chelating agents is an important topic (Domingo, 1998). For some chelating agents, teratogenic or fetotoxic effects have been reported at doses higher than those currently used to treat poisoning with toxic metals. The teratogenic potential of some other agents is due to induced trace element deficiencies, at least in part. Hence it is important that pregnant women given chelation therapy also receive adequate doses of mineral supplements (Domingo, 1998).

■ CHAPTER 2 ■

Chelation therapy – toxic metals I

- The aim is to administer a non-toxic compound that binds metal ions more strongly than cell macromolecules and forms a water-soluble compound which can be excreted
- A chelate is a coordination compound in which the central atom (usually a metal) is covalently bonded to two or more other atoms
- Heterocyclic rings are formed with the metal atom as part of each ring
- The most stable rings are five- or six-membered
- Ligands offering two groups for attachment to the metal ion are termed bidentate, those offering three groups tridentate, etc.
- A fundamental concern is the risk of enhancing toxicity by forming complexes that favour absorption and/or distribution of the metal ion to tissues
- There may be a risk of trace element depletion if chelating agents are given for prolonged periods

---

Chelation therapy – toxic metals II

- Chelation therapy is used to treat:
  - poisoning with metal ions
  - metal storage diseases, notably Wilson's disease (genetic caeruloplasmin deficiency) and haemochromatosis
- Sometimes used to aid elimination of metallic radionuclides
- Treatment is most effective if given while the metal ion is still in the extracellular compartment
- Important to maintain constant excess of chelating agent to minimize dissociation of the chelate
- Haemodialysis may be necessary to remove the chelate if renal function is impaired, although chelators such as DMSA probably chelate metal ions in the gut, facilitating faecal elimination

---

2.2 AGENTS USED TO TREAT POISONING WITH LEAD AND OTHER TOXIC METALS

2.2.1 Overview of the clinical features of lead poisoning

Lead toxicity remains an important issue, even in countries where much has been done to minimize exposure. Lead distributes to three compartments in man: blood, vascular tissues and bone (Rabinowitz *et al.*, 1976; Figures 2.1 and 2.2). Absorbed lead that is not retained in bone or soft tissues is excreted in urine (65 %) and in bile (35 %) (Goyer, 1993). Lead from blood and vascular tissues can be readily removed from the body. However, animal studies indicate that, even when powerful chelators such as edetate (EDTA) are used, the bone lead store is not directly chelatable (Doniec *et al.*,

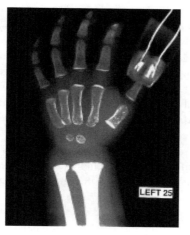

Figure 2.1: Radiograph of the left hand of a 3-year-old girl showing metaphyseal radio-opacity due to lead deposition ('lead lines')

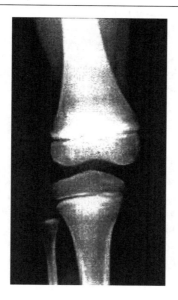

Figure 2.2: Radiograph of the knee of a 43-year-old man showing radio-opacity at growing surfaces due to lead deposition

■ CHAPTER 2 ■

1983). Bone lead leaches out into blood in the days that follow chelation therapy and post-treatment increases in blood lead concentrations are well recognized by those who treat lead poisoning.

Accumulation of Δ-aminolaevulinic acid in blood and urine is the earliest easily measurable marker of lead toxicity, other than measurement of blood lead. This occurs at blood lead concentrations > 100 μg/L (10 μg/dL, 0.5 μmol/L). The commonest scenarios for clinical effects of lead poisoning to occur are as a result of chronic environmental exposure in children or chronic occupational exposure in adults. Although the benefit of chelation therapy for acute lead poisoning is clear, the optimum use of such therapy for 'low-level' lead poisoning, with the aim in children being to safeguard against possible developmental retardation, remains to be evaluated.

In children, acute lead encephalopathy is usually associated with blood lead concentrations > 1,000 µg/L, although it has been reported with concentrations as low as 700 µg/L. The incidence of death or permanent neurological damage including mental impairment, seizures, blindness and hemiparesis after encephalopathy was 25–35 % before the introduction chelation therapy (Chisolm, 1968). With blood lead concentrations between 500 and 700 µg/L a child often shows evidence of hyperirritable behaviour with decreased interest in play. They may even become labelled as 'difficult'. Intermittent vomiting, abdominal pain and anorexia may occur subsequently or concurrently.

In adults, early symptoms of chronic lead exposure (blood lead concentrations 400–800 µg/L) include increased tiredness, readiness to fall asleep and irritability. Subclinical effects on reproductive function and hypertension may also be seen. As exposure increases (blood lead concentrations > 800 µg/L), symptoms include headache, memory loss, insomnia, metallic taste, abdominal pain with guarding and tenderness, decreased appetite, weight loss and constipation (Goyer, 1996). As exposure increases further, the frequency of abdominal colicky pain increases, anaemia worsens and the patient is at substantial risk of encephalopathy or peripheral neuropathy with dominant hand or wrist weakness. In encephalopathy (blood lead concentrations > 1,500 µg/L), coma and papilloedema are usually present. Interestingly, patients with tetraethyl lead toxicity do not become anaemic and blood lead concentrations are not necessarily elevated, even in affected patients.

2.2.1.1 Management of lead poisoning in children

The baseline excretion of lead in urine is not considered a sensitive biomarker of lead exposure. A blood lead concentration of 100 µg/L has been defined as the 'intervention level' for children in the USA (Centers for Disease Control and Prevention, 1991) and 250 µg/L is the corresponding figure used in the UK. It is noteworthy that current evidence points to cognitive deficits at a blood lead concentration well below 250 µg/L in children. The most important aspect of the management of lead poisoning in children is removal from continuing exposure to lead in domestic drinking water, paint, dust and other sources such as ayurevic products (Indian cosmetics) containing high concentrations of toxic metal ions (Landrigan, 1983; Lanphear et al., 1999; Matte, 1999).

Use of chelation therapy is a relatively inefficient process, with a course of therapy perhaps decreasing body lead burden by as little as 1–2 % (Mortensen and Walson, 1993). The need for chelation therapy is determined by the child's age, clinical features of toxicity and blood lead concentration (Table 2.2). Dimercaprol (British anti-lewisite, BAL) and calcium disodium edetate (calcium disodium EDTA) are used parenterally in more severe cases. Succimer (dimercaptosuccinic acid, DMSA) is available for oral therapy (Dart et al., 1994). Full details of the use of each of these antidotes are given in subsequent sections. DMSA is effective in removing lead from the body when given by mouth, and this makes it tempting to prescribe this routinely for all paediatric outpatients. However, some evidence from animal work suggests that DMSA may enhance lead absorption from the gastrointestinal tract, and therefore it is prudent to

TABLE 2.2
Guidelines for the use of chelation therapy in treating lead poisoning in children (modified after Henretig, 1998)

Clinical state	Dose and therapy indicated	Notes
Encephalopathy	Dimercaprol 450 mg m^{-2} d^{-1} + calcium disodium edetate 1,500 mg m^{-2} d^{-1}	75 mg m^{-2} i.m. 4-hourly (5 days) + continuous infusion, or 2–4 divided i.v. doses (5 days, start 4 h after dimercaprol), with subsequent courses based on blood lead concentration and clinical features
Symptomatic (blood lead above 700 µg/L)	Dimercaprol 300–450 mg m^{-2} d^{-1} + calcium disodium edetate 1,000–1,500 mg m^{-2} d^{-1}	50–75 mg/m^2 i.m. 4-hourly (3–5 days) + continuous infusion, or 2–4 divided i.v. doses (5 days, start 4 h after dimercaprol), with subsequent courses based on blood lead concentration and clinical features
Asymptomatic (blood lead 450–690 µg/L)	Succimer (DMSA) 700–1,050 mg m^{-2} d^{-1} or calcium disodium edetate 1,000 mg m^{-2} d^{-1} (or, rarely, D-penicillamine)	350 mg/m^2 8-hourly (5 days), then twice daily (14 days); continuous infusion, or 2–4 divided i.v. doses (5 days), with subsequent courses based on blood lead concentration and clinical features
Blood lead 200–440 µg/L	Controversial (American Academy of Pediatrics, 1995). Routine chelation not indicated, but consider DMSA if blood lead > 350 µg/L in a child < 2 years old and rising despite aggressive exposure reduction measures	350 mg/m^2 8-hourly (5 days), then twice daily (14 days)
Blood lead less than 200 µg/L	Chelation not indicated, attempt exposure reduction	

protect children from continued lead exposure during treatment with this compound (Chisolm, 1992, 2000). After initial chelation therapy, decisions to repeat courses of treatment are based on both clinical features and blood lead concentrations. In children with milder degrees of plumbism, i.e. asymptomatic or with blood lead concentrations < 700 µg/L, it is reasonable to allow 10–14 days of re-equilibration before restarting chelation therapy (American Academy of Pediatrics, 1995). D-Penicillamine has also been used to treat children with mild/moderate lead poisoning, but it has now largely been replaced by DMSA.

Chelation therapy effectively reduces blood lead, but remarkably it is still unclear whether it reduces total or critical body burdens of lead in asymptomatic children with moderately elevated blood lead concentrations (Kosnett, 1992; Markowitz et al., 1993; Mortensen and Walsen, 1993). There is fear that chelation therapy may merely redistribute metal from less vulnerable sites such as bone to more vulnerable target organs such as brain (Chisolm, 1987; Kosnett, 1992). However, effective chelation clearly reduced the morbidity and mortality of clinically overt lead poisoning in the 1960s (Chisolm, 1968). In the USA and UK, the majority of children with blood lead concentrations of 250–450 µg/L do not receive either calcium disodium edetate or DMSA (Norman and Bordley, 1995). Where treatment of lead poisoning with a chelating agent is required, oral DMSA is now more commonly used than i.v. calcium disodium edetate.

DMSA forms soluble complexes with lead that are excreted by the kidneys. In the USA, DMSA is approved only for the treatment of children with blood lead concentrations > 450 µg/L (2.17 µmol/L). However, it is equally effective at lowering blood lead in children with concentrations of this element < 450 µg/L (Liebelt et al., 1994; Besunder et al., 1995). DMSA is well tolerated and toxicity is infrequent. It is a relatively specific chelating agent for lead, producing less undesired excretion of zinc, copper, iron and calcium than calcium disodium edetate (Graziano, 1993). Few studies have examined the effect of chelation treatment on neurobehavioural outcomes, particularly in low-level chronic lead exposure in children, although it is theoretically appealing. In one clinical trial, Ruff et al. (1993) showed that, after treatment with calcium disodium edetate, improvements in performance were related to decreases in blood lead concentrations. Standardized mental development scores increased 1 point for every 30 µg/L (0.14 µmol/L) decrease in blood lead. Unfortunately, in the major centres that provide care for lead-poisoned children in the UK and in other parts of Europe, and in the USA, there is no consensus on the use of chelation therapy for treating 'low-level' lead poisoning. Poisons information centres will advise on the appropriate management of individual cases.

Children with acute encephalopathy, anaemia and either lead lines or evidence of recent pica on abdominal radiographs need immediate chelation therapy for lead poisoning. Confirmation of elevated blood lead should not need to occur before treatment is instituted if this may cause unnecessary delay. Acute bacterial meningitis or herpetic encephalitis must of course first be excluded, but lumbar puncture in the presence of lead encephalopathy is dangerous because of the likelihood that the intracranial pressure will be raised. Encephalopathy requires treatment by a combination of parenteral chelation therapy, maximal dose dimercaprol and calcium disodium edetate, and meticulous supportive care (Table 2.2) (American Academy of Pediatrics, 1995). If there is radiological evidence of residual gut lead, whole-bowel irrigation with polyethylene glycol to remove this has been advocated (American Academy of Pediatrics, 1995). Fluids and electrolytes should be closely monitored. Seizure control is achieved by use of diazepam (0.1–0.3 mg/kg) or phenytoin (loading dose 15–20 mg/kg, then 5–10 mg/kg). Hyperventilation, osmotic diuretics and steroids have not been rigorously evaluated but might offer pragmatic approaches to reduction of intracerebral pressure (American Academy of Pediatrics, 1995). Patients with encephalopathy or with initial blood lead concentrations > 1,000 µg/L will often require repeated courses of treatment. It is suggested that at least 2 days elapse before restarting chelation therapy after the first course to allow equilibration from other compartments into the vascular compartment to take place.

Studies to investigate the benefits of combining calcium disodium edetate with DMSA or dimercaptopropanesulphonate (DMPS; section 2.2.7) have been performed in rats, and the combination seems more effective in enhancing urine and faecal excretion and lowering concentrations of lead in blood and the liver but may increase the incidence of nephrotoxicity and zinc depletion (Tandon *et al.*, 1994; Flora *et al.*, 1995a). The appropriate clinical application of this work remains to be elucidated.

2.2.1.2 Management of lead poisoning in adults

The most important aspect of management of lead poisoning is removal from sources of exposure to lead. Chelation therapy should never be given prophylactically (Seward, 1996). The decision to give chelation therapy to treat lead poisoning is influenced by the clinical features of toxicity and blood lead concentration, as discussed for children. However, the threshold for use of chelation therapy is at higher blood lead concentrations in adults than in children because children's brains are growing and developing and are thus thought to be more susceptible to lead-induced toxicity (Table 2.3).

A patient who presents with acute lead encephalopathy, with an occupational history of lead exposure and laboratory findings such as anaemia, basophilic stippling, elevated red blood cell protoporphyrin, especially if > 0.44 µmol/L (250 µg/L) and abnormal urinalysis requires urgent treatment for lead poisoning. Delay in administration of chelation therapy while waiting for the result of a blood lead measurement is unacceptable. On the other hand, treatment of patients with poisoning due to tetraethyl lead is largely supportive, with sedation as necessary. If blood lead concentrations are very high, chelation therapy may be considered but has not been found efficacious as yet (Saryan and Zenz, 1994).

TABLE 2.3

Guidelines for the use of chelation therapy in treating lead poisoning in adults (modified after Henretig, 1998)

Clinical state	Dose and therapy indicated	Notes
Encephalopathy	Dimercaprol 450 mg m^{-2} d^{-1} + calcium disodium edetate 1,500 mg m^{-2} d^{-1}	75 mg/m^2 i.m. 4-hourly (5 days) + continuous infusion, or 2–4 divided i.v. doses (5 days, start 4 h after dimercaprol), with subsequent courses based on blood lead concentration and clinical features
Symptomatic, blood lead concentration above 1,000 µg/L	Dimercaprol 300–450 mg m^{-2} d^{-1} + calcium disodium edetate 1,000–1,500 mg m^{-2} d^{-1}	50–75 mg/m^2 i.m. 4-hourly (3–5 days) + continuous infusion, or 2–4 divided i.v. doses (5 days, start 4 h after dimercaprol), with subsequent courses based on blood lead concentration and clinical features
Mild features of toxicity, or blood lead concentration 700–1,000 µg/L	DMSA 700–1,050 mg m^{-2} d^{-1}	350 mg/m^2 thrice daily (5 days), then twice daily (14 days), with subsequent courses based on blood lead concentration and clinical features
Asymptomatic (blood lead below 700 µg/L)	Usually not indicated	Remove from exposure

2.2.2 Calcium disodium edetate (calcium disodium EDTA)

Disodium edetate (sodium edetate, sodium EDTA) has a strong affinity for calcium and other divalent cations (Schwarzenbach and Ackermann, 1948). However, disodium edetate can cause tetany if given i.v. because it chelates calcium. Calcium disodium edetate (sodium calciumedetate; sodium calcium edetate; calcium disodium EDTA; calcium disodium ethylenediaminetetra-acetic acid; calcium disodium versenate; edathamil calcium disodium; Ledclair, Sinclair; Sequestrene) (Figure 2.3) forms water-soluble complexes with polyvalent metal ions that have a higher affinity for EDTA than calcium such as lead, iron, copper, cobalt and zinc (Anonymous, 1953). Striking increases in urinary lead excretion followed i.v. injection of calcium disodium edetate in patients with chronic lead poisoning (Hardy *et al.*, 1954). Oral administration is less effective in removing lead from the body in such patients as judged post dose by urinary and faecal lead excretion (Bell *et al.*, 1956), probably because the oral bioavailability of the drug is less than 5 % (Lilis and Fischbein, 1976).

Calcium disodium edetate is rapidly absorbed if given intramuscularly (i.m.). However, it is so painful when given by this route that it is always given i.v. It has a plasma half-life of 20–60 min, exhibits first-order elimination kinetics, is 10 % bound to plasma protein and distributes to extracellular space with a volume of distribution (V_D) of some 0.2 L/kg (Klaasen, 1996). It has been estimated that only around 5 % of the plasma concentration is found in CSF (Foreman and Trujilo, 1954). Calcium disodium edetate is excreted rapidly in urine, if renal function is normal, at a rate that equates to the glomerular filtration rate (Morgan, 1975). Some 70 % of an i.v. dose appears in urine within 2 h, and 90 % within 6 h (Osterloh and Becker, 1986). A reduced dose is needed in patients with impaired renal function such as in those with lead nephropathy (Morgan, 1975; Osterloh and Becker, 1986).

Calcium disodium edetate

CAS registry number	62-33-9 (anhydrous)
Relative formula mass	374.3 (anhydrous)
Oral absorption (%)	< 5
Plasma half-life (min)	20–60
Volume of distribution (L/kg)	0.2
Plasma protein binding (%)	10
Urinary excretion (% unchanged)	70 (2 h post dose)

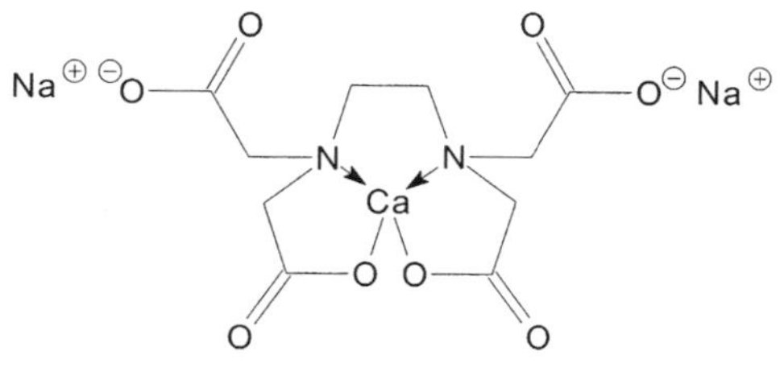

Figure 2.3: Molecular formula of calcium disodium edetate (calcium disodium EDTA)

TABLE 2.4

Approximate stability constants of some metal ion–EDTA complexes (Martell and Calvin, 1953)

Metal ion	Stability constant ($\log_{10}$)
Na^+	1.7
Li^+	2.8
Ba^{2+}	7.8
Sr^{2+}	8.6
Mg^{2+}	8.7
Ca^{2+}	10.6
Mn^{2+}	13.4
Fe^{2+}	14.4
La^{3+}	15.4
Co^{2+}	16.1
Zn^{2+}	16.1
Cd^{2+}	16.4
Pb^{2+}	18.2
Cu^{2+}	18.3
Ni^{2+}	18.4
Fe^{3+}	25.1

CHAPTER 2

The affinity constant of a metal for edetate is a measure of the stability of the resultant complex. A metal with a given affinity constant will displace a metal with a lower affinity constant (Table 2.4). Thus, the affinity constant of the lead complex is 10^7 times greater than that of the calcium complex, and therefore the principal clinical role for calcium disodium edetate is in the treatment of lead poisoning. Castellino and Aloj (1965) showed in rats a biphasic pattern of lead excretion after EDTA weakly bound extracellular lead being excreted rapidly, with lead complexed within cells being removed very slowly. Hammond (1971) further showed that bone provides the primary source of intracellular lead, which is chelated by EDTA only once it has entered the blood. There is limited evidence to suggest that folate, pyridoxine and thiamine may increase the efficacy of calcium disodium edetate treatment of lead poisoning (Tandon et al., 1987).

Mercury forms a complex with EDTA that is even more stable than that formed by lead. Unfortunately, this has no clinical application because mercury binds to sulphydryl groups of intracellular enzymes, and EDTA, which is ionized at physiological pH, penetrates cell membranes poorly (Osterloh and Becker, 1986). Calcium disodium edetate also chelates zinc and, to a lesser extent, iron, copper, manganese and cadmium. However, EDTA is ineffective in iron poisoning because it has less affinity for iron than transferrin and other iron-binding proteins.

2.2.2.1 Clinical use of calcium disodium edetate

The primary use of calcium disodium edetate is in the management of lead poisoning in children and adults (Tables 2.2 and 2.3). It has also been used to treat plutonium intoxication.

After use of EDTA, urinary lead excretion is increased 20- to 50-fold. Calcium disodium edetate should be given parenterally to treat lead poisoning because oral administration may enhance lead absorption from the gut. The dose is calculated using the body surface area or weight of the patient taking into account the severity of poisoning. Usually the total daily dose is given i.v. as a single prolonged daily infusion over 8–24 h for up to 5 days, followed by a rest period of at least 2–4 days. The rest period allows time for the lead to redistribute, for example from bone. It is important that before a follow-up blood lead concentration is measured, the edetate infusion should be interrupted for at least 1 h to avoid a falsely elevated value. The dose of calcium disodium edetate is 30–40 mg kg^{-1} d^{-1} or 1,500 mg m^{-2} d^{-1}. For infusion, every 2 g Ledclair should be diluted with 250 mL of 0.9 % (w/v) sodium chloride or 5 % (w/v) D-glucose; it is not compatible with other solutions such as sodium bicarbonate. Alternatively, the daily dose may be divided into two i.m. injections provided that procaine 0.5 % is added to reduce the pain at the injection site (Klaasen, 1996). After not less than 2 days (to allow for redistribution of lead between intra- and extracellular compartments) the course may be repeated. In theory each 0.5 g of calcium disodium edetate should result in the excretion of 260 mg lead, but the efficiency is only 0.5 % or so, probably because release of lead from tissue binding sites is slow.

It is important to monitor renal function closely during calcium disodium edetate administration and to adjust the dose and dosage schedule should renal dysfunction be present (Morgan, 1975; Osterloh and Becker, 1986). Induction of nephrotoxicity is reduced by keeping the total daily dose to 1 g in children or 2 g in adults, though doses may need to be higher than this, particularly if encephalopathy is present. Small doses, widely spaced with adequate hydration, increase the efficacy of therapy and decrease the chance of nephrotoxicity (Morgan, 1975). However, patients with encephalopathy should not be given large volumes of fluid too rapidly as this may worsen cerebral oedema and raise intracranial pressure.

There is some evidence that giving dimercaprol by deep i.m. injection (4-hourly, 24 h) enhances the efficacy of calcium disodium edetate in increasing urinary lead excretion in children and may prevent the effects of lead on haemoglobin synthesis and limit progression of toxicity (American Academy of Pediatrics, 1995). It has become accepted that for children or adults with lead encephalopathy or blood lead concentrations greater than 700 or 1000 μg/L, respectively, treatment should start with dimercaprol (5 mg/kg or 50–75 mg/m^2 i.m.), a second i.m. dose being given 4 h later. This should be followed immediately by an infusion of calcium disodium edetate (Tables 2.2 and 2.3). This is much more effective than starting calcium disodium edetate before or at the same time as dimercaprol in children with acute lead encephalopathy, probably because EDTA alone promotes redistribution of lead from soft tissue to brain (Cory-Slechta *et al.*, 1987; American Academy of Pediatrics, 1995; Cory-Slechta, 1995).

Combined use of parenteral calcium disodium edetate and dimercaprol increased urinary lead excretion over 5 days in 20 male patients admitted with petrol-sniffing encephalopathy (Burns and Currie, 1995). This report is especially interesting as alkyl lead petrol additives are not themselves chelatable. However, there is concern that dimercaprol may enhance brain lead and arsenic uptake (Chisolm, 1970; Hoover and Aposhian, 1983; Kreppel *et al.*, 1990). On the other hand, calcium disodium edetate itself may enhance brain lead uptake (Cory-Slechta *et al.*, 1987; Kosnett, 1992); comparable findings have been obtained with bismuth (Slikkerveer *et al.*, 1992).

The use of calcium disodium edetate challenge in diagnosing subacute lead poisoning has been described previously (Brangstrup Hansen *et al.*, 1981; Saenger *et al.*, 1982). For example, a dose of 25 mg/kg was given i.v. over 90 min, or 75 mg/kg was given i.m. with procaine in three equal parts 8-hourly. Urine was collected over 24 h for lead measurement, a urinary lead excretion after EDTA of more than 650 µg/d suggesting the presence of potentially toxic amounts of lead in the body. However, the test is expensive, relatively difficult to perform, may redistribute lead to the brain in rats, offers no real advantage over blood lead measurement and is now considered obsolete (Chisolm, 1987; American Academy of Pediatrics, 1995).

A patient with beryllium poisoning tolerated doses of 10 g/d calcium disodium edetate up to a total of 99 g. Calcium disodium edetate ointment is valuable in treating ulceration of the skin and nasal septum caused by hexavalent chromium (Anonymous, 1963; Maloof, 1965) and may also be useful after topical exposure to salts of other metals.

2.2.2.2 *Adverse effects of calcium disodium edetate*

The principal toxicity of calcium disodium edetate relates to the metal chelate, and in lead poisoning this affects the proximal tubule, distal tubule and glomerulus of the kidney as lead is released from the chelate in the kidneys (Klaasen, 1996). Cases of anuria have been reported when EDTA has been used to treat lead poisoning (Ohlsson, 1962; Tolot *et al.*, 1978). Such chelate-induced renal damage is reversible (Moel and Kumar, 1982) and probably results not from the chelate directly, but from reabsorption of the toxic metal in the tubule (Dally, 1992). Of 130 children receiving dimercaprol and calcium disodium edetate, 3 % developed acute renal failure, which did not need haemodialysis, and 13 % had biochemical evidence of nephrotoxicity (Moel and Kumar, 1982). In this context it should be remembered that lead poisoning can also cause renal damage independent of any chelation therapy. In another series of 122 patients given EDTA, none showed a post-treatment increase in plasma creatinine (Wedeen *et al.*, 1983).

Reversible mild increases in plasma hepatic aminotransferase activities are frequently reported after calcium disodium edetate. Extravasation may result in development of painful calcinosis at the injection site (Schumacher *et al.*, 1987). Prolonged systemic therapy with calcium disodium edetate may cause zinc and vitamin B$_6$ deficiency (Cantilena and Klaasen, 1982; Thomas and Chisolm, 1986). Febrile reactions with headache, myalgia, nausea and vomiting, and lachrymation, nasal, mucocutaneous lesions, glycosuria, hypotension, and electrocardiographic (ECG) abnormalities have also been reported.

The safety of calcium disodium edetate in pregnancy is not established, but in rats more live fetuses resulted when EDTA was used to treat lead poisoning (Flora and Tandon, 1987). However, in rats that did not have lead poisoning, increases in submucous clefts, cleft palate, syndactyly, adactyly, abnormal ribs and vertebrae occurred with doses of EDTA comparable to those used in man and without noticeable changes in the mother (Brownie *et al.*, 1986). Use of zinc calcium edetate caused no teratogenicity at low doses, and therefore it has been proposed that zinc calcium edetate should be available for use in pregnancy (Brownie *et al.*, 1986).

CHAPTER 2

■ 49

Calcium disodium edetate (Ledclair, Sequestrene)

- Chelates many polyvalent metal ions [Fe(III), Hg, Cu, Ni, Pb, Zn, Cd, Co, Fe(II), Mn, Ca, etc.]
- Principal role is in the treatment of lead poisoning (Ca^{2+} salt used as sodium edetate causes tetany)
- Ineffective in iron poisoning as less affinity for iron than iron-binding proteins
- Not useful in mercury poisoning as mercury is protein bound and EDTA does not cross cell membranes
- Given i.v. because oral dosage may enhance absorption of lead from the gastrointestinal tract
- Dimercaprol sometimes used as adjunct in lead encephalopathy in children

---

2.2.3 Calcium trisodium diethylenetriaminepenta-acetate (DTPA)

Diethylenetriaminepenta-acetic acid (pentetic acid; DTPA; CAS 67-43-6) is a synthetic polyaminocarboxylic acid with properties similar to those of EDTA (Hammond, 1971). As with all chelating agents, calcium trisodium DTPA (CAS 12111-24-9) is most effective if administered shortly after exposure. Oral calcium trisodium DTPA (Figure 2.4) has been used to treat iron-overloaded patients (Muller-Eberhard *et al.*, 1963; Constantoulakis *et al.*, 1974). DTPA may be more effective than EDTA in treating acute poisoning with cobalt salts (Llobet *et al.*, 1985), but appears to have no advantage over EDTA in treating lead poisoning, at least in mice (Jones, 1991).

Measures to enhance the excretion of plutonium and other actinides such as americium have been studied extensively. Plutonium-238 can be accidentally inhaled after accidents in the nuclear power industry. The plutonium(IV) ion complexes with transferrin in serum and may follow a metabolic path similar to that of iron(III). Deferoxamine is effective in removing plutonium, but DTPA can be given orally and is therefore the drug of choice for enhancing plutonium elimination (Truhaut *et al.*, 1966; Jones, 1991). Long-term zinc DTPA protected against the carcinogenicity of [239]Pu(IV) in mice (Jones *et al.*, 1986). A number of other chelating agents for plutonium have been investigated, but none has been found to be more effective than DTPA in removing Pu(IV) from tissues (Jones, 1991). Inhaled plutonium is difficult to remove with oral DTPA, and bronchoalveolar lavage with the chelating agent should enhance removal in such cases.

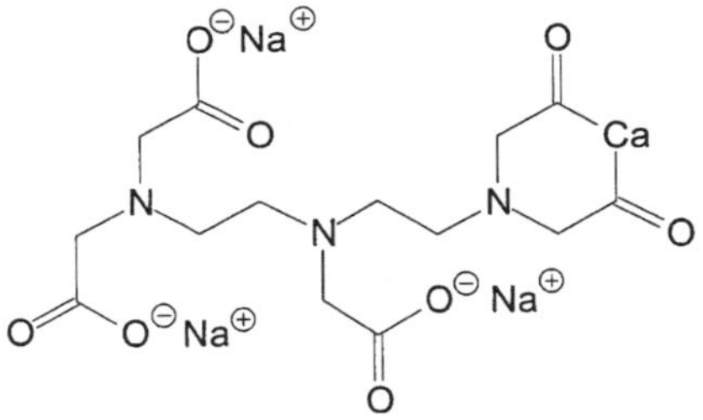

Figure 2.4: Molecular formula of calcium trisodium diethylenetriaminepenta-acetate (DTPA)

DTPA is provided as a white powder, which is made up in 0.9 % (w/v) sodium chloride for i.v. use. DTPA is given in a dose range of about 1 g/d (about 30 μmol/kg/d) by slow i.v. infusion over a few hours. In some cases, treatment has been carried out for one or more years intermittently and without adverse effect, and with enhanced excretion of small amounts of plutonium and americium. Combined treatment with early inhaled DTPA followed by repeated i.v. injection is thought likely to be the most effective treatment after inhalation of actinides (Stather *et al.*, 1985). DTPA can also be given additionally as an aerosolized solution (2 μmol/kg) in the case of inhalation of radionuclides (Dally, 1992). DTPA has side-effects similar to those of EDTA, especially loss of essential divalent cations such as calcium, copper, iron, zinc and magnesium. At high dose, renal toxicity is seen, probably due to tubular reabsorption of the metal, rather than the chelate itself (Dally, 1992). It has been suggested that, during chronic therapy, calcium DTPA should be replaced by zinc DTPA in the later stages of long-term DTPA treatment as zinc DTPA does not deplete the body of zinc and manganese (Taylor and Volf, 1980; Mays *et al.*, 1981).

Puchel [12,15,18,21,24-penta-azapentatriacontanedioic acid, 15,18,21-tris-(carboxymethyl)-13,21-dioxo; CAS 75977-88-7 (pentasodium salt); Figure 2.5], a lipophilic analogue of DTPA, was developed with the aim of enhancing the clearance of plutonium from intracellular sites (Stradling and Bulman, 1981).

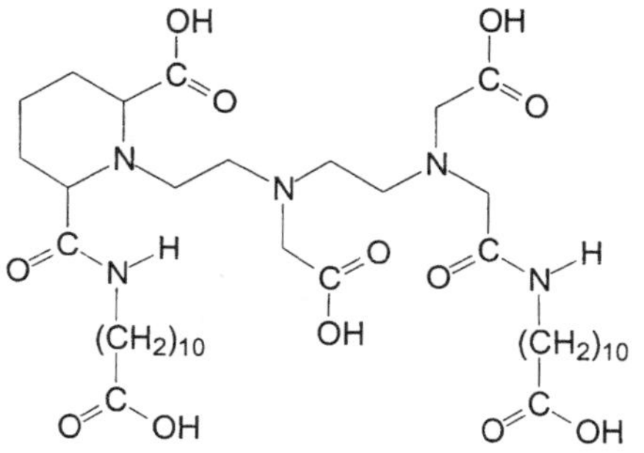

Figure 2.5: Structural formula of Puchel

2.2.4 Dimercaprol

Dimercaprol (2,3-dimercaptopropanol; Figure 2.6), the first chelating agent to be used clinically, was designed to treat poisoning with the arsenical chemical warfare agent lewisite [dichloro(2-chlorovinyl)arsine] (Peters *et al.*, 1945 – see section 7.5.1), hence its original name, British anti-lewisite (BAL). Currently, dimercaprol is sometimes still used to treat arsenic (Eagle and Magnuson, 1946), inorganic mercury (Longcope and Leutscher, 1946) and gold intoxication, and as an adjunct to calcium disodium edetate in severe lead poisoning. In the treatment of poisoning with arsenic or with mercury, dimercaprol has been largely superseded by DMPS and DMSA in many countries (Mückter *et al.*, 1997). It is thought that all of these compounds form stable, relatively water-soluble 1,2,5-arsadithiolane derivatives with bifunctional arsenicals (Figure 2.7).

Dimercaprol

CAS registry number	59-52-9
Relative formula mass	124.2
Oral absorption	Negligible
t_{max} (i.m.) (min)	30
Plasma half-life (h)	< 2
Urinary excretion (% dose)	90+ (4 h)

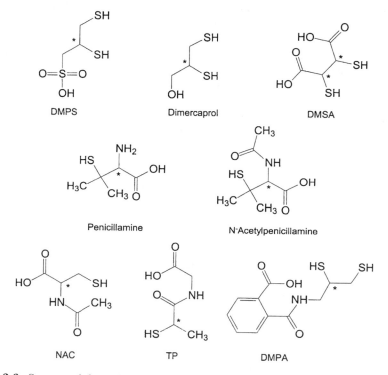

Figure 2.6: Structural formulae of some thiols used as chelating agents (DMPA = N-(2,3-dimercaptopropyl)phthalamidic acid, DMPS = 2,3-dimercaptopropanesulphonic acid, DMSA = 2,3-dimercaptosuccinic acid, NAC = N-acetyl-L-cysteine, TP = thiopronine [N-(2-mercaptopropionyl)glycine]). *Chiral centre

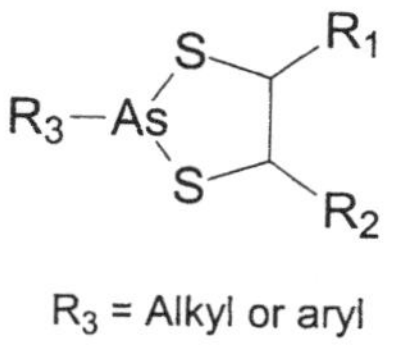

	R_1	R_2	
	H	CH_2OH	Dimercaprol
	H	CH_2SO_3H	DMPS
	CO_2H	CO_2H	DMSA

R_3 = Alkyl or aryl

Figure 2.7: Proposed structures of organoarsenic complexes with dimercaprol, DMPS and DMSA

In lead encephalopathy it is important to administer the dimercaprol first and the EDTA several hours later with the second dose of dimercaprol to prevent EDTA increasing the distribution of lead into the brain. Dimercaprol may also be useful in antimony, bismuth, chromium, nickel, tungsten and zinc poisoning (Braun *et al.*, 1946; Petersilge, 1947). It has been employed to chelate copper in Wilson's disease and may still have a role in patients allergic to D-penicillamine. Dimercaprol is widely used in developing countries, possibly because it is cheap and readily available.

Dimercaprol is said not to cause trace element depletion. However, it is not generally used in adult lead poisoning, and dimercaprol alone is contraindicated in poisoning with cadmium, iron, selenium, tellurium and organomercurials as it may increase tissue uptake of the poison. In sodium selenate poisoning, however, use of ascorbic acid (1 g i.m. and then 4 g/d orally) together with dimercaprol (initially 150 mg 6-hourly i.v.) has been reported to be effective (Civil and McDonald, 1978). Dimercaprol should not be used in patients with hepatic damage as rats with damaged livers showed toxicity with dimercaprol and arsenic (Peters *et al.*, 1945). Haemolytic anaemia may occur in patients with glucose-6-phosphate dehydrogenase (G6PDH) deficiency, but many G6PDH deficiencies are partial in nature, so it is not absolutely contraindicated in this group (Janakiraman *et al.*, 1978). Dimercaprol is known to inactivate the succinate oxidase system via a specific interaction with the Rieske iron–sulphur cluster in the respiratory chain of submitochondrial particles (Slater and de Vries, 1980).

Dimercaprol forms relatively stable dimercaptides with the metal ions mentioned above. Optimal effect seems to be obtained if dimercaprol concentrations sufficient to favour the formation of a 2:1 dimercaprol–metal complex are maintained and if the dimercaprol is administered as soon as possible after the exposure (Eagle and Magnuson, 1946). The hydroxyl moiety of dimercaprol confers some water solubility and helps excretion of the dimercaprol–metal complex in urine and bile. Dimercaprol–metal chelates are thought to be more stable at higher pH values, and thus maintenance of alkaline urine may protect the kidney from renal liberation of the metal (Dally, 1992). Dimercaprol did not impair arsenic clearance during haemodialysis in a patient poisoned with sodium arsenate (Mathieu *et al.*, 1992). The dimercaprol–mercury complex is removed by dialysis (Giunta *et al.*, 1983).

Dimercaprol is available in 200-mg ampoules. Although dimercaprol is soluble in water, the resulting solution is not stable. Secondly, dimercaprol bioavailability is negligible after oral dosage. Thus, dimercaprol is usually administered in a lipid solvent (arachis or vegetable oil) by deep i.m. injection to minimize pain and sterile abscess formation. Sometimes it is formulated in groundnut (peanut) oil and therefore the patient should be evaluated for nut allergy prior to administration to avoid anaphylaxis. Studies using ^{35}S-labelled dimercaprol have shown that it is rapidly absorbed from the injection site, peak blood concentrations occurring within 30 min, and persists for at least 12 h (Vale and Meredith, 1986). After 1 h approximately 80 %, and after 6 h nearly 90 %, of a dose is absorbed. Hepatic metabolism (by glucuronidation and sulphation) and excretion are essentially complete within 4 h. This explains the need for repetitive injections in general every 6 h to achieve therapeutic effect. Dimercaprol is the only commonly used chelating agent that readily crosses cell membranes. The concentration in some organs (liver, kidney, small intestine) can be up to five times that in blood.

Dimercaprol is given exclusively by the i.m. route. The usual dose is 2.5–5 mg/kg by deep i.m. injection 4-hourly for 2 days, then 2.5 mg/kg 12-hourly on day 3, and once or twice daily thereafter for 1–2 weeks depending upon the response; 36 mg/kg daily for 6 weeks has been given to rabbits (Dalhamn and Friberg, 1955). It is thought that dimercaprol may only be effective up to 9 days after acute poisoning with inorganic arsenic (Mahieu *et al.*, 1981). The injection is often very painful and pain over the injection site may persist. Rarely, sterile abscesses have been formed (Dally, 1992).

Dimercaprol is the most toxic of the currently used chelating agents – median lethal dose (LD_{50}) *c.* 1 mmol/kg (Jones, 1991). In clinical use it causes dose-related increases in both systolic and diastolic blood pressure up to 50 mmHg, and thus blood pressure should be monitored regularly, as should the pulse because of the possibility of tachycardia. Dimercaprol toxicity is dose dependent, and when 4 mg/kg and 5 mg/kg were given the incidence of adverse effects rose from 14 % to 65 % (Eagle and Magnuson, 1946). Such effects include nausea, vomiting, abdominal pain, tachycardia, headache, hypertension, sweating, lachrymation, muscle pain and spasm, a burning sensation in the lips, mouth, throat and eyes, with rhinorrhoea and salivation, and a feeling of constriction in the throat, chest or hands. These effects are maximal within 10–30 min and usually settle within 1 h (Eagle and Magnuson, 1946). Febrile reactions sometimes occur, especially in children, and these often persist during therapy. Convulsions and coma have been described, and in some cases have related more to the contamination with trimercaptopropane than to the dimercaprol itself. Haemodialysis or haemodiafiltration may be required to remove the dimercaprol–metal chelate in the presence of renal failure (Vaziri *et al.*, 1980; Mathieu *et al.*, 1992).

Dimercaprol (2,3-dimercaptopropanol, BAL)

- Designed to treat poisoning with the war gas lewisite [dichloro(2-chlorovinyl)arsine], hence known as British anti-lewisite (BAL)
- Now used to treat poisoning with arsenic, mercury and gold, and sometimes as adjunct to calcium disodium edetate to treat lead encephalopathy in children
- Sometimes used in Wilson's disease (copper storage disease) in patients allergic to D-penicillamine
- Given by deep i.m. injection as oral bioavailability is low. Check that the patient is not allergic to nuts before injection as it is sometimes formulated in groundnut oil
- Not used in adult lead poisoning and contraindicated in cadmium, iron, selenium and tellurium poisoning as it increases tissue uptake of the metal ion

---

2.2.5 *meso*-2,3-Dimercaptosuccinic acid (DMSA)

meso-2,3-Dimercaptosuccinic acid (DMSA; succimer; Chemet, McNeil) is a water-soluble analogue of dimercaprol (Figure 2.6). It is both less toxic than dimercaprol as evidenced by animal studies (Table 2.5) and more effective when given orally than either dimercaprol or calcium disodium edetate as an antidote for heavy metal poisoning (Aposhian, 1983; Graziano, 1986; Fournier *et al.*, 1988; Aposhian and Aposhian, 1990; Aposhian *et al.*, 1995). It is a relatively specific chelator that, unlike calcium disodium edetate, does not cause depletion of essential elements such as copper, iron and zinc. Although iron supplementation cannot be given concomitantly with dimercaprol because meso-*2,3-Dimercaptosuccinic acid (DMSA)*

CAS registry number	304-55-2
Relative formula mass	182.2
Presystemic metabolism	Extensive
t_{max} (oral) (h)	3
Plasma half-life (total DMSA) (h)	2
Plasma protein binding (%)	95
Urinary excretion (% dose)	30

TABLE 2.5

Toxicity of dimercaprol, DMPS and DMSA in mice (Aposhian *et al.*, 1984)

Compound	LD_{50} (mmol/kg)	Range (95 % confidence interval)
Dimercaprol	1.48	1.11–1.97
DMPS	6.53	5.49–7.41
meso-DMSA	13.72	11.36–15.22

the dimercaprol–iron complex is such a potent emetic, iron has been given with DMSA without such effects (Haust *et al.*, 1989). The acceptability of DMSA to patients makes it the antidote of choice for a variety of chronic heavy metal poisonings. For children, DMSA capsules can be opened immediately before use and mixed with fruit juice (Chisolm, 2000). Unlike D-penicillamine, DMSA does not increase, and may even decrease, the gastrointestinal absorption of lead (Kapoor *et al.*, 1989). Whereas dimercaprol can cause haemolysis in patients with G6PDH deficiency, DMSA has been given to two such patients with no resultant haemolysis.

DMSA was first synthesized as a potential water-soluble chelating agent for arsenic (Owen and Sultanbawa, 1949). It was subsequently studied with the aim of increasing antimony uptake during schistosomiasis therapy (Stohler and Frey, 1964), and was also proposed as an antidote for poisoning with lead or mercury (Wang *et al.*, 1965). DMSA has two chiral centres. The optically inactive form, *meso*-DMSA, is commonly used as a chelating agent and has been shown to be as effective as D,L-DMSA in chelating arsenic, cadmium, mercury and zinc (Egorova *et al.*, 1971; Aposhian *et al.*, 1983). Racemic DMSA (race-DMSA), however, is more water-soluble (Fang and Fernando, 1994). DMSA has an unpleasant 'egg-like' taste and smells of hydrogen sulphide. This can be disguised by co-administrations with food.

After an oral dose, most of the drug is absorbed via the stomach, with a peak plasma concentration being attained at up to 4 h (Dart *et al.*, 1994). Most (95 %) DMSA in plasma is protein bound. More than 90 % is present in urine as a disulphide in which each of the sulphur atoms of DMSA is linked to an L-cysteine molecule (Aposhian *et al.*, 1992, 1995). DMSA does not cross cell membranes extensively, despite the fact that it can be given orally (Gabard, 1978; Aposhian *et al.*, 1992). It is possible that metal chelation after DMSA occurs primarily in the kidney. *In vitro* Cd^{2+} and Pb^{2+} form a coordination complex with adjacent hydroxyl and thiol moieties of DMSA while Hg^{2+} forms a complex with adjacent thiols (Rivera *et al.*, 1989). No such complexes have been isolated from human urine after DMSA administration, however. Of course, the excretion of complexes with two DMSA molecules or with DMSA and other thiols such as L-cysteine is also possible. The half-life of total DMSA (parent drug plus oxidized metabolites) is longer in lead-poisoned children than in lead-poisoned or healthy adults, and renal clearance of DMSA metabolites is greater in healthy adults than in poisoned patients (Dart *et al.*, 1994). DMSA undergoes enterohepatic circulation, and a DMSA metabolite may be an active chelator (Asiedu *et al.*, 1995). Some 95 % of the drug is eliminated within 24 h of administration: 16 % in urine, 70 % in faeces and 1.6 % as carbon dioxide (Dally, 1992). In contrast, if given i.v. 82 % is found in the urine and only 0.3 % in faeces.

DMSA is as effective as calcium disodium EDTA in treating chronic lead poisoning, and as effective as DMPS in treating chronic mercury poisoning, as judged by urinary metal excretion (Wang *et al.*, 1965). In a more recent study, DMSA was given for 6 days to five lead-poisoned smelter workers (Friedheim *et al.*, 1978). DMSA treatment consisted of 8–13 mg kg^{-1} d^{-1} by mouth on day 1 with increases to 28–42 mg kg^{-1} d^{-1} on the last day. DMSA increased lead excretion and the blood lead concentration fell from 970 to 430 µg/L. The urinary excretion of iron, zinc and other essential trace elements was only minimally increased. Controlled trials of DMSA in 18 men with occupational lead poisoning found a 5-day course of 30 mg kg^{-1} d^{-1} (in three divided doses daily) to be more effective than 10–20 mg kg^{-1} d^{-1} (Graziano *et al.*, 1985). Blood concentrations fell from a mean of 790 to 230 µg/L in response to the drug and there were no clinically significant effects on excretion of calcium, magnesium, iron, copper and zinc. DMSA has also been used to treat systemic lead poisoning arising from fragments of lead bullets (Meggs *et al.*, 1994).

DMSA has been found to be effective in treating chronic lead poisoning in children (Graziano *et al.*, 1992). DMSA (10 mg/kg 8-hourly for 5 days, followed by 10 mg/kg 12-hourly for 14 days or 1,050 mg m^{-2} d^{-1}, for 5 days, followed by 700 mg m^{-2} d^{-1}) has been recommended as the sole chelation treatment for children with blood lead concentrations in the range 450–700 µg/L and in the absence of symptoms suggesting encephalopathy (Mortensen and Walson, 1983; Graziano *et al.*, 1988; American Academy of Pediatrics, 1995). The DMSA was well tolerated and no adverse effects were found. More recently, a regime using 1,050 mg m^{-2} d^{-1}, in three divided doses for 5 days, followed by the same regime after a drug-free interval of 7 days, has been proposed and is an acceptable alternative (Farrar *et al.*, 1999). Chisolm (2000) has reported that oral DMSA (initially 1,050 mg m^{-2} d^{-1}, 5 days) for 26–28 days was effective in lowering mean whole-blood lead concentrations in children (initial blood lead concentrations 250–660 µg/L) from 400 to 230 µg/L if re-exposure was prevented. Urinary copper and zinc excretion was not enhanced. Combination therapy with i.m. dimercaprol and calcium disodium edetate is recommended for children with severe lead poisoning, however, as use of DMSA alone may exacerbate encephalopathy. Thus, clinical studies of DMSA indicate that a 5-day course of 30 mg kg^{-1} d^{-1} in adults, or the dosage regime given above for children, is safe and effective in treating lead poisoning. However, as with other chelating agents, a rebound increase in blood lead concentration occurs following completion of the 5-day course (Graziano, 1986).

DMSA was found to be useful in treating a 46-year-old man who ingested 2 g of arsenic in a suicide attempt (Lenz *et al.*, 1981). Treatment with 300 mg of DMSA orally every 6 h for 3 days caused an increase in the urinary excretion of arsenic. The patient recovered. DMSA was more effective than *N*-acetyl-D,L-penicillamine in promoting the excretion of mercury in 53 patients poisoned by elemental mercury, but as the chelation therapy was continued for only 2 weeks the clinical benefit could not be evaluated

(Bluhm *et al.*, 1992). DMSA was also used to treat a 20-year-old man who had ingested approximately 0.5 L of a 16 % (w/v) solution of monosodium methylarsenate. The patient made a full recovery after four courses of oral DMSA (30 mg kg^{-1} d^{-1}, 5 days) (Shum *et al.*, 1995).

Both DMSA and DMPS have been used in the former Soviet Union and in China to enhance urinary excretion of copper in the treatment of Wilson's disease (Konovaloff *et al.*, 1957; Aposhian, 1983). D-Penicillamine, though, remains the treatment of choice in the Western world. Either DMSA or DMPS may be the agent of choice for treating acute bismuth poisoning (Basinger *et al.*, 1983a; Playford *et al.*, 1990; Slikkerveer *et al.*, 1992). However, DMPS, but not DMSA, appears to have beneficial effects in experimental beryllium intoxication in rats (Flora *et al.*, 1995b). DMSA has also been reported to protect against the testicular toxicity of nickel in mice (Xie *et al.*, 1995).

Minor adverse effects such as nausea and rash, especially in the mouth and other mucous membranes, have been reported in patients treated with DMSA (Grandjean *et al.*, 1991). Transient elevation of serum aminotransferase activity has been reported in adults given DMSA, but such effects may in fact be lead related rather than due to DMSA (Graziano, 1986). Reported adverse effects in children include nausea, vomiting, diarrhoea, loose stools, appetite loss and foul-smelling urine and/or stools. The occurrence of an anaphylactoid reaction when starting a second course of DMSA in one child and dramatic increases in serum alkaline phosphatase activity of bone origin in two further children have been described previously (Mortensen and Walson, 1993). The serum alkaline phosphatase returned to normal 5 weeks after the end of DMSA therapy in both cases. Trace element depletion is not a common problem in man, except for zinc (Fournier *et al.*, 1988). As DMSA has been introduced into clinical practice in Europe and North America only in the last decade, there is limited clinical experience with the drug, particularly with regard to long-term administration. Effects on the fetus have been found in mice at doses above 410 mg/kg/d s.c. (Domingo *et al.*, 1988). Thus, administration in pregnancy is a balance between risk to the fetus from the antidote and risk to both mother and child from the heavy metal.

DMSA mono- and dimethyl esters and the zinc chelate of dimethyl DMSA have been studied experimentally with the aim of enhancing tissue uptake of chelating agent (Aposhian *et al.*, 1992). Use of monoalkyl esters (methyl, ethyl, propyl, isopropyl, butyl, isobutyl, pentyl, isopentyl and hexyl) of DMSA to mobilize cadmium and lead from tissues has also been investigated in mice (Jones *et al.*, 1992; Walker *et al.*, 1992). All of these analogues were more effective than DMSA itself in lowering hepatic and renal cadmium and brain lead concentrations. However, the LD$_{50}$ of DMSA monoisopentyl ester, the most active analogue, was estimated to be 750 mg/kg (the reported LD$_{50}$ of DMSA is 3 g/kg).

2.2.6 D-Penicillamine

D-Penicillamine (penicillamine, 3,3-dimethyl-D-cysteine; Cuprimine; Distamine; Figure 2.6) can chelate arsenic, mercury, lead, nickel, copper, zinc, bismuth, cadmium, cobalt, iron and manganese, but its principal clinical use is in the treatment of Wilson's disease characterized by abnormal liver function test results, Kayser–Fleischer rings and haemolysis (Walshe, 1956; Joyce, 1989). The ability of penicillamine to reduce Cu^{2+} to Cu^+, which is less tightly complexed to protein ligands, may be important in its ability

D-Penicillamine	
CAS registry number	52-67-5
Relative formula mass	149.2
pK_a	1.8, 7.9, 10.5
Oral absorption (%)	40
t_{max} (oral) (h)	1–2
Plasma half-life	
α (h) (range)	1 (1–6)
β (d)	c. 8
Volume of distribution (L/kg)	0.8
Plasma protein binding (%)	85

to mobilize plasma protein-bound copper (Joyce, 1989). After 5 days the metal-mobilizing ability of penicillamine is said to decline – this could be due to removal of metal from extracellular spaces and limited ability to mobilize metal from tissues. Penicillamine seems to be ineffective in treating poisoning with bismuth (Nwokolo and Pounder, 1990; Slikkerveer et al., 1992).

Penicillamine for drug use is derived from the controlled hydrolysis of penicillin and consists of D-penicillamine only. Penicillamine is absorbed from the gastrointestinal tract although bioavailability is only about 40 % (Netter et al., 1987). Food, antacids and iron salts reduce penicillamine absorption from the gut and therefore it should be taken on an empty stomach (Rudge and Perrett, 1988). Peak blood concentrations are usually achieved within 1–2 h. Penicillamine in plasma is largely protein bound (up to 85 %), but also occurs as disulphides with itself and with cysteine and homocysteine, and as S-methylpenicillamine (Perrett, 1981). It is excreted in urine mainly as metabolites. Its initial plasma half-life after either oral or i.v. administration is about 1 h (range 1–6 h), and its terminal half-life is about 8 days (Rudge and Perrett, 1988). Pharmacokinetic studies in patients acutely poisoned with copper, lead, mercury and zinc have not been performed, and the recommended adult oral dose of penicillamine (0.25–2 g/d in divided doses for 5 days) is based on clinical response and on measurement of the amount of metal ion excreted in urine (Vale and Meredith, 1986). The penicillamine dose in children is 20 mg/kg daily in divided doses.

Chelation therapy in Wilson's disease is often achieved by use of penicillamine, but this agent would not be clinically useful in the case of deliberate ingestion of copper or copper-containing salts, particularly if renal failure were present. In such circumstances, dimercaprol might be of value (section 2.2.4). In Wilson's disease penicillamine is given in divided doses of 1.5–2.0 g/d before food. The maximum dose is 2 g daily for 1 year.

With acute arsenic poisoning, chelation therapy should begin as soon as acute toxicity is suspected and should not be withheld pending laboratory confirmation of a diagnosis of arsenic poisoning. In chronic toxicity, chelation therapy should be withheld until there is laboratory confirmation of excessive arsenic accumulation. The recommended dose of penicillamine is 25 mg/kg 6-hourly until the urinary arsenic concentration is less than 50 µg/L in 24 h (maximum penicillamine dose 1 g/d). However, a comparison of the effectiveness of penicillamine, dimercaprol, DMPS and DMSA in animal models found penicillamine to be ineffective in removing arsenic (Kreppel et al., 1989).

Penicillamine has been used in patients with mild or moderate lead body burden

(Ohlsson, 1962), but since 1990 it has been largely superseded in this role by DMSA. A typical dose regime is 10 mg kg^{-1} d^{-1} for 1 week increased to 20 mg kg^{-1} d^{-1} (two divided doses) for a further week. Subsequently a maximum of 30 mg kg^{-1} d^{-1} (in three divided doses) is maintained until a satisfactory reduction in blood lead concentration is achieved (Liebelt and Shannon, 1994). The American Academy of Pediatrics (1995) recommends penicillamine use only when unacceptable adverse reactions to both DMSA and i.v. calcium disodium edetate have occurred and yet it remains important to continue chelation therapy.

In chelating mercury penicillamine has been largely replaced by DMSA. If penicillamine is used, the duration of therapy should be guided by serial mercury concentrations in urine, and by clinical evaluation. If prolonged therapy is required, it has been recommended that treatment courses of 1–2 weeks should alternate with brief interruptions to minimize the risk of adverse events, particularly haematological toxicity. Penicillamine should be administered only after complete gastrointestinal decontamination, as the absorption of mercury may be theoretically enhanced after chelation with penicillamine.

Penicillamine is contraindicated in patients allergic to penicillin but seems to be safe in pregnancy (Miranda and Villagra, 1997). Adverse reactions include nausea, vomiting, fever, haematuria, proteinuria, rash, life-threatening bone marrow depression with leucopenia and thrombocytopenia, haemolytic anaemia, gastrointestinal distress, reversible renal and hepatic dysfunction, taste disorders and, rarely, autoimmune diseases (Goodpasture's syndrome, myasthenia gravis, polymyositis, systemic lupus erythematosus) (Gordon and Burnside, 1977; Hill, 1979; Hall *et al.*, 1988). Such adverse effects have generally been reported in adults on high-dose treatment. In children, milder gastrointestinal and renal effects tend to predominate (Liebelt and Shannon, 1994). Pyridoxine (vitamin B$_6$; section 4.12) (10–25 mg/d) should be given concurrently because penicillamine inhibits pyridoxine-dependent enzymes. Only about 10 % of patients under treatment for Wilson's disease develop penicillamine-related side-effects even though the doses used are much higher than in rheumatoid arthritis (Scheinberg, 1981).

CHAPTER 2

D-Penicillamine (Cuprimine, Distamine)

- Chelates arsenic, mercury, lead, nickel, copper, zinc, bismuth, cadmium, cobalt, iron and maganese
- Major clinical use is in the treatment of Wilson's disease (copper storage disease)
- Given orally although bioavailability is only *c.* 40 %. Food antacids and iron salts reduce absorption
- Pyridoxine (vitamin B$_6$) should be given concurrently
- Contraindicated in patients allergic to penicillin
- Adverse reactions occur in some 10 % of patients – severe toxic effects such as autoimmune manifestations are rare
- Other toxic effects may include fever, rash, haematuria, proteinuria, bone marrow depression, gastrointestinal effects, renal and hepatic dysfunction, taste disorders

2.2.6.1 Triethylenetetramine (TETA)

Triethylenetetramine (trientine; trien; TETA; TECZA; Cuprid; CAS 112-24-3; Figure 2.8) is an orally active chelating agent that has been used successfully in Wilson's disease and is indicated if intolerance to D-penicillamine develops (Walshe, 1982). Each TETA molecule is theoretically capable of chelating two copper atoms to form five-membered rings via the lone pairs on the adjacent primary and secondary amine moieties. It is given orally. Maximum daily doses of 2 g (adults) or 1.5 g (children) are taken in 2–4 divided portions on an empty stomach. When given at equivalent doses, TETA is less effective than cyclic analogues, namely Cyclam (1,4,8,11-tetra-azocyclotetradecane; CAS 295-37-4) and Cyclam 5, a hexamethylated Cyclam derivative (5,7,7′,12,14,14′-hexamethyl-1,4,8,11-tetra-azocyclotetradecane; CAS not available; Figure 2.8) in protecting against acute nickel chloride toxicity in rats (Athar et al., 1987).

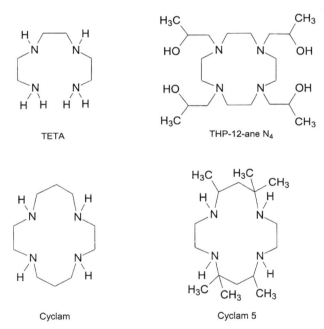

Figure 2.8: Structural formulae of triethylenetetramine (TETA), N,N',N'',N'''-tetrakis(2-hydroxypropyl)1,4,7,10-tetraazacyclododecane (THP-12-ane N_4), 1,4,8,11-tetra-azocyclotetradecane (Cyclam) and 5,7,7′,12,14,14′-hexamethyl-1,4,8,11-tetra-azocyclotetradecane (Cyclam 5)

2.2.7 Sodium dimercaptopropanesulphonate (DMPS)

Sodium D,L-2,3-dimercaptopropanesulphonate (DMPS; unithiol; unitiol; Dimaval, Heyl; CAS 4076-02-2) is a water-soluble analogue of dimercaprol (Figure 2.6). Like DMSA, DMPS was first synthesized as a potential water-soluble chelating agent for arsenic poisoning (Johary and Owen, 1955). Some of the metal-binding properties of DMPS were reported by Petrunkin (1956). It has been used to treat Wilson's disease in a patient intolerant of both D-penicillamine and TETA (Walshe, 1985). DMPS is both less toxic than dimercaprol (Table 2.5) and more effective when given orally than either dimercaprol or calcium disodium EDTA as an antidote for heavy metal poisoning (Aposhian, 1983; Hruby and Donner, 1987; Aposhian *et al.*, 1995). However, DMPS is more toxic than DMSA when administered to laboratory animals (Jones, 1991). Its main use is in treating mercury or arsenic poisoning (Aposhian, 1983; Campbell *et al.*, 1986; Kruszewska *et al.*, 1996). Combined with continuous veno-venous haemo-diafiltration it can remove as much as 12.7 % of an ingested dose of mercuric sulphate (Dargan *et al.*, 1999).

DMPS may be given orally or parenterally. Plasma protein binding is about 90 % (Aposhian, 1983). In acute poisoning 250 mg is given i.v. every 3–4 h initially, reducing in subsequent days. Hypotension is possible after bolus i.v. dosage of DMPS, and thus such injections should be given over at least 5 min (Aposhian *et al.*, 1995). In chronic poisoning 100 mg is given orally three times per day. The metabolism and pharmacokinetics of DMPS have been studied extensively (Aposhian *et al.*, 1995). After DMPS, acyclic and cyclic disulphides of DMPS are found in urine. As with DMSA, DMPS does not cross cell membranes extensively (Gabard, 1978; Aposhian *et al.*, 1992). Allergic reactions to DMPS occurred in 26 of 168 patients with scleroderma who were receiving receiving DMPS. Eleven patients felt sick, four felt dizzy and three developed itch. No renal complications were observed (Dally, 1992). After a therapeutic error (100 mg/kg was given instead of 5 mg/kg), cutaneous necrosis was found at the injection site (Dally, 1992).

Like DMSA, DMPS has been found to be effective in arsenic poisoning in man (Aposhian, 1983; Moore *et al.*, 1994), and in the former Soviet Union it was reported to be the drug of choice (Aposhian *et al.*, 1984). The relative effectiveness or therapeutic indices of these compounds, compared with dimercaprol, have been studied in mice by assessing the protection achieved against an LD_{99} of sodium arsenite (Aposhian *et al.*, 1984). The relative efficacy recorded was DMSA > DMPS > dimercaprol in the ratios 42:14:1. Use of intraperitoneal (i.p.) DMPS together with oral DMPS and cholestyramine was found to enhance faecal arsenic excretion in guinea pigs (Reichl *et al.*, 1995). It was thought that the enterohepatic recirculation of arsenic had been interrupted. DMPS and DMSA are more effective than dimercaprol in treating systemic poisoning with lewisite in rabbits (Inns and Rice, 1993). Like dimercaprol, DMPS is contraindicated in arsine poisoning.

The successful treatment with DMPS of 60 men with chronic lead poisoning has been reported from the former Soviet Union (Aposhian, 1983). The patients were given 250 mg/d for 20 days, with a resultant gradual reduction in the clinical features of lead toxicity. Treatment with DMPS does not redistribute lead or mercury to the brain of rats (Aposhian *et al.*, 1996). However, clinical experience suggests that DMPS is not appropriate for use in lead poisoning in children (Chisolm, 1992).

Various metal-binding agents were used to treat victims of the 1971–72 methylmercury poisoning disaster in Iraq (Clarkson *et al.*, 1981). The elimination half-life of methylmercury from the blood was used as an indication of efficacy. The mean half-lives obtained were as follows: no treatment, 63 days; DMPS, 10 days; thiolated resin, 20 days; D-penicillamine, 26 days; and NAPA, 24 days. Thus, DMPS administration led to a striking reduction of the blood elimination half-life of mercury. Clinical improvement was not seen in any treatment group, but it seems reasonable to postulate that reducing the total body burden of methylmercury may limit the progression of CNS toxicity. DMPS has also been given in inorganic mercury poisoning following the inhalation of mercury vapour (six patients) and the ingestion of mercuric oxide (one patient) and was associated with enhanced urinary mercury excretion (Mant, 1985). Fluid replacement and DMPS (250 mg i.v. 4-hourly for 60 h, and then twice daily for 18 d) were used to treat a 53-year-old male patient who had ingested approximately 50 g of mercuric iodide (Anderson *et al.*, 1996). DMPS was commenced approximately 8 h post ingestion and the patient made an uneventful recovery, his renal function and other biochemical parameters remaining within normal limits.

In animals, DMSA is more effective than DMPS in removing organomercurials from the body (Aposhian, 1983), whereas DMPS removes more inorganic mercury. A combination of DMSA and DMPS removes most types of mercury from most organs. Although further studies are necessary, DMSA will probably prove to be the treatment of choice for methylmercury poisoning because of its low toxicity and reported efficacy in animal studies. Urinary mercury excretion after DMPS challenge (300 mg orally after an 11-h fast) may be a better indicator of low-level mercurialism than unchallenged urinary mercury excretion after exposure to mercury vapour, and to mercurous and mercuric salts (Aposhian *et al.*, 1992, 1995; Maiorino *et al.*, 1996). However, the clinical relevance of these observations is unclear as yet. Neurological sequelae, particularly those resulting from exposure to organomercurials, remain a largely irreversible problem despite progress in chelation therapies.

DMPS (unithiol) and DMSA (succimer)

- Water-soluble analogues of dimercaprol that are less toxic and more effective in treating heavy metal poisoning
- Relative efficacies DMSA > DMPS > dimercaprol 42:14:1 in protecting against arsenic toxicity in mice
- DMSA is given orally (250–500 mg t.d.s.); DMPS is given either orally or parenterally
- DMSA has been shown to chelate arsenic, cadmium, copper, mercury, lead and zinc
- Allergic reactions such as rash reported with both drugs

2.2.8 Other agents used to treat poisoning with toxic metals

A large number of chelating agents have been studied in recent years with the aim of improving treatment of poisoning with metal ions. Areas studied include the use of dithiocarbamates in treating chronic cadmium poisoning.

2.2.8.1 N-Acetyl-L-cysteine (NAC)

N-Acetyl-L-cysteine (NAC; CAS 616-91-1; Figure 2.6) is able to chelate heavy metal ions (Henderson *et al.*, 1985; Girardi and Elias, 1991; Livardjani *et al.*, 1991; Ballatori *et al.*, 1998). Potential advantages over other chelating agents are that NAC is relatively safe and can be given orally and in relatively large amounts. Moreover, high tissue concentrations are achieved. One concern in using NAC is that tissue absorption of metal ions might be enhanced. Clinical studies that demonstrate the efficacy of NAC as a chelating agent for heavy metals are sparse (see Lund *et al.*, 1984), and more effective agents such as DMSA and DMPS are now available.

NAC is a monodentate ligand whose adducts with arsenic are not as stable as those formed by dithiols such as dimercaprol or DMSA. However, in rats NAC is more effective than calcium disodium EDTA or DMSA in increasing elimination of chromium and boron (Banner *et al.*, 1986), and in animals both cysteine and NAC have ameliorated arsenic toxicity (Shum *et al.*, 1981; Baker and Czarnecki-Maulden, 1987). A 25-year-old patient survived after ingesting 16 g of a hexavalent chromium salt when NAC and haemodialysis were used (Vassallo and Howland, 1988). Thus, in similar patients with hexavalent chromium poisoning, i.v. ascorbate (1 g initially every 10 min and repeated frequently) and NAC orally or i.v. in doses equivalent to those used routinely for the management of paracetamol (acetaminophen) poisoning (section 4.16.1) should be employed together with haemodialysis. Similarly, oral NAC seems to be effective in removing methylmercury in mice (Ballatori *et al.*, 1998), although it also appears to have a complicated effect on uptake of mercuric ions by the different parts of the renal tubule (Zalups and Barfuss, 1998). NAC is not thought to protect against the nephrotoxicity of cisplatin (*cis*-diaminedichloroplatinum(II), *cis*-$[(NH_3)_2PtCl_2]$) (Dorr, 1996).

There seems to have been no studies of combined treatment with NAC and a second, more water-soluble, chelating agent such as DMSA. Parenteral dimercaprol and i.v. NAC have been used succesfully to treat acute poisoning with sodium arsenate (Martin *et al.*, 1990) and arsenic pentoxide (Gjonovich *et al.*, 1990). It has been suggested that i.v. NAC might enhance gold excretion in patients with sodium aurothiomalate-induced aplastic anaemia. However, 1.2 kg NAC over 4 months was associated with the excretion of only 48 mg gold in a patient given more than 7 g gold over the previous 5 years (Hansen *et al.*, 1985). Oral NAC (600 mg/d, 2 weeks) did not enhance the excretion of iron, zinc or copper in healthy volunteers (Hjortsø *et al.*, 1990).

2.2.8.2 N-Acetyl-D,L-penicillamine (NAPA)

N-Acetyl-D,L-penicillamine (NAPA; CAS 15537-71-0; Figure 2.6) is more effective than D-penicillamine in protecting against the toxic effects of mercury (Aposhian and Aposhian, 1959). However, NAPA (250 mg 6-hourly) was less effective than DMSA in promoting the excretion of mercury in patients poisoned by elemental mercury (Bluhm *et al.*, 1992), and it has now been superseded by DMSA and DMPS.

2.2.8.3 Aurintricarboxylic acid (ATA)

Aurintricarboxylic acid (5-((3-carboxy-4-hydroxyphenyl)(3-carboxy-4-oxo-2,5-cyclohexadien-1-ylidene)methyl)-2-hydroxybenzoic acid; ATA; CAS 4431-00-9; Figure 2.9) has been listed for use in the treatment of beryllium poisoning (Meredith *et al.*, 1993).

2.2.8.4 N-(2,3-Dimercaptopropyl)phthalamidic acid (DMPA)

N-(2,3-Dimercaptopropyl)phthalamidic acid (DMPA; CAS 13312-78-2; Figure 2.6) was synthesized by Portnyagina and Morgun (1966). Subsequently, Yonaga and Morita (1981) demonstrated the ability of this substance to increase bile flow and the excretion of

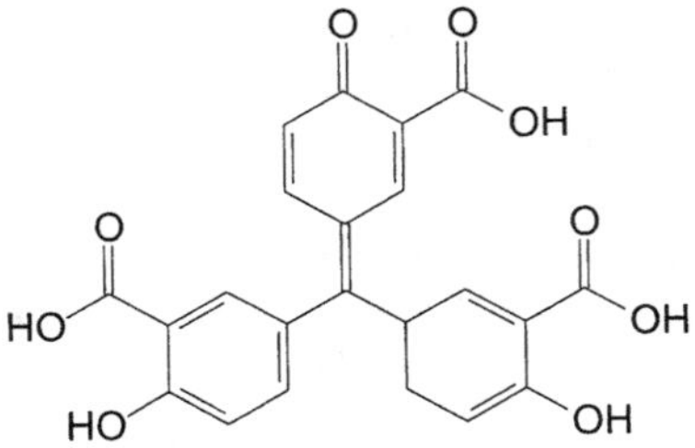

Figure 2.9: Structural formula of aurintricarboxylic acid.

mercury by this route in mice. DMPA was also shown to be more effective than dimercaprol for the mobilization and excretion of mercury. DMPA has been investigated as an antidote for arsenic poisoning in mice, but was less effective than either DMSA or DMPS (Aposhian *et al.*, 1984). DMPA is neither easy to prepare nor readily available commercially.

2.2.8.5 Dithiocarbamates

Sodium diethyldithiocarbamate (DEDTC; DDTC; dithiocarb; ditiocarb; CAS 148-18-5; Figure 2.10), the active metabolite of disulfiram, greatly increases the urinary excretion of nickel in acute nickel tetracarbonyl [Ni(CO)$_4$] poisoning (Sunderman, 1979, 1990). DEDTC can be given orally in moderately severe nickel poisoning, initially at a rate of 50 mg/kg in divided doses. At the low pH of the stomach, DEDTC decomposes to ethylamine and carbon disulphide. This can be minimized by the concomitant oral administration of 2 g sodium bicarbonate. Alternatively, the drug may be administered in gelatin capsules or i.v. at a dose of 4 g/m^2 body surface area. DEDTC undergoes hepatic metabolism to give a glucuronide that is excreted renally.

Studies in rodents have shown that DEDTC can ameliorate the nephrotoxicity and myelosuppression caused by cisplatin while enhancing the elimination of platinum. Clinical studies with 4 g/m^2 DEDTC as a 1.5–3.5 h infusion 45 min after cisplatin demonstrated reduced renal toxicity (DeGregorio *et al.*, 1989). DEDTC has been shown

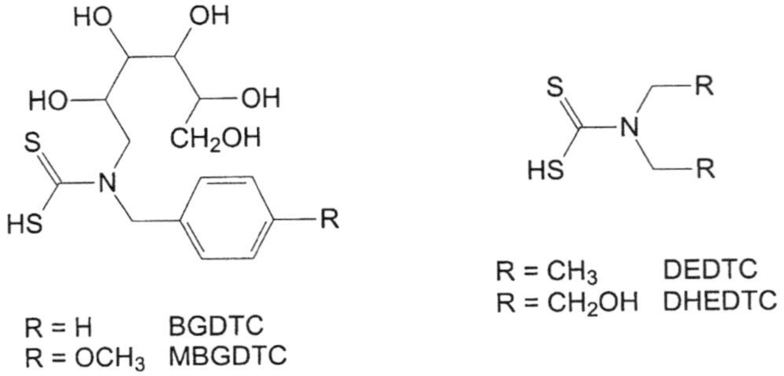

Figure 2.10: Structural formulae of some dithiocarbamates used as chelating agents (BGDTC = N-benzyl-N-D-glucaminedithiocarbamate, DEDTC = diethyldithiocarbamate, DHEDTC = dihydroxyethyldithiocarbamate; MBGDTC = N-(4-methoxybenzyl)-N-D-glucamine-dithiocarbamate)

to enhance platinum biliary excretion 30-fold in rats (Basinger *et al.*, 1989). However, more recent clinical studies with this agent have shown that, at tolerable doses, DEDTC has no major benefits when given with platinum-containing anti-cancer drugs (Dorr, 1996). It could, however, be considered in a cisplatin overdose. Physiologically, induction of a chloride diuresis encourages platinum exchange at the distal convoluted tubule.

DEDTC given up to 4 h after cadmium administration to mice can provide some protection against the toxicity of this ion (Gale *et al.*, 1981), but was associated with increased total brain cadmium concentrations. Sodium (dihydroxyethyl)dithio-carbamate (DHEDTC; CAS 1528-72-9; Figure 2.10) is as effective as DEDTC in enhancing cadmium excretion and does not enhance cadmium transport to the brain (Jones, 1991). A range of additional dithiocarbamates has been synthesized and found to have enhanced cadmium-mobilizing ability in rodents. Jones *et al.* (1991), for example, studied the effects of treatment with dimercaprol, DMPA and sodium *N*-(4-methoxybenzyl)-*N*-D-glucaminedithiocarbamate (MBGDTC; CAS 115459-35-3; Figure 2.10) on biliary cadmium excretion in rats. MBGDTC treatment increased the biliary cadmium concentration 580-fold compared with controls. It remains to be seen whether MBGDTC or other thiocarbamates (Jones, 1991) will prove effective in treating chronic cadmium poisoning in humans.

Xie *et al.* (1995) studied ammonium DHEDTC and sodium *N*-benzyl-*N*-D-glucaminedithiocarbamate (BGDTC; CAS 110771-92-1; Figure 2.10) in addition to DEDTC and DMSA in mice poisoned with nickel chloride. Treatment with either BGDTC or DMSA was equally effective, and DHED and DEDTC were both less effective, in decreasing testicular nickel concentrations.

The principal toxicity of DEDTC occurs with concomitant ethanol ingestion. This results in the classic 'Antabuse reaction' of facial flushing, headache, nausea, vomiting, weakness, blurred vision and hypotension. In the absence of ethanol, adverse reactions to the drug are very rare.

2.2.8.6 *Etidronic acid (EHDP)*

Etidronic acid (ethane-1-hydroxy-1,1-diphosphonate, EHDP; ethane-1-hydroxy-1,1-biphosphonate, EHBP; 1-hydroxy-1,1-diphosphonoethane; CAS 2809-21-4; Figure 2.11) has been shown to protect against acute uranium toxicity in rats (Ubios *et al.*, 1994).

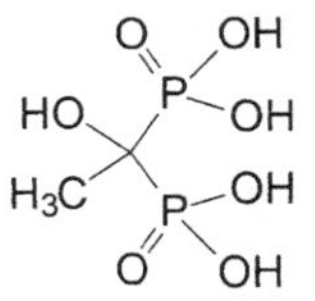

Figure 2.11: Structural formula of etidronic acid

2.2.8.7 *1,2-Cyclohexanediaminetetra-acetic acid (CDTA)*

1,2-Cyclohexanediaminetetra-acetic acid (CDTA; CAS 482-54-2; Figure 2.12) has been reported to be more effective than DEDTC in removing nickel from heart and brain of rats after nickel(II) sulphate administration (Tandon and Mathur, 1976). However,

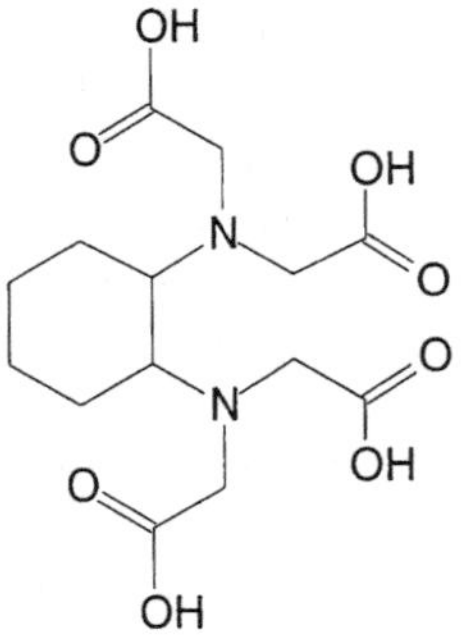

Figure 2.12: Structural formula of 1,2-cyclohexanediaminetetra-acetic acid (CDTA)

CDTA was less effective than DMSA or BGDTC in decreasing testicular nickel in mice after nickel chloride administration (Xie *et al.*, 1995).

2.2.8.8 N,N′,N″,N‴-Tetrakis(2-hydroxypropyl)1,4,7,10-tetraazacyclododecane

N,N′,N″,N‴-Tetrakis(2-hydroxypropyl)1,4,7,10-tetraazacyclododecane (THP-12-ane N$_4$; CAS 119167-08-7; Figure 2.8) has been designed with the aid of computer simulation. Animal experiments have suggested that this agent could be useful in treating poisoning with mercury and with cadmium (Gulumian *et al.*, 1993).

2.2.8.9 Thiopronine (TP)

Thiopronine [*N*-(2-mercaptopropionyl)glycine; tiopronin; Thiola; TP; CAS 1953-02-2; Figure 2.6) has been used as an adjunct to dimercaprol in treating acute poisoning with mercuric chloride (Giunta *et al.*, 1983). It has also been evaluated for use in treating acute bismuth poisoning (Slikkerveer *et al.*, 1992).

2.3 DEFEROXAMINE AND OTHER IRON/ALUMINIUM CHELATORS

2.3.1 Overview of acute iron poisoning and the role of deferoxamine

Iron salts are used for the treatment or prophylaxis of iron-deficiency anaemia. Oral iron preparations may be tablets or capsules in immediate-release or modified-release form, or liquids. Parenteral preparations are also available. In addition, iron is available in combination with folic acid and vitamins. There are many different iron preparations, each containing a different amount of ferrous (Fe^{2+}) or ferric (Fe^{3+}) iron; it is the content of this element that determines toxicity.

Toxic doses of *elemental* iron in man are (Proudfoot *et al.*, 1986):

- < 30 mg/kg – mild toxicity
- > 30 mg/kg – moderate toxicity
- > 60 mg/kg – severe toxicity

> 150 mg/kg – usually death

Absorbed iron is rapidly cleared from the extracellular space by uptake into parenchymal cells, particularly in the liver. It can cause mitochondrial damage and cellular dysfunction, resulting in metabolic acidosis and necrosis (Link *et al.*, 1998). Eventually widespread organ damage may become apparent and death from hepatic failure with hypoglycaemia and coagulopathy may ensue.

The early features of iron poisoning are due to the corrosive effects of iron salts, while later effects are largely due to the disruption of cellular processes (Proudfoot *et al.*, 1986). Iron tablets may adhere to the stomach, causing irritation and, in severe cases, haemorrhage and necrosis (Pestaner *et al.*, 1999). The consequential fluid and blood loss may be substantial and result in severe hypovolaemia. This in turn can lead to tissue hypoxia, lactic acidosis and circulatory collapse (Proudfoot *et al.*, 1986).

The clinical course of acute iron poisoning may be divided into four phases (Table 2.6). Blood should be taken at approximately 4–6 h post ingestion for measurement of the serum iron concentration, as iron absorption peaks at this time. It is important to take the sample carefully to avoid haemolysis. If deferoxamine (DFO) is to be given before 4–6 h because the history or clinical features suggest that a large dose of iron has been ingested, then blood should be taken for serum iron measurement before administration of DFO. Prior administration of the chelating agent renders serum iron assays uninterpretable. If DFO is not given, measurement in a sample taken after 6 h post ingestion may underestimate the body burden of elemental iron because distribution from blood into tissues may have occurred. On the other hand, if a modified-release preparation has been taken, serum iron should be measured at 4 h and again at 8 h post ingestion. It is essential to interpret the serum iron concentration in the context of the patient's clinical condition and an accurate history. Measurement of the total iron-binding capacity is of no value (Proudfoot *et al.*, 1986). In patients who present more than 8 h post ingestion, the serum iron should be measured on arrival. In such

TABLE 2.6
Possible clinical course of acute iron poisoning (Proudfoot *et al.*, 1986)

Phase	Time post ingestion	Clinical features and progress
1	30 min to several hours	Toxicity is due to the corrosive effects of iron. Haematemesis, diarrhoea, melaena and abdominal pain may occur. In severe cases gastrointestinal haemorrhage can result in shock, metabolic acidosis and renal failure
2	6–24 h	Either the features of poisoning resolve and the patient recovers or severe toxicity ensues
3	12–48 h	Severe lethargy, coma, convulsions, gastrointestinal haemorrhage, shock, cardiovascular collapse, metabolic acidosis, hepatic failure with hypoglycaemia, coagulopathy, pulmonary oedema and renal failure may occur
4	2–5 weeks	Scarring from the initial corrosive damage can result in small bowel strictures and pyloric stenosis

patients a low iron concentration cannot be interpreted, while a high concentration indicates potential toxicity. If serum iron measurements are not available, the presence of nausea, vomiting, leucocytosis ($> 15 \times 10^9/L$) and hyperglycaemia (blood glucose > 8.3 mmol/L) suggests ingestion of a potentially toxic amount of iron in children but not necessarily in adults (Palatnick and Tenenbein, 1996).

If < 30 mg/kg of elemental iron has been ingested, patients are unlikely to require active treatment but may vomit. If vomiting is severe, rehydration may be necessary. If > 30 mg/kg of elemental iron has been ingested, an abdominal radiograph should be performed to assess the need for gut decontamination. If undissolved iron tablets are visible then gastric lavage (if tablets are present in the stomach – see Figure 2.13) or whole-bowel irrigation (if tablets are seen in the small bowel) with polyethylene glycol electrolyte lavage solution should be undertaken (Everson *et al.*, 1991; AACT/EAPCCT, 1997). (Note that dissolved iron is not visible on radiographs.) In addition, the patient's serum iron concentration should be measured. The decision to give parenteral DFO is based on assessment of the patient's clinical condition and on the results of serum iron measurements (Proudfoot *et al.*, 1986):

- Patients with a serum iron concentration of 3–5 mg/L (55–90 μmol/L) should be observed for 24–48 h. They do not require chelation therapy unless they develop features of serious toxicity such as haematemesis or melaena (Proudfoot, 1995).
- Intravenous DFO should be given urgently to any patient with hypotension, shock, severe lethargy, coma or convulsions, or a serum iron concentration of > 5 mg/L (> 90 μmol/L). The decision to treat is based not only on the serum iron concentration, but also on the clinical condition of the patient.

DFO should be continued until the urine colour has returned to normal, clinical features of toxicity have resolved and no tablets are detectable on abdominal radiographs. Haemodialysis may be needed to remove the iron–DFO complex in patients with renal failure. Measurement of uncomplexed iron in serum is helpful in deciding when to stop DFO (Chapter 9).

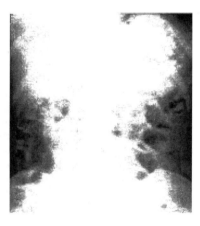

Figure 2.13: Abdominal radiograph of a 24-year-old patient who had ingested approximately 30 ferrous sulphate tablets 1 h previously – note the radio-opaque tablets in the stomach

2.3.2 Clinical pharmacology of deferoxamine

Deferoxamine (desferrioxamine; DFO) mesilate (Desferal, Novartis; Figure 2.14) is at present the agent of choice in the treatment of acute iron poisoning and is commonly used in treating transfusion haemosiderosis and other iron storage diseases (Proudfoot *et al.*, 1986; Kontoghiorghes, 1995a). DFO is also effective in controlling haemochromatosis (Cutler, 1989) and has been used for the treatment of aluminium toxicity in dialysis patients. DFO is a sideramine produced by *Streptomyces pilosus* (Actinomycetes), and was introduced to clinical practice in 1963. It is a water-soluble, aliphatic compound containing three hydroxylamine moieties and one free amine group. It is relatively expensive.

DFO has a very high affinity for ferric iron [iron(III), Fe^{3+}; complex formation constant, $K_a = 10^{31}$] coupled with a very low affinity for divalent cations such as calcium ($K_a = 10^2$), ferrous iron [iron(II), Fe^{2+}], copper or magnesium ($K_a = 10^{14}$ or below).

Deferoxamine mesilate	
CAS registry number	138-14-7
Relative formula mass (free base)	656.7 (560.7)
Oral absorption	Poor
Presystemic metabolism	Negligible
Plasma half-life	
(α) (h)	1
(β) (h)	6
Volume of distribution (L/kg)	2.9

■ CHAPTER 2 ■

DFO also has a high affinity for trivalent aluminium (Al^{3+}; $K_a = 10^{25}$) and is of value in removing aluminium (Ackrill *et al.*, 1980, 1986; Malluche *et al.*, 1984) as well as iron(III) (Baker *et al.*, 1976) from the body in patients undergoing chronic dialysis. Recently, treatment of aluminium overload using a cartridge containing immobilized DFO has been reported (Anthone *et al.*, 1995).

DFO is theoretically capable of binding iron and aluminium in a 1:1 molar ratio; thus, 100 mg DFO can bind approximately 8.5 mg iron(III) and 4.1 mg aluminium. In practice, the amount of iron excreted in patients with iron storage disease under treatment with i.v. DFO is much less than that predicted by theory. DFO can remove iron from haemosiderin and ferritin when present in tissues in excessive amounts, and to a lesser extent from transferrin, but not from haemoglobin or cytochrome oxidases. DFO does not significantly enhance iron or aluminium excretion in healthy individuals. Early use of DFO in an amount proportional to the transfusional iron load reduces the body iron burden and helps protect against iron toxicity in patients with thalassaemia major (Brittenham *et al.*, 1994). A cardioprotective effect of DFO has been reported (Bel *et al.*, 1996).

The red DFO–ferric iron complex (ferrioxamine; Figure 2.14) is soluble in water and is slowly metabolized (Porter, 2001). However, unless renal failure is present, some 50 % is rapidly excreted unchanged in urine, to which it imparts an orange/red

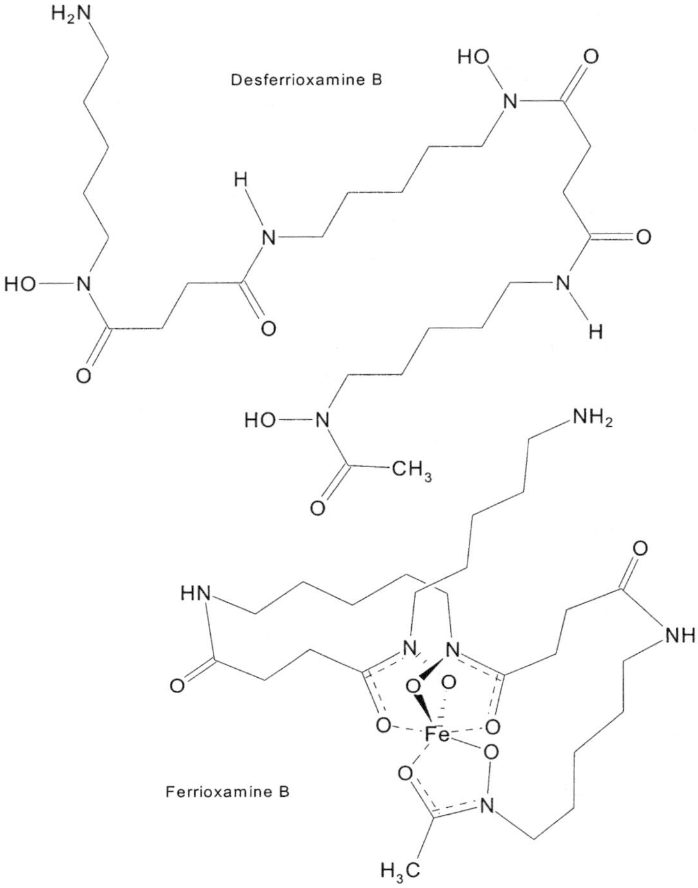

Figure 2.14: Structural formulae of desferrioxamine B and ferrioxamine B

colouration, with the remainder being excreted in bile (Pippard *et al.*, 1982). The DFO–aluminium chelate (aluminoxamine) is treated similarly. It is thought that the basic primary amine moiety at the end of the pentyl chain of ferrioxamine and aluminoxamine confers water solubility on the molecules, thereby facilitating renal and biliary excretion. Oral ascorbate, up to 200 mg/d in divided doses, can increase urinary iron excretion in patients with iron storage disease under treatment with DFO (Cohen *et al.*, 1981; Nienhuis, 1981; Pippard *et al.*, 1982). However, ascorbate administration in such patients is not without risk (Hershko, 1988).

2.3.3 Clinical use of deferoxamine

Animal studies have established that DFO reduces morbidity and mortality in acute iron poisoning, but no controlled trials in human poisoning have been performed (Lovejoy, 1983; Proudfoot *et al.*, 1986). Many anecdotal reports testify to its value, however, although it is not always effective in preventing serious sequelae such as acute liver failure (Kozaki *et al.*, 1995). The mechanism(s) by which DFO protects against acute iron poisoning remain uncertain (Lovejoy, 1983). Clinical studies suggest that DFO does not exert its beneficial action simply by increasing iron elimination as relatively trivial amounts are recovered in urine (Proudfoot *et al.*, 1986). It is possible that DFO binds sufficient free iron to prevent interference with mitochondrial enzyme systems or disruption of mitochondrial membranes without directly affecting the iron bound in haemoglobin, haemosiderin and ferritin.

DFO is poorly absorbed after oral administration (Kattamis *et al.*, 1981), but ferrioxamine is thought to be more readily absorbed. Thus, parenteral DFO administration is preferred. Nevertheless, although there is no clear evidence of efficacy, oral DFO (5–10 g in 50–100 mL of water) has been given after gastric aspiration and lavage (Henretig and Karl, 1983). High-formula-mass chelators for i.v. use have been obtained by covalently bonding DFO to dextran or hydroxyethylstarch. These compounds are reported to be much more effective antagonists for acute iron intoxication than DFO itself and have the advantage of not exacerbating the hypotension usually apparent in acute iron poisoning (Mahoney *et al.*, 1989). However, these compounds are not widely available.

Within 3 min of an i.v. infusion of DFO [10 mg (15.24 μmol) per kg] to six volunteers and seven patients with iron overload, peak DFO concentrations of 4.5–7.3 mg/L (80–130 μmol/L) were achieved (Summers *et al.*, 1979). There was rapid clearance from the blood, with the DFO concentration falling to half the initial value in 10–60 min (Summers *et al.*, 1979; Allain *et al.*, 1987a). This is probably the result of different processes, including penetration into both intra- and extracellular spaces, renal excretion and metabolism. Four DFO metabolites have been isolated in urine from patients with iron overload. Ferrioxamine is eliminated at a similar rate to DFO, but has a low V_D and remains in the extracellular space.

During a 24-h s.c. infusion of DFO (100 mg/kg) to 29 subjects, 21 of whom had iron overload, plasma DFO concentrations rose at different rates in different individuals, but a plateau was almost always reached by 12 h (Summers *et al.*, 1979). The height of the plateau appeared to be directly related to the degree of iron overload, so that heavily loaded subjects had relatively low concentrations of DFO in the plasma. The half-life of DFO in healthy subjects is about 1 h, but is about 19 h in patients with renal failure (Allain *et al.*, 1987b) – this may be advantageous in enhancing aluminium removal in such patients. DFO alone is not dialysable to any great extent.

No pharmacokinetic studies have been carried out in patients following oral overdosage of iron salts (Vale and Meredith, 1986), and thus the currently recommended DFO dosage regimens are based on clinical observation alone. It is now unusual to give the previously recommended doses of 2 g for an adult and 1 g for a child i.m., combined with an i.v. infusion at a rate which does not exceed 15 mg kg^{-1} h^{-1}, although some would still advocate such a regimen for 'mild to moderate' poisoning. The compelling argument against i.m. dosing is that more stable plasma concentrations are achieved with infusions (Propper *et al.*, 1976; Tenenbein, 1996). It is now much more common to give DFO at a dose of 15 mg/kg over at least 5 h to avoid hypotension, repeated as necessary until free iron is no longer detectable in plasma (Jones and Dargan, 2001).

The total i.v. DFO dose should not exceed 80 mg/kg in 24 h, though this is based on theoretical calculations rather than clinical data and higher doses have been used successfully (Howland, 1996; Tenenbein, 1996). One patient in particular was given DFO 425 mg/kg i.v. over 24 h without adverse events, although the increase in urinary

CHAPTER 2

iron excretion seen when the DFO dose was increased may not have been clinically important (Propper *et al.*, 1976). Severely poisoned patients probably require higher i.v. dosing for 24 h, whereas mildly poisoned patients are often given excessive DFO doses (Howland, 1996). DFO should be stopped when the condition of the patient has improved, free iron is no longer present in the plasma or no iron is detectable in urine. If oliguria develops, haemodialysis or peritoneal dialysis may be required to aid excretion of ferrioxamine (Stivelman *et al.*, 1989). DFO (6–12 g/d i.v.) has been successful in reducing serum, liver, cardiac and other tissue iron concentrations in individuals with severe iron overload with no adverse effects (Cohen *et al.*, 1989). Cardiac abnormalities associated with iron overload were also reversed.

2.3.4 The deferoxamine challenge test

In cases of suspected iron overload when the results of serum ferritin measurements were equivocal, measurement of urinary iron excretion over 6 h after DFO (500 mg i.v.) followed by a light breakfast and ingestion of 400 mL fluid was used as a diagnostic test (DFO challenge test). Excretion of 1–1.5 mg (18–27 µmol) iron per kilogram body weight over the 6-h period has been said to confirm a diagnosis of iron overload. If the amount of iron excreted exceeded 1.5 mg/kg, pathological iron deposition was said to be confirmed (Baldus *et al.*, 1978). However, the appearance of the orange/red colour of ferrioxamine in urine after DFO administration (50 mg/kg up to a maximum of 1 g) is not a reliable diagnostic aid in acute iron poisoning (Klein-Schwartz *et al.*, 1990; Proudfoot, 1995).

A variant of the DFO challenge test (5 mg/kg DFO i.v. during the last hour of a haemodialysis session in patients with serum aluminium > 60 µg/L associated with serum ferritin > 100 µg/L) may be used to test for aluminium overload. The test was considered positive if the post-test serum aluminium was more than 150 µg/L above the pre-test value (Anonymous, 1993; De Broe *et al.*, 1993). More recently, D'Haese *et al.* (1995) suggested that an increase in the serum aluminium of more than 50 µg/L associated with an initial serum immunoreactive parathyroid hormone (iPTH) concentration of < 150 ng/L was indicative of aluminium overload.

2.3.5 Toxicity of deferoxamine

Rapid i.v. administration of DFO may cause flushing, erythema, urticaria, hypotension and cardiovascular shock. The patent's blood pressure should therefore be monitored throughout the infusion. Histamine release is probably responsible at least in part for infusion rate-related hypotension, although intravascular volume depletion due to iron poisoning almost certainly also contributes. Pulmonary toxicity (adult respiratory distress syndrome, ARDS) has been described in acute iron overdose or haemosiderosis following i.v. DFO at doses of 15 mg kg^{-1} h^{-1} for more than 24 h (Tenenbein *et al.*, 1992). The underlying mechanism is unknown but may result from chelation of intracellular iron, free radical toxicity or from direct toxicity of the iron itself (Howland, 1996; Tenenbein, 1996). Use of a DFO infusion rate of no more than 15 mg kg^{-1} h^{-1} minimizes the risk of adverse reactions (Westlin, 1971; Tenenbein, 1996).

Cataract formation and renal failure (Cianciulli *et al.*, 1994) have been reported in patients undergoing prolonged DFO therapy such as those with thalassaemia.

Sensorineural hearing loss, night blindness, visual field defects, toxic retinal pigmentary degeneration, optic neuropathy and acute visual loss have been associated with chronic DFO therapy in such patients (Olivieri *et al.*, 1986; Bentur *et al.*, 1991; Kanno *et al.*, 1995). It is possible that these effects are due to reaction of DFO with superoxide free radical (O_2^{-}) to form the relatively stable nitroxide free radical. However, these effects have not been observed in patients treated for *acute* iron intoxication. There is no evidence of trace element depletion in patients treated with DFO, although not only iron, but also copper and zinc, excretion is increased in such patients (Davies *et al.*, 1983; Pall *et al.*, 1989; Uysal *et al.*, 1993).

Deferoxamine (desferrioxamine, DFO, *Desferal*)

- DFO is a siderochrome produced by *Streptomyces pilosus*. It is an aliphatic compound with three hydroxylamine groups and one primary amine
- DFO has a very high affinity for iron(III) and aluminium, but low affinity for calcium, copper, iron(II) and magnesium
- The red DFO–iron(III) complex (ferrioxamine) is water-soluble and is normally excreted in urine and bile. The DFO–aluminium complex (aluminoxamine) behaves similarly
- DFO can remove iron from haemosiderin and ferritin, but not from haemoglobin or cytochrome oxidases
- DFO does not increase excretion of iron(III) or aluminium from healthy individuals
- DFO is used to treat acute iron poisoning and transfusion-related iron overload

---

Clinical use of deferoxamine (DFO)

- DFO probably acts by binding free iron as well as enhancing excretion of iron(III)
- DFO is given parenterally as it has poor oral bioavailability (ferrioxamine readily absorbed)
- Flushing, erythema, urticaria, hypotension and shock may follow rapid i.v. dosage – monitor blood pressure and do not infuse at a rate greater than 15 mg kg^{-1} h^{-1}
- A daily dose of no more than 80 mg/kg should be used, except in severe iron poisoning
- Range of eye problems observed in patients undergoing long-term DFO therapy – use cautiously
- DFO half-life prolonged in renal failure – an advantage when DFO used to remove aluminium in dialysis encephalopathy

2.3.6 Overview of the role of deferoxamine in acute iron poisoning

Acute poisoning with preparations containing iron salts is common, especially in children. Although deaths have resulted when relatively large amounts of elemental iron have been ingested, in general mortality is low when the dose of iron ingested has not exceeded 60 mg ferric or ferrous iron per kilogram body weight (a 200-mg tablet of ferrous sulphate contains 60 mg of ferrous iron). Acute iron overdose in pregnancy is also common, and concern over possible teratogenic effects of DFO should not be a reason for witholding DFO in serious cases (McElhatton *et al.*, 1991). Parenteral DFO is the treatment of choice for severe iron poisoning, and indeed clinical experience suggests that survival may depend upon DFO administration at the earliest opportunity. DFO is widely used despite the fact that there are no controlled studies of efficacy in severe iron poisoning. Calcium trisodium DTPA (section 2.2.3) has been suggested for use in iron-overloaded patients who become intolerant to DFO.

Parenteral DFO should be given without awaiting the result of a serum iron measurement if it is clear that poisoning is severe, i.e. if coma or shock are present. Otherwise, the decision to treat iron poisoning with DFO is based on the clinical features of poisoning and the serum iron concentration. Initial serum iron concentrations in poisoned children correlate with clinical features such as shock or coma that suggest a poor prognosis. It has thus been recommended that an initial serum concentration greater than 5 mg/L (90 µmol/L) is an indication for DFO treatment. The kinetics of iron after acute overdose in humans remain to be investigated, but probably the peak serum concentration is achieved within 4–6 h post ingestion. Therefore, low serum iron concentrations 6 h or more post ingestion are uninterpretable, except after ingestion of a sustained-release formulation.

2.3.7 Other iron/aluminium chelators

A large number of chelating agents have been studied with the aim of producing a cheap, orally effective, non-toxic alternative to DFO (Jones, 1991; Porter, 1996). By analogy with DFO, these compounds may also be effective in enhancing aluminium and possibly plutonium excretion (Durbin *et al.*, 1989).

2.3.7.1 Deferiprone

Deferiprone (1,2-dimethyl-3-hydroxypyridin-4-one; L1; CP20; DMHP; CGP 37 391; CAS 30652-11-0; Figure 2.15) is one of a group of orally active iron chelators that form water-soluble, coloured, stable (stability constant 10^{36}), 3:1 [chelator–iron(III)] molar ratio complexes at physiological pH (Kontoghiorghes, 1985; Porter *et al.*, 1989a; Barman Balfour and Foster, 1999). These compounds are uncharged at pH 7.4 and are thus able to cross cell membranes more easily than negatively charged species. Maximal efficacy in chelating iron(III) from isolated hepatocytes was associated with an octanol–pH 7.4 buffer partition constant of 1 or thereabouts (Porter *et al.*, 1988).

Deferiprone has an iron-binding constant (10^{19}) similar to that of transferrin (10^{20}) and has proved as effective as DFO in treating experimental iron overload in animals. Deferiprone (0.5–3 g daily by mouth) enhanced urinary iron excretion, but not the

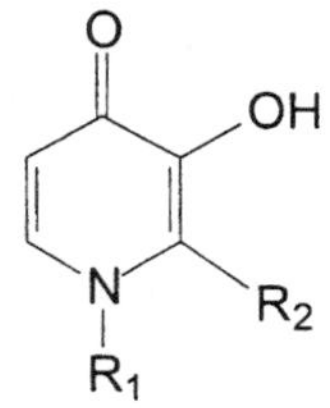

	R_1	R_2	
	CH_3	CH_3	Deferiprone (CP20, L1)
	C_2H_5	CH_3	CP21
	$(CH_2)_2OCH_3$	CH_3	CP51
	C_2H_5	C_2H_5	CP94

Figure 2.15: Structural formulae of deferiprone, CP21, CP51 and CP94

excretion of calcium, magnesium or zinc, in three patients with iron overload (Kontoghiorghes *et al.*, 1987). Oral deferiprone (75 mg/kg daily) showed similar efficacy to s.c. DFO in 26 patients with transfusion-related iron overload (Olivieri *et al.*, 1990). It is rapidly absorbed from the stomach. Peak plasma deferiprone concentrations were attained at 45–60 min post dose in 14 thalassaemia patients given the drug either with or without food (Matsui *et al.*, 1991). Deferiprone is excreted as a glucuronide and as an iron complex in the urine (Kontoghiorghes *et al.*, 1990). The plasma half-life of deferiprone is in the range 0.8–2.3 h.

There are major concerns as to the safety of deferiprone (Kontoghiorghes *et al.*, 2000). Eye toxicity and reduction of blood haemoglobin and white cell count have been reported in mice and in rats (Kontoghiorghes *et al.*, 1989; Porter *et al.*, 1989b), and preclinical studies showed a pattern of toxicities typical of a cytotoxic (antiproliferative) compound at doses similar to those used to treat thalassaemia in humans (Berdoukas *et al.*, 1993; Pfannkuch *et al.*, 1993). Embryotoxicity and teratogenicity at doses as low as 25 mg/kg were observed in rats and rabbits. Deferiprone may interfere with cell proliferation by removing intracellular iron needed for this process (Berdoukas *et al.*, 1993).

In humans, the development of reversible neutropenia and agranulocytosis during deferiprone therapy was described in one patient in 1989 (Hoffbrand *et al.*, 1989) and there have been further reports (Berdoukas *et al.*, 1993; Hershko, 1993). In addition, use of deferiprone has been associated with arthralgias and arthritis, and possibly with induction of systemic lupus erythematosus (Berdoukas, 1991; Mehta *et al.*, 1991, 1993). Arthropathy in 3 of 16 thalassaemia patients receiving deferiprone has been described previously (Berkovitch *et al.*, 1994), and visual and auditory toxicity has also been reported, although deferiprone is undoubtedly effective in decreasing and sustaining lower hepatic iron concentrations in this condition (Olivieri *et al.*, 1995). Deferiprone may thus only be of value in iron-overloaded patients who are unable or unwilling to receive i.v. DFO but who have potentially life-threatening serum iron concentrations or serious iron toxicity such as coma or metabolic acidosis (Hershko, 1993; Olivieri *et al.*, 1995). Deferiprone may also be valuable when used in combination with DFO (Richardson, 2001). Frequent haematological monitoring is mandatory, however, and embryotoxicity and teratogenicity are major concerns and therefore a negative pregnancy test must be obtained before deferiprone is given to a woman of child-bearing age.

Kontoghiorghes (1995b) reported on over 600 patients given oral deferiprone in over 15 countries. In most iron-loaded patients doses of 55–100 mg/kg deferiprone were associated with iron excretion greater than accumulation from transfusion (25–35 mg/d) and reduction in plasma ferritin and liver iron to near normal. Aluminium was removed from aluminium-loaded patients at similar deferiprone doses. Adverse

CHAPTER 2

effects included (reversible) agranulocytosis (six patients), musculoskeletal and joint pain (up to 30 % of patients), gastric intolerance (up to 6 %) and zinc deficiency (up to 2 %).

All of the 3-hydroxypyridin-4-ones studied are equally effective in binding iron *in vitro*, but their pharmacological properties differ according to the substituents at the 1 and 2 positions. Other 3-hydroxypyridin-4-ones which are possibly less toxic than deferiprone are thus being studied (Porter *et al.*, 1989a), notably the 1-ethyl- (CP21; CAS 30652-12-1) and 1-(2-methoxyethyl)- (CP51; CAS 118178-79-3) and 1,2-diethyl- (CP94; CAS 115900-75-9) analogues (Figure 2.15).

2.3.7.2 Dexrazoxane

Esters and lactones of aminocarboxylic acids have been studied as prodrugs for iron removal (Pitt *et al.*, 1986). Notable in this group is dexrazoxane [(+)-(S)-4,4'-propylenebis-2,6-piperazinedione; ADR-529; ICRF-187; Cardioxane; Eucardion; CAS 24584-09-6; Figure 2.16], a cyclized analogue of EDTA, which undergoes extra- and intracellular hydrolysis to yield a bidentate chelator. This compound can protect against doxorubicin-induced cardiac toxicity, thus permitting higher, longer doxorubicin dosage in women with breast cancer (Speyer *et al.*, 1992). Dexrazoxane is thought to act by chelating iron required by doxorubicin for the generation of free radicals (Lewis, 1994). It is given parenterally. It is thought not to compromise the anti-cancer activity of co-administered anthracyclines, and has relatively mild toxicity at the doses used as a cardioprotectant (Lewis, 1994).

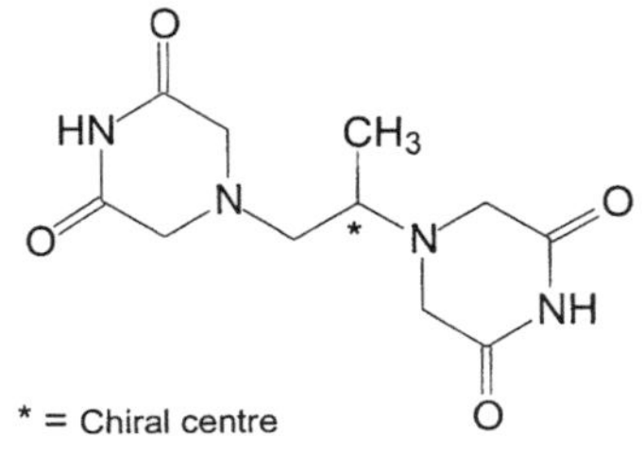

* = Chiral centre

Figure 2.16: Structural formula of razoxane

2.3.7.3 4,5-Dihydroxy-1,3-benzenedisulphonic acid

Sodium 4,5-dihydroxy-1,3-benzenedisulphonate (sodium catechol-3,5-disulphonate; tiron; CAS 149-45-1; Figure 2.17) is as effective as some other agents in protecting against acute uranyl acetate poisoning in mice (Basinger *et al.*, 1983b), and as effective as DFO in protecting against vanadium toxicity and in enhancing vanadium excretion in mice (Domingo *et al.*, 1986). In a further study, tiron, gallic acid (3,4,5-trihydroxybenzoic acid; CAS 149-91-7), and DTPA were more effective than other agents in protecting against acute uranyl acetate poisoning (Ortega *et al.*, 1989). The efficacy of a number of novel chelating agents based on carboxylic acid derivatives of catechol, for example catecholamic acid [catechol-3,6-bis(methyleneiminodiacetate); CAS 82773-07-7], in enhancing uranium excretion after chronic exposure has been studied (Jones, 1991).

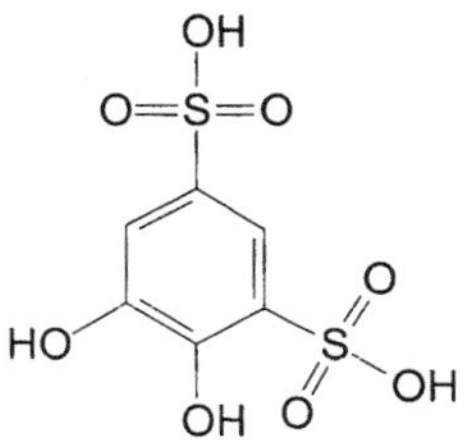

Figure 2.17: Structural formula of 4,5-dihydroxy-1,3-benzenedisulphonic acid

2.3.7.4 2,3-Dihydroxybenzoic acid

2,3-Dihydroxybenzoate (3-hydroxysalicylic acid; CAS 303-38-8) and its derivatives have been studied as orally active iron chelators. Although 2,3-dihydroxybenzoate itself has proved ineffective in clinical trials, a large number of derivatives including 2,3-dihydroxyterephthalamides have been studied. Analogues of enterobactin such as TRENCAM (CAS not available; Figure 2.18), whose iron(III) complex has a formation constant of $10^{43.6}$, have also been prepared (Rodgers *et al.*, 1987).

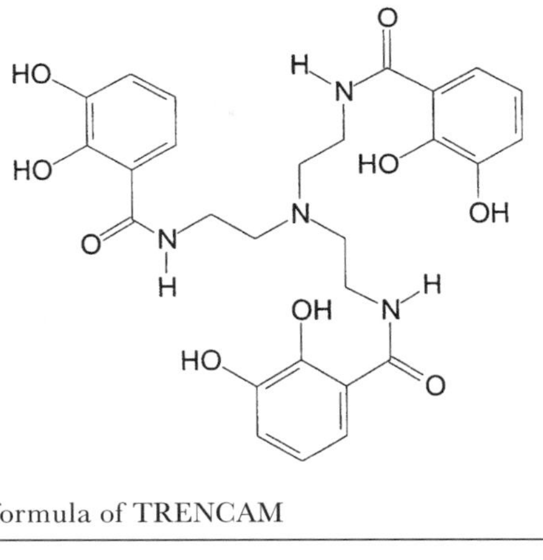

Figure 2.18: Structural formula of TRENCAM

2.3.7.5 Ethylenebis-2-hydroxyphenylglycine

N,N′-Ethylenebis[2-(2-hydroxyphenyl)glycine] (EHPG; CAS 1170-02-1; Figure 2.19) has been studied as an iron chelator. The iron(III) complex with this agent has a stability constant of $10^{33.9}$, which is greater than the corresponding value for EDTA by about 9 log units. A related compound, *N,N′*-bis(2-hydroxybenzyl)ethylenediamine-*N,N′*-diacetic acid (HBED; CAS 35998-29-9; Figure 2.19), forms a complex with iron(III) with a stability constant of $10^{39.68}$. Both of these compounds are effective in enhancing the urinary excretion of iron, but EHPG is superior *in vivo* and can be given orally (Pitt, 1981). However, interest in these compounds has waned in recent years.

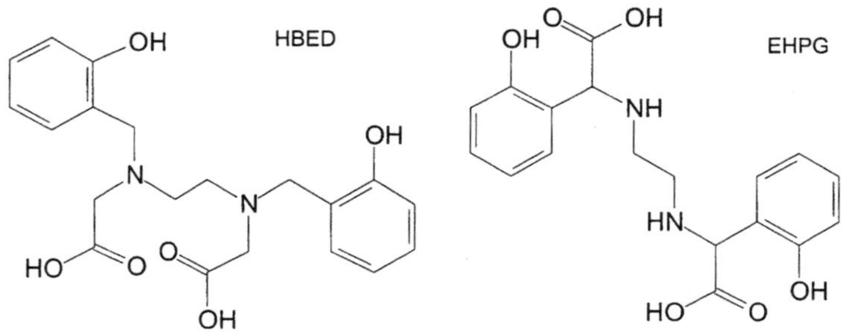

Figure 2.19: Structural formulae of *N,N'*-bis(2-hydroxybenzyl)ethylenediamine-*N,N'*-diacetic acid (HBED) and *N,N'*-ethylenebis[2-(2-hydroxyphenyl)glycine] (EHPG)

2.3.7.6 Phosphorothioate oligodeoxynucleotides

Phosphorothioate oligodeoxynucleotides (PS-ODNs) are modified DNA molecules that have a sulphur atom incorporated into the deoxyribose chain in place of one of the non-bridging oxygen atoms of the phosphate moiety. This creates polyanionic molecules that may have a role as heavy metal chelators, although other therapeutic possibilities are also under investigation. Continuous low-dose i.v. infusion (0.05 mg/kg hourly) of a PS-ODN known as OL(1)p53 increased the urinary excretion of iron 7.5-fold in a group of 16 patients being given the drug primarily for other purposes (Mata *et al.*, 2000).

2.3.7.7 Pyridoxal isonicotinoyl hydrazone (PIH)

Pyridoxal isonicotinoyl hydrazone (PIH; CAS 737-86-0; Figure 2.20) and its analogues, and related Schiff bases, have been studied extensively as iron chelators (Williams *et al.*, 1982). PIH itself has been given orally to patients, with complete recovery (Brittenham, 1990). Some of the PIH analogues studied, notably pyridoxal 2-pyrimidinylethoxycarbonyl methbromide (CAS not available), seem to be more effective than PIH itself (Hershko, 1988; Hershko and Weatherall, 1988).

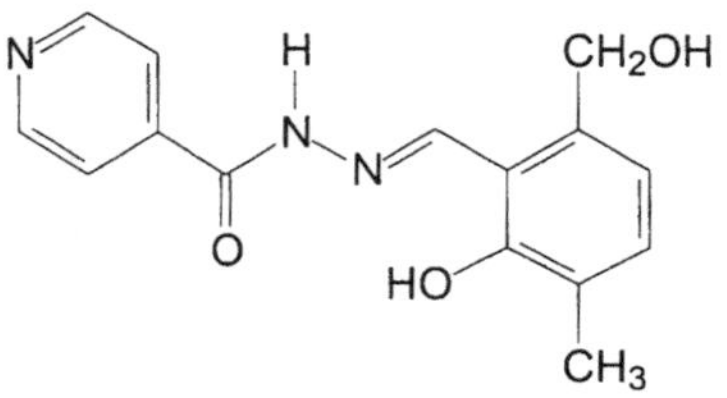

Figure 2.20: Structural formula of pyridoxal isonicotinoyl hydrazone (PIH)

2.3.7.8 Rhodotorulic acid

Natural and synthetic siderophores and hydroxamic acids such as rhodotorulic acid (CAS 18928-00-2; Figure 2.21) have been studied as oral iron chelators (Jones, 1991). In general, these compounds have been found to be not only unstable in the gastrointestinal tract, but also too toxic for clinical use.

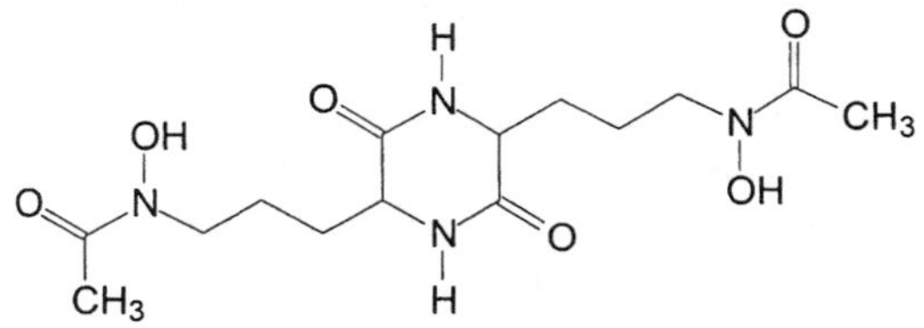

Figure 2.21: Structural formula of rhodotorulic acid

2.4 METAL-COMPLEXING AGENTS

2.4.1 Potassium iron(III) hexacyanoferrate(II) (Prussian Blue)

Potassium iron(III) hexacyanoferrate(II) (potassium ferric ferrocyanide; Iron Blue; Prussian Blue; Berlin Blue; CAS 12240-15-2; Figure 2.22) is used to treat poisoning with thallium. It is not a chelating agent, and indeed thallium does not respond to traditional chelation therapy such as EDTA, dimercaprol, D-penicillamine or DTPA. Ingested thallium (Tl^+) is absorbed and distributed rapidly. Like potassium, thallium is excreted via the kidneys and into the gastrointestinal tract via saliva and bile, and through the intestinal mucosa, across which a secretion/reabsorption cycle operates.

Oral Prussian Blue (250 mg/kg daily in 2–4 divided doses) given via a fine-bore nasogastric tube prevents reabsorption of the thallium ion – thallium is exchanged for potassium in the Prussian Blue crystal lattice and is then excreted in the faeces (Heydlauf, 1969). 'Prussian Blue' is available in a variety of preparations that differ in efficacy. The colloid or 'soluble' form (CAS 12240-15-2) is more effective than the insoluble form [iron(III) hexacyanoferrate(II); $Fe_4[Fe(CN)_6]_3$; CAS 14038-43-8] (Stevens et al., 1974). Adsorption of thallium to Prussian Blue is dependent on the size of the crystal lattice of the particular batch of the material used (Kravzov et al., 1993).

While some reports suggest that oral Prussian Blue is not absorbed (Stevens et al., 1974), this is difficult to reconcile with the observation of bluish sweat and tears in patients receiving oral therapy. Oral potassium supplements should not be given at the same time as Prussian Blue as they compete for entry into the matrix of the antidote. The exchange in the lattice is favoured by the smaller ionic radius of thallium, creating

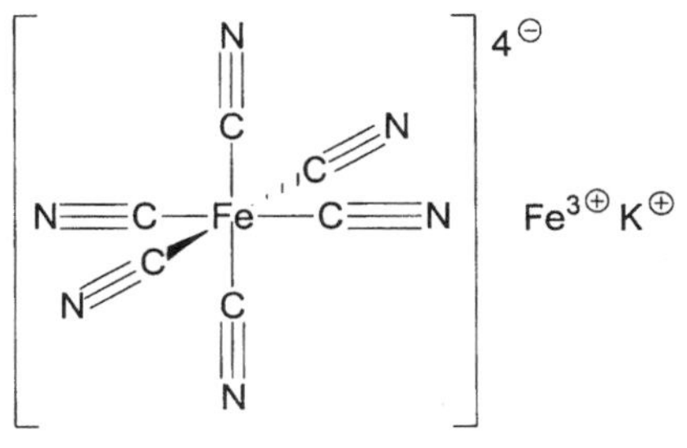

Figure 2.22: Molecular formula of potassium iron(III) hexacyanoferrate(II)

CHAPTER 2

'sink' conditions analogous to those created by repeat-dose oral activated charcoal (see section 1.4.4.1). In essence, Prussian Blue acts as an ion exchanger for univalent cations, its affinity increasing with increasing atomic radius of the cation. Oral Prussian Blue thus also enhances the faecal elimination of caesium (Iinuma *et al.*, 1971) and rubidium (Schäfer and Forth, 1983). A nickel iron(II)cyanide–anion exchange resin has been developed for oral administration to enhance elimination of ^{137}Cs (Iinuma *et al.*, 1971).

Prussian Blue is the antidote of choice for the treatment of thallium poisoning (Stevens *et al.*, 1974), although for ethical reasons there are no controlled trials that compare Prussian Blue with other agents. During treatment with Prussian Blue, plasma thallium concentrations fall and urinary thallium excretion declines exponentially (Kamerbeek *et al.*, 1971; Stevens *et al.*, 1974). In contrast, faecal excretion of thallium is detectable even when urinary thallium excretion is not measureable. Administration of Prussian Blue should therefore be continued until thallium can no longer be detected in the faeces, or at least until urinary thallium excretion is < 0.5 mg/d. Oral Prussian Blue may be combined with other forms of therapy to enhance thallium excretion (Thompson, 1981; de Groot *et al.*, 1987), but probably use of haemodialysis is no better than diuresis as the amount of thallium removed by such methods is trivial (De Backer *et al.*, 1982). The elimination half-life of thallium in man is reduced by treatment with Prussian Blue alone from more than a week to 3.0 ± 0.7 days; the addition of forced diuresis further reduces the half-life to 2.0 ± 0.3 days. Charcoal haemoperfusion may also be of value, especially within 2 days of exposure. Thallotoxicosis is commonly associated with intestinal stasis and severe constipation, and thus a laxative such as mannitol or lactulose should be co-administered regularly. Prussian Blue, 10 g in 100 mL 15 % (w/v) mannitol, is convenient.

2.4.2 Ammonium tetrathiomolybdate

Ammonium tetrathiomolybdate (CAS 15060-55-6; Figure 2.23) aids the elimination of copper and is under investigation for the initial reduction of plasma copper concentrations in the treatment of Wilson's disease (Brewer, 1995). When taken with food, ammonium tetrathiomolybdate, which can form a complex with protein and copper, prevents copper absorption. When given between meals it is absorbed and combines with albumin- and caeruloplasmin-bound copper. It may be particularly suitable for patients with impaired neurological function (Brewer *et al.*, 1994). Reversible bone marrow depression has been reported in two patients treated with ammonium tetrathiomolybdate (Harper and Walshe, 1986).

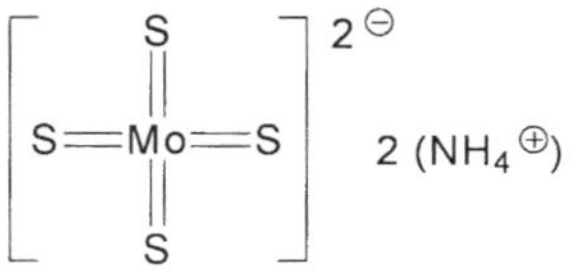

Figure 2.23: Molecular formula of ammonium tetrathiomolybdate

REFERENCES

AACT/EAPCCT (American Academy of Clinical Toxicology and European Association of Poisons Centres). Position statement: Whole bowel irrigation. *J Toxicol Clin Toxicol* 1997; 35: 753–62.

Aaseth J. Recent advances in the therapy of metal poisonings with chelating agents. *Hum Toxicol* 1983; 2: 257–72.

Ackrill P, Ralston AJ, Day JP, Hodge KC. Successful removal of aluminium from patient with dialysis encephalopathy [letter]. *Lancet* 1980; ii: 692–3.

Ackrill P, Ralston AJ, Day JP. Role of desferrioxamine in the treatment of dialysis encephalopathy. *Kidney Int* 1986; 29 (Suppl 18): S104–7.

Allain P, Mauras Y, Chaleil D, Simon P, Ang KS, Cam G, Le Mignon L, Simon M. Pharmacokinetics and renal elimination of desferrioxamine and ferrioxamine in healthy subjects and patients with haemochromatosis. *Br J Clin Pharmacol* 1987a; 24: 207–12.

Allain P, Chaleil D, Mauras Y, Beaudeau G, Varin MC, Poignet JL, Ciancioni C, Ang KS, Cam G, Simon P. Pharmacokinetics of desferrioxamine and of its iron and aluminium chelates in patients on haemodialysis. *Clin Chim Acta* 1987b; 170: 331–8.

American Academy of Pediatrics. Committee on Drugs. Treatment guidelines for lead exposure in childen. *Pediatrics* 1995; 96: 155–60.

Anderson RA, McAllister WAC, Taylor A. Acute mercuric iodide poisoning. *Ann Clin Biochem* 1996; 33: 468–70.

Anonymous. Use of calcium ethylenediaminetetraacetate in treating heavy-metal poisoning. Report of a conference held at Massachusetts General Hospital. *Arch Ind Hyg Occup Med* 1953; 7: 137–47.

Anonymous. Chrome ulceration of the nasal septum. *Br Med J* 1963; 1: 1364–5.

Anonymous. Consensus conference. Diagnosis and treatment of aluminium overload in end-stage renal failure patients. *Nephrol Dial Transplant* 1993; Suppl 1: 1–4.

Anthone S, Ambrus CM, Kohli R, Min R, Anthone A, Stadler A, Stadler I, Vladutiu A. Treatment of aluminium overload using a cartridge with immobilized desferrioxamine. *J Am Soc Nephrol* 1995; 6: 1271–7.

Aposhian HV. DMSA and DMPS – water soluble antidotes for heavy metal poisoning. *Annu Rev Pharmacol Toxicol* 1983; 23: 193–215.

Aposhian HV, Aposhian MM. N-Acetyl-D,L-penicillamine, a new oral protective agent against the lethal effects of mercuric chloride. *J Pharmacol Exp Ther* 1959; 126: 131–5.

Aposhian HV, Aposhian MM. *meso*-2,3-Dimercaptosuccinic acid: chemical, pharmacological and toxicological properties of an orally effective metal chelating agent. *Annu Rev Pharmacol Toxicol* 1990; 30: 279–306.

Aposhian HV, Hsu C-A, Hoover TD. DL- and *meso*-Dimercaptosuccinic acid: *in vitro* and *in vivo* studies with sodium arsenite. *Toxicol Appl Pharmacol* 1983; 69: 206–13.

Aposhian HV, Carter DE, Hoover TD, Hsu C-A, Maiorino RM, Stine E. DMSA, DMPS, and DMPA – as arsenic antidotes. *Fundam Appl Toxicol* 1984; 4: S58–70.

Aposhian HV, Maiorino RM, Rivera M, Bruce DC, Dart RC, Hurlbut KM, Levine DJ, Zheng W, Fernando Q, Carter D, Aposhian MM. Human studies with the chelating agents DMPS and DMSA. *Clin Toxicol* 1992; 30: 505–28.

Aposhian HV, Maiorino RM, Gonzalez-Ramirez D, Zuniga-Charles M, Xu Z, Hurlbut KM, Junco-Munoz P, Dart RC, Aposhian MM. Mobilization of heavy metals by newer, therapeutically useful chelating agents. *Toxicology* 1995; 97: 23–38.

Aposhian MM, Maiorino RM, Xu Z, Aposhian HV. Sodium 2,3-dimercapto-1-propanesulphonate (DMPS) treatment does not redistribute lead or mercury to the brain of rats. *Toxicology* 1996; 109: 49–55.

Asiedu P, Moulton T, Blum CB, Roldan E, Lolacono NJ, Graziano JH. Metabolism of meso-2,3-dimercaptosuccinic acid in lead-poisoned children and normal adults. *Environ Hlth Perspect* 1995; 103: 734–9.

Athar M, Misra M, Srivastava RC. Evaluation of chelating drugs on the toxicity, excretion and distribution of nickel in poisoned rats. *Fundam Appl Toxicol* 1987; 9: 26–33.

Baker DH, Czarnecki-Maulden GL. Pharmacologic role of cysteine in ameliorating or exacerbating mineral toxicities. *J Nutr* 1987; 117: 1003–10.

Baker LRI, Barnett MD, Brozovic B, Cattell WR, Ackrill P, McAlister J, Nimmon C. Hemosiderosis in a patient on regular haemodialysis: treatment by desferrioxamine. *Clin Nephrol* 1976; 6: 326–8.

Baldus WP, Fairbanks VF, Dickson ER, Baggenstoss AH. Deferoxamine-chelatable iron in hemochromatosis and other disorders of iron overload. *Mayo Clinic Proc* 1978; 53: 157–65.

Ballatori N, Lieberman MW, Wang W. N-Acetylcystine as an antidote in methylmercury poisoning. *Env Hlth Perspect* 1998; 106: 267–71.

Banner W, Koch M, Capin DM, Hopf SB, Chang S, Tong TG. Experimental chelation therapy in chromium, lead and boron intoxication with N-acetylcysteine and other compounds. *Toxicol Appl Pharmacol* 1986; 83: 142–7.

Barman Balfour JA, Foster RH. Deferiprone: a review of its clinical potential in iron overload in β-thallassaemia major and other transfusion-dependent diseases. *Drugs* 1999; 58: 553–78.

Basinger MA, Jones MM, McCroskey SA. Antidotes for acute bismuth intoxication. *J Toxicol Clin Toxicol* 1983a; 20: 159–65.

Basinger MA, Forti RL, Burka LT, Jones MM, Mitchell WM, Johnson JE, Gibbs SJ. Phenolic chelating agents as antidotes for acute uranyl acetate intoxication in mice. *J Toxicol Environ Hlth* 1983b; 11: 237–46.

Basinger MA, Jones MM, Gilbreath SG, Walker EM, Fody EP, Mayhue MA. Dithiocarbamate-induced biliary platinum excretion and the control of cis-platinum nephrotoxicity. *Toxicol Appl Pharmacol* 1989; 97: 279–88.

Bel A, Martinod E, Menasché P. Cardioprotective effect of desferrioxamine. *Acta Haematol* 1996; 95: 63–5.

Bell RF, Gilliland JC, Boland JR, Sullivan BR. Effect of oral edathamil calcium-disodium on urinary and fecal lead excretion. *Arch Ind Hlth* 1956; 13: 366–71.

Bentur Y, McGuigan M, Koren G. Deferoxamine (desferrioxamine): new toxicities for an old drug. *Drug Safety* 1991; 6: 37–46.

Berdoukas V. Antinuclear antibodies in patients taking L1 [letter]. *Lancet* 1991; 337: 672.

Berdoukas V, Bentley P, Frost H, Schnebli HP. Toxicity of oral iron chelator L1 [letter]. *Lancet* 1993; 341: 1088.

Berkovitch M, Laxer RM, Inman R, Koren G, Pritzker KPH, Fritzler MJ, Olivieri NF. Arthropathy in thalassaemia patients receiving deferiprone. *Lancet* 1994; 343: 1471–2.

Besunder JB, Anderson RL, Super DM. Short-term efficacy of oral dimercaptosuccinic acid in children with low to moderate lead intoxication. *Pediatrics* 1995; 96: 683–7.

Bluhm RE, Bobbitt RG, Welch LW, Wood AJJ, Bonfiglio JF, Sarzen C, Heath AJ, Branch RA. Elemental mercury vapour toxicity, treatment, and prognosis after acute, intensive exposure in chloralkali plant workers. Part I. History, neuropsychological findings and chelator effects. *Hum Exp Toxicol* 1992; 11: 201–10.

Brangstrup Hansen JP, Døssing M, Paulev P-E. Chelatable lead body burden (by calcium-disodium EDTA) and blood lead concentration in man. *J Occup Med* 1981; 23: 39–43.

Braun HA, Lusky LM, Calvery HO. The efficacy of 2,3-dimercaptopropanol (BAL) in the therapy of poisoning by compounds of antimony, bismuth, chromium, mercury and nickel. *J Pharmacol Exp Ther* 1946; 87 (Suppl 1): 119–25.

Brewer GJ. Practical recommendations and new therapies for Wilson's disease. *Drugs* 1995; 50: 240–9.

Brewer GJ, Dick RD, Johnson V, Wang Y, Yuzbasiyan-Gurkan V, Kluin K, Fink JK, Aisen A. Treatment of Wilson's disease with ammonium tetrathiomolybdate. I. Initial therapy in 17 neurologically affected patients. *Arch Neurol* 1994; 51: 545–54.

Brittenham GM. Pyridoxal isonicotinoyl hydrazone: an effective iron-chelator after oral administration. *Semin Haematol* 1990; 27: 112–16.

Brittenham GM, Griffith PM, Nienhuis AW, McLaren CE, Young NS, Tucker EE, Allen CJ, Farrell DE, Harris JW. Efficacy of deferoxamine in preventing complications of iron overload in patients with thalassemia major. *N Engl J Med* 1994; 331: 567–73.

Brownie CF, Brownie C, Noden D, Krook L, Haluska M, Aronson AL. Teratogenic effect of calcium edatate (CaEDTA) in rats and the protective effect of zinc. *Toxicol Appl Pharmacol* 1986; 82: 426–43.

Burns CB, Currie B. The efficacy of chelation therapy and factors influencing mortality in lead intoxicated petrol sniffers. *Aust NZ J Med* 1995; 25: 197–203.

Campbell JR, Clarkson TW, Omar MD. The therapeutic use of 2,3-dimercaptopropane-1-sulfonate in two cases of inorganic mercury poisoning. *J Am Med Assoc* 1986; 256: 3127–30.

Cantilena LR, Klaassen CD. The effect of chelating agents on the excretion of endogenous metals. *Toxicol Appl Pharmacol* 1982; 63: 344–50.

Castellino N, Aloj S. Effects of calcium sodium ethylenediaminetetra-acetate on the kinetics of distribution and excretion of lead in the rat. *Br J Industr Med* 1965; 22: 172–80.

Centers for Disease Control and Prevention. *Preventing Lead Poisoning in Young Children: a statement by the Centers for Disease Control*. Atlanta: US Department of Health and Human Services, Public Health Service, 1991.

Chisolm JJ. The use of chelating agents in the treatment of acute and chronic lead intoxication in childhood. *J Pediatr* 1968; 73: 1–38.

Chisolm JJ. Poisoning due to heavy metals. *Pediat Clin N Am* 1970; 17: 591–615.

Chisolm JJ. Mobilization of lead by calcium disodium edetate: a reappraisal. *Am J Dis Child* 1987; 141: 1256–7.

Chisolm JJ. BAL, EDTA, DMSA and DMPS in the treatment of lead poisoning in chidren. *Clin Toxicol* 1992; 30: 493–504.

Chisolm JJ. Safety and efficacy of meso-2,3-dimercaptosuccinic (DMSA) in children with elevated blood lead concentrations. *J Toxicol Clin Toxicol* 2000; 38: 365–75.

Cianciulli P, Sollecito D, Sorrentino F, Forte L, Gilardi E, Massa A, Papa G, Carta S. Early detection of nephrotoxic effects in thalassemic patients receiving desferrioxamine therapy. *Kidney Int* 1994; 46: 467–70.

Civil IDS, McDonald MJA. Acute selenium poisoning: Case report. *NZ Med J* 1978; 87: 354–6.

Clarkson TW, Magos L, Cox C, Greenwood MR, Amin-Zaki L, Majeed MA, AL-Damluji SF. Tests of efficacy of antidotes for removal of methylmercury in human poisoning during the Iraq outbreak. *J Pharmacol Exp Ther* 1981; 218: 74–83.

Cohen A, Cohen IJ, Schwartz E. Scurvy and altered iron stores in thalassemia major. *N Engl J Med* 1981; 304: 158–60.

Cohen AR, Mizanin J, Schwartz E. Rapid removal of excessive iron with daily, high-dose intravenous chelation therapy. *J Pediatr* 1989; 115: 151–5.

Constantoulakis M, Economidou J, Karagiorga M, Katsantoni A, Gyftaki E. Combined long-term treatment of hemosiderosis with desferrioxamine and DTPA in homozygous β-thalassemia. *Ann NY Acad Sci* 1974; 232: 193–200.

Cory-Slechta DA. Relationships between lead-induced learning impairments and changes in dopaminergic, cholinergic, and glutaminergic neurotransmitter system functions. *Annu Rev Pharmacol Toxicol* 1995; 35: 391–415.

Cory-Slechta DA, Weiss B, Cox C. Mobilization and redistribution of lead over the course of calcium disodium ethylenediamine tetraacetate chelation therapy. *J Pharmacol Exp Ther* 1987; 243: 804–13.

Cutler P. Deferoxamine therapy in high-ferritin diabetes. *Diabetes* 1989; 38: 1207–10.

Dalhamn T, Friberg L. Dimercaprol (2,3-dimercaptopropanol) in chronic cadmium poisoning. *Acta Pharmacol Toxicol* 1955; 11: 68–71.

Dally S. Les chélateurs. In: *Les Antidotes*. Baud F, Barriot P, Riou B (eds). Paris: Masson, 1992: 43–62.

Dargan PI, Giles L, House IM, Murphy N, Wallace C, Jones AL, Beale R. A case of severe mercuric sulfate ingestion treated with 2,3-dimercaptopropane-1-sulphonate (DMPS) and hi-flow hemodiafiltration [abstract]. *J Toxicol Clin Toxicol* 1999; 37: 622–3.

Dart RC, Hurlbut KM, Maiorino RM, Mayersohn M, Aposhian HV, Hassen VB. Pharmacokinetics of meso-2,3-dimercaptosuccinic acid in patients with lead poisoning and in healthy adults. *J Pediatr* 1994; 125: 309–16.

Davies SC, Hungerford JL, Arden GB, Marcus RE, Miller MH, Huehns ER. Ocular toxicity of high dose intravenous desferrioxamine. *Lancet* 1983; ii: 181–4.

De Backer W, Zachee P, Verpooten GA, Majelyne W, Vanheule A, De Broe ME. Thallium intoxication treated with combined hemoperfusion-hemodialysis. *J Toxicol Clin Toxicol* 1982; 19: 259–64.

De Broe ME, D'Haese PC, Couttenye M-M, Van Landeghem GF, Lamberts LV. New insights and strategies in the diagnosis and treatment of aluminium overload in dialysis patients. *Nephrol Dial Transplant* 1993; Suppl 1: 47–50.

DeGregorio MW, Gandara DR, Holleran WM, Perez EA, King CC, Wold HG, Montine TJ, Borch RF. High-dose cisplatin with diethyldithiocarbamate (DDTC) rescue therapy: preliminary pharmacologic observations. *Cancer Chemother Pharmacol* 1989; 23: 276–8.

D'Haese PC, Couttenye M-M, Goodman WG, Lemoniatou E, Digenis P, Sotornik I, Fagalde A, Barsoum RS, Lamberts LV, De Broe ME. Use of the low-dose desferrioxamine test to diagnose and differentiate between patients with aluminium-related bone disease, increased risk for aluminium toxicity, or aluminium overload. *Nephrol Dial Transplant* 1995; 10: 1874–84.

Domingo JL. Developmental toxicity of metal chelating agents. *Reprod Toxicol* 1998; 12: 499–510.

Domingo JL, Llobet JM, Tomas JM, Corbella J. Influence of chelating agents on the toxicity, distribution and excretion of vanadium in mice. *J Appl Toxicol* 1986; 6: 337–41.

Domingo JL, Paternain JL, Llobet JM, Corbella J. Developmental toxicity of subcutaneously administered meso-2,3-dimercaptosuccinic acid in mice. *Fundam Appl Toxicol* 1988; 11: 715–22.

Doniec J, Trojanowska B, Trzcinka-Ochocka M, Garlicka I. Effects of $Na_2CaEDTA$ on lead deposits in rabbit osseous tissue. *Toxicol Lett* 1983; 19: 1–5.

Dorr RT. A review of the modulation of cisplatin toxicities by chemoprotectants. In: *Platinum and Other Metal Coordination Compounds in Cancer Chemotherapy 2*. Pinedo HM, Schornagel JH (eds). New York: Plenum, 1996: 131–54.

Durbin PW, Jeung N, Rodgers SJ, Turowski PN, Weitl FL, White DL, Raymond KN. Removal of [238]Pu(IV) from mice by polycatecholate, -hydroxamate, or -hydroxypyridinonate ligands. *Rad Prot Dosimet* 1989; 26: 351–8.

Eagle H, Magnuson HJ. The systemic treatment of 227 cases of arsenic poisoning (encephalitis, dermatitis, blood dyscrasias, jaundice, fever) with 2,3-dimercaptopropanol (BAL). *Am J Syph Gonor Vener Dis* 1946; 30: 420–41.

Egorova LG, Okonishnikova IE, Nirenburg VL, Postovskiy IY. Comparative study of the interaction of spatial isomers of dimercaptosuccinic acid with some metals. *Khim Farm Zh* 1971; 5: 26–30.

Everson GW, Bertaccini EJ, O'Leary J. Use of whole bowel irrigation in an infant following iron overdose. *Am J Emerg Med* 1991; 9: 366–9.

Fang X, Fernando Q. Synthesis, structure, and properties of *rac*-dimercaptosuccinic acid, a potentially useful chelating agent for toxic metals. *Chem Res Toxicol* 1994; 7: 148–56.

Farrar HC, McLeane LR, Wallace M, White K, Watson J. A comparison of two dosing regimens of succimer in children with chronic lead poisoning. *J Clin Pharmacol* 1999; 39: 180–3.

Flora GJS, Mathur S, Mathur R. Effects of *meso*-2,3-dimercaptosuccinic acid or 2,3-dimercaptopropane 1-sulphonate on beryllium-induced biochemical alterations and metal concentration in male rats. *Toxicology* 1995a; 95: 167–75.

Flora GJS, Seth PK, Prakash AO, Mathur R. Therapeutic efficacy of combined meso 2,3-dimercaptosuccinic acid and calcium disodium edetate treatment during acute lead intoxication in rats. *Hum Exp Toxicol* 1995b; 14: 410–13.

Flora SJS, Tandon SK. Influence of calcium disodium edetate on the toxic effects of lead administration in pregnant rats. *Ind J Physiol Pharmacol* 1987; 31: 267–72.

Foreman H, Trujilo TT. The metabolism of C[14] labeled ethylenediaminetetraacetic acid in human beings. *J Lab Clin Med* 1954; 43: 566–71.

Fournier L, Thomas G, Garnier R, Buisine A, Houze P, Pradier F, Dally S. 2,3-Dimercaptosuccinic acid treatment of heavy metal poisoning in humans. *Med Toxicol Adverse Drug Exp* 1988; 3: 499–504.

Friedheim E, Graziano JH, Popovac D, Dragovic D, Kaul B. Treatment of lead poisoning by 2,3-dimercaptosuccinic acid. *Lancet* 1978; ii: 1234–6.

Funk F, Lenders J-P, Crichton RR, Schneider W. Reductive mobilisation of ferritin iron. *Eur J Biochem* 1985; 152: 167–72.

Gabard B. Distribution and excretion of the mercury chelating agent sodium 2,3-dimercaptopropane-1-sulfonate in the rat. *Arch Toxicol* 1978; 39: 289–98.

Gale GR, Smith AB, Walker EM. Diethyldithiocarbamate in treatment of acute cadmium poisoning. *Ann Clin Lab Sci* 1981; 11: 476–83.

Girardi G, Elias MM. Effectiveness of N-acetylcysteine in protecting against mercuric chloride-induced nephrotoxicity. *Toxicology* 1991; 67: 155–64.

Giunta F, Di Landro D, Chiaranda M, Zanardi L, Del Palù A, Giron GP, Bressa G, Cima L. Severe acute poisoning from the ingestion of a permanent wave solution of mercuric chloride. *Hum Toxicol* 1983; 2: 243–6.

Gjonovich A, Del Monte D, Petolillo M, Capolongo F, Carrara M, Cima L. Differences in toxicological pattern of acute poisoning from arsenite and arsenate in the light of an extremely rare case of arsenic pentoxide ingestion [abstract]. *Trace Element Med* 1990; 7: 63.

Gordon RA, Burnside JW. D-Penicillamine-induced myasthenia gravis in rheumatoid arthritis. *Ann Intern Med* 1977; 87: 578–9.

Goyer RA. Lead toxicity: current concerns. *Environ Hlth Perspect* 1993; 100: 177–87.

Goyer RA. Toxic effects of metals. In: *Casarett and Doull's Toxicology: The Basic Science of Poisons*, 5th edn. Klassen CD, Amdur MO, Doull J (eds). New York: McGraw-Hill, 1996: 691–736.

Grandjean P, Jacobsen IA, Jørgenson PJ. Chronic lead poisoning treated with dimercaptosuccinic acid. *Pharmacol Toxicol* 1991; 68: 266–9.

Graziano JH. Role of 2,3-dimercaptosuccinic acid in the treatment of heavy metal poisoning. *Med Toxicol Adverse Drug Exp* 1986; 1: 155–62.

Graziano JH. Conceptual and practical advances in the measurement and clinical management of lead toxicity. *Neurotoxicology* 1993; 14: 219–24.

Graziano JH, Siris ES, Lolacono N, Silverberg SJ, Turgeon L. 2,3-Dimercaptosuccinic acid as an antidote for lead intoxication. *Clin Pharmacol Ther* 1985; 37: 431–8.

Graziano JH, Lolacono NJ, Meyer P. Dose–response study of oral 2,3-dimercaptosuccinic acid in children with elevated blood lead concentrations. *J Pediatr* 1988; 113: 751–7.

Graziano JH, Lolacono NJ, Moulton T, Mitchell ME, Slavkovich V, Zarate C. Controlled study of meso-2,3-dimercaptosuccinic acid for the management of childhood lead intoxication. *J Pediatr* 1992; 120: 133–9.

de Groot G, Savelkoul TJF, Remmert HP, Wubs KL, Cardozo BL, van Alphen D. No evidence for general thallium poisoning in Guyana [letter]. *Lancet* 1987; i: 1084.

Gulumian M, Casimiro E, Linder PW, Rama DBK, Hancock RD. Evaluation of a new chelating agent for cadmium: a preliminary report. *Hum Exp Toxicol* 1993; 12: 247–51.

Hall CL, Jawad S, Harrison PR, MacKenzie JC, Bacon PA, Klouda PT, MacIver AG. Natural course of penicillamine nephropathy: a long term study of 33 patients. *Br Med J* 1988; 296: 1083–6.

Hammond PB. The effects of chelating agents on the tissue distribution and excretion of lead. *Toxicol Appl Pharmacol* 1971; 18: 296–310.

Hansen RM, Csuka ME, McCarty DJ, Saryan LA. Gold induced aplastic anaemia. Complete response to corticosteroids, plasmapheresis, and N-acetylcysteine infusion. *J Rheumatol* 1985; 12: 794–7.

Hardy HL, Elkins HB, Ruotolo BPW, Quinby J, Baker WH. Use of monocalcium disodium ethylene diamine tetra-acetate in lead poisoning. *J Am Med Assoc* 1954; 154: 1171–5.

Harper PL, Walshe JM. Reversible pancytopenia secondary to treatment with tetrathiomolybdate. *Br J Haematol* 1986; 64: 851–3.

Harris WR. Kinetics of the removal of ferric ion from transferrin by aminoalkylphosphonic acids. *J Inorg Biochem* 1984; 21: 263–76.

Harris WR, Rezvani AB, Bali PK. Removal of iron from transferrin by pyrophosphate and tripodal phosphonate ligands. *Inorg Chem* 1987; 26: 2711–16.

Haust HL, Inwood M, Spence JD, Poon HC, Peter F. Intramuscular administration of iron during long-term chelation therapy with 2,3-dimercaptosuccinic acid in a man with severe lead poisoning. *Clin Biochem* 1989; 22: 189–96.

Henderson P, Hale TW, Shum S, Habersang RW. N-Acetylcysteine therapy of acute heavy metal poisoning in mice. *Vet Hum Toxicol* 1985; 27: 522–5.

Henretig FM. Lead. In: *Goldfrank's Toxicologic Emergencies*, 6th edn. Goldfrank LR, Flomenbaum NE, Lewin NA, Weisman RS, Howland MA, Hoffman RS (eds). Stamford: Appleton and Lange, 1998: 1277–309.

Henretig FM, Karl SR. Severe iron poisoning treated with enteral and intravenous deferoxamine. *Ann Emerg Med* 1983; 12: 306–9.

Hershko C. Oral iron chelating drugs: coming but not yet ready for clinical use. *Br Med J* 1988; 296: 1081–2.

Hershko C. Development of oral iron chelator L1. *Lancet* 1993; 341: 1088–9.

Hershko C, Weatherall DJ. Iron-chelating therapy. *Crit Rev Clin Lab Sci* 1988; 26: 303–45.

Heydlauf H. Ferric-cyanoferrate (II): an effective antidote in thallium poisoning. *Eur J Pharmacol* 1969; 6: 340–4.

Hill HFH. Penicillamine in rheumatoid arthritis. Adverse effects. *Scand J Rheumatol* 1979; 28 (Suppl): 94–9.

Hjortsø E, Fomsgaard JS, Fogh-Andersen N. Does N-acetylcysteine increase the excretion of trace metals (calcium, magnesium, iron, zinc and copper) when given orally? *Eur J Clin Pharmacol* 1990; 39: 29–31.

Hoffbrand AV, Bartlett AN, Veys PA, O'Connor NTJ, Kontoghiorghes GJ. Agranulocytosis and thrombocytopenia in patient with Blackfan-Diamond anaemia during oral chelator trial [letter]. *Lancet* 1989; ii: 457.

Hoover TD, Aposhian HV. BAL Increases the arsenic-74 content of rabbit brain. *Toxicol Appl Pharmacol* 1983; 70: 160–2.

Howland MA. Risks of parenteral deferoxamine for acute iron poisoning. *J Toxicol Clin Toxicol* 1996; 34: 491–7.

Hruby K, Donner A. 2,3-Dimercapto-1-propanesulphonate in heavy metal poisoning. *Med Toxicol Adverse Drug Exp* 1987; 2: 317–23.

Iinuma TA, Izawa M, Watari K, Enomoto Y, Matsusaka N, Inaba J, Kasuga T, Nagai T. Application of metal ferrocyanide-anion exchange resin to the enhancement of elimination of ^{137}Cs from human body. *Hlth Phys* 1971; 20: 11–21.

Inns RH, Rice P. Efficacy of dimercapto chelating agents for the treatment of poisoning by percutaneously applied dichloro(2-chlorovinyl)arsine in rabbits. *Hum Exp Toxicol* 1993; 12: 241–6.

Janakiraman N, Seeler RA, Royal JE, Chen MF. Haemolysis during BAL chelation therapy for high blood lead levels in two G6PD deficient children. *Clin Pediatr* 1978; 17: 485–7.

Johary NS, Owen LN. Dithiols. XVIII. Some water soluble derivatives containing the sulphonic acid group. *J Chem Soc* 1955: 1307–11.

Jones AL, Dargan PI. *Textbook of Toxicology*. Edinburgh: Churchill Livingstone, 2001: 54–7.

Jones CW, Mays CW, Taylor GN, Lloyd RD, Packer SM. Reducing the cancer risk of [239]Pu by chelation therapy. *Radiat Res* 1986; 107: 296–306.

Jones MM. New developments in therapeutic chelating agents as antidotes for metal poisoning. *Crit Rev Toxicol* 1991; 21: 209–33.

Jones MM, Cherian MG. The search for chelate antagonists for chronic cadmium intoxication. *Toxicology* 1990; 62: 1–25.

Jones MM, Cherian MG, Singh PK, Basinger MA, Jones SG. A comparative study of the influence of vicinal dithiols and a dithiocarbamate on the biliary excretion of cadmium in rat. *Toxicol Appl Pharmacol* 1991; 110: 241–50.

Jones MM, Singh PK, Gale GR, Smith AB, Atkins LM. Cadmium mobilization *in vivo* by intraperitoneal or oral administration of monoalkyl esters of *meso*-2,3-dimercaptosuccinic acid in the mouse. *Pharmacol Toxicol* 1992; 70: 336–43.

Joyce DA. D-Penicillamine pharmacokinetics and pharmacodynamics in man. *Pharmacol Ther* 1989; 42: 405–27.

Kamerbeek HH, Rauws AG, ten Ham M, van Heijst ANP. Prussian Blue in therapy of thallotoxicosis. *Acta Med Scand* 1971; 189: 321–4.

Kanno H, Yamanobe S, Rybak LP. The ototoxicity of deferoxamine mesylate. *Am J Otolaryngol* 1995; 16: 148–52.

Kapoor SC, Wielopolski L, Graziano JH, LoIacono NJ. Influence of 2,3-dimercaptosuccinic acid on gastrointestinal lead absorption and whole-body lead retention. *Toxicol Appl Pharmacol* 1989; 97: 525–9.

Kattamis C, Fitsialos J, Sinopoulou C. Oral desferrioxamine in young patients with thalassaemia [letter]. *Lancet* 1981; i: 51.

Klaassen CD. Heavy metals and heavy-metal antagonists. In: *Goodman and Gilman's The Pharmacological Basis of Therapeutics*, 9th edn. Hardman JG, Limbird LE, Molinoff PB, Ruddon RW (eds). New York: McGraw-Hill, 1996: 1649–71.

Klein-Schwartz W, Oderda GM, Gorman RL, Favin F, Rose SR. Assessment of management guidelines. Acute iron ingestion. *Clin Pediatr* 1990; 29: 316–21.

Konovaloff NV, Mittelstedt AA, Bauman LK, Gotovtseva EV. Copper metabolism in hepatolenticular degeneration in its treatment with thiol preparations. *Zh Neuropat Psikhiatr* 1957; 57: 39–48.

Kontoghiorghes GJ. New orally active iron chelators [letter]. *Lancet* 1985; i: 817.

Kontoghiorghes GJ. Comparative efficacy and toxicity of desferrioxamine, deferiprone and other iron and aluminium chelating drugs. *Toxicol Lett* 1995a; 80: 1–18.

Kontoghiorghes GJ. New concepts of iron and aluminium chelation therapy with oral L1 (deferiprone) and other chelators: a review. *Analyst* 1995b; 120: 845–51.

Kontoghiorghes GJ, Sheppard L, Aldouri MA, Hoffbrand AV. 1,2-Dimethyl-3-hydroxypyrid-4-one, an orally active chelator for treatment of iron overload. *Lancet* 1987; i: 1294–5.

Kontoghiorghes GJ, Nasseri-Sina P, Goddard JG, Barr JM, Nortey P, Sheppard LN. Safety of oral iron chelator L1. *Lancet* 1989; ii: 457–8.

Kontoghiorghes GJ, Goddard JG, Bartlett AN, Sheppard L. Pharmacokinetic studies in humans with the oral iron chelator 1,2-dimethyl-3-hydroxypyrid-4-one. *Clin Pharmacol Ther* 1990; 48: 255–61.

Kontoghiorghes GJ, Pattichi K, Hadjigavriel M, Kolnagou, A. Transfusional iron overload and chelation therapy with deferoxamine and deferiprone (L1). *Transfus Sci* 2000; 23: 211–23.

Kosnett MJ. Unanswered questions in metal chelation. *Clin Toxicol* 1992; 30: 529–47.

Kozaki K, Egawa H, Garcia-Kennedy R, Cox KL, Lindsay J, Esquivel CO. Hepatic failure due to massive iron ingestion successfully treated with liver transplantation. *Clin Transplant* 1995; 9: 85–7.

Kravzov J, Rios C, Altagracia M, Monroy-Noyola A, López F. Relationship between physicochemical properties of Prussian Blue and its efficacy as antidote against thallium poisoning. *J Appl Toxicol* 1993; 13: 213–16.

Kreppel H, Reichl FX, Forth W, Fichtl B. Lack of effectiveness of D-penicillamine in experimental arsenic poisoning. *Vet Hum Toxicol* 1989; 31: 1–5.

Kreppel H, Reichl F-X, Szinicz L, Fichtl B, Forth W. Efficacy of various dithiol compounds in acute As_2O_3 poisoning in mice. *Arch Toxicol* 1990; 64: 387–92.

■ CHAPTER 2 ■

Kruszewska S, Wiese M, Kolacinski Z, Mielczarska J. The use of haemodialysis and 2,3 propanesulphonate (DMPS) to manage acute oral poisoning by lethal dose of arsenic trioxide. *Int J Occup Med Environ Hlth* 1996; 9: 111–15.

Landrigan PJ. Occupational and paediatric aspects of lead toxicity. *Vet Hum Toxicol* 1983; 25 (Suppl 1): 1–6

Lanphear BP, Howard C, Eberly S, Auinger P, Kolassa J, Weitzman M, Schaffer SJ, Alexander K. Primary prevention of childhood lead exposure: a randomized trial of dust control. *Pediatrics* 1999; 103: 772–7.

Lenz K, Hruby K, Druml W, Eder A, Gaszner A, Kleinberger G, Pichler M, Weiser M. 2,3-Dimercaptosuccinic acid in human arsenic poisoning. *Arch Toxicol* 1981; 47: 241–3.

Lewis C. A review of the use of chemoprotectants in cancer chemotherapy. *Drug Safety* 1994; 11: 153–62.

Liebelt EL, Shannon MW. Oral chelators for childhood lead poisoning. *Pediatr Ann* 1994; 23: 616–26.

Liebelt EL, Shannon M, Graef JW. Efficacy of oral meso-2,3-dimercaptosuccinic acid therapy for low-level childhood plumbism. *J Pediatr* 1994; 124: 313–17.

Lilis R, Fischbein A. Chelation therapy in workers exposed to lead: a critical review. *J Am Med Assoc* 1976; 235: 2823–4.

Link G, Saada A, Pinson A, Konijn AM, Hershko C. Mitochondrial respiratory enzymes are a major target of iron toxicity in rat heart cells. *J Lab Clin Med* 1998; 131: 466–74.

Livardjani F, Ledig M, Kopp P, Dahlet M, Leroy M, Jaeger A. Lung and blood superoxide dismutase activity in mercury vapour exposed rats: effect of N-acetylcysteine treatment. *Toxicology* 1991; 66: 289–95.

Llobet JM, Domingo JL, Corbella J. Comparison of antidotal efficacy of chelating agents upon acute toxicity of Co(II) in mice. *Res Comm Chem Pathol Pharmacol* 1985; 50: 305–8.

Longcope WT, Luetscher JA. Clinical uses of 2,3-dimercaptopropanol (BAL). XI. The treatment of acute mercury poisoning by BAL. *J Clin Invest* 1946; 25: 557–67.

Lovejoy FH. Chelation therapy in iron poisoning. *J Toxicol Clin Toxicol* 1983; 19: 871–4.

Lund ME, Banner W, Clarkson TW, Berlin M. Treatment of acute methylmercury ingestion by haemodialysis with N-acetylcysteine (Mucomyst) infusion and 2,3-dimercaptopropane-sulphonate. *J Toxicol Clin Toxicol* 1984; 22: 31–49.

McElhatton PR, Roberts JC, Sullivan FM. The consequences of iron overdose and its treatment with desferrioxamine in pregnancy. *Hum Exp Toxicol* 1991; 10: 251–9.

Mahieu P, Buchet JP, Roels HA, Lauwerys R. The metabolism of arsenic in humans acutely intoxicated by As_2O_3: its significance for the duration of BAL therapy. *J Toxicol Clin Toxicol* 1981; 18: 1067–75.

Mahoney JR, Hallaway PE, Hedlund BE, Eaton JW. Acute iron poisoning: rescue with macromolecular chelators. *J Clin Invest* 1989; 84: 1362–6.

Maiorino RM, Gonzalez-Ramirez D, Zuniga-Charles M, Xu Z, Hurlbut KM, Aposhian MM, Dart RC, Woods JS, Ostrosky-Wegman P, Gonsebatt ME, Aposhian HV. Sodium 2,3-dimercaptopropane-1-sulphonate challenge test for mercury in humans. III. Urinary mercury after exposure to mercurous chloride. *J Pharmacol Exp Ther* 1996; 277: 938–44.

Malluche HH, Smith AJ, Abreo K, Faugere M-C. The use of deferoxamine in the management of aluminium accumulation in bone in patients with renal failure. *N Engl J Med* 1984; 311: 140–4.

Maloof CC. The use of Edathamil calcium in the treatment of chronic ulcers of the skin. *Arch Industr Hlth* 1965; 2: 123–5.

Mant TGK. Clinical studies with dimercaptopropane sulphonate in mercury poisoning [abstract]. *Hum Toxicol* 1985; 4: 346.

Markowitz ME, Bijur PE, Ruff H, Rosen JF. Effects of calcium disodium versenate (CaNa$_2$EDTA) chelation in moderate childhood lead poisoning. *Pediatrics* 1993; 92: 265–71.

Martell AE, Calvin M. *Chemistry of the Metal Chelate Compounds.* New York: Prentice-Hall, 1953: 192, 445, 537–8.

Martin DS, Willis SE, Cline DM. N-Acetylcysteine in the treatment of human arsenic poisoning. *J Am Board Fam Pract* 1990; 3: 293–6.

Mata JE, Bishop MR, Tarantolo SR, Angle CR, Swanson SA, Iverson PL. Evidence of enhanced iron excretion during systemic phosphorothioate oligodeoxynuleotide treatment. *J Toxicol Clin Toxicol* 2000; 38: 383–7.

Mathieu D, Mathieu-Nolf M, Germain-Alonso M, Neviere R, Furon D, Wattel F. Massive arsenic poisoning – effect of hemodialysis and dimercaprol on arsenic kinetics. *Inten Care Med* 1992; 18: 47–50.

Matsui D, Klein J, Hermann C, Grunau V, McClelland R, Chung D, St-Louis P, Oliveri N, Koren G. Relationship between the pharmacokinetics and iron excretion pharmacodynamics of the new oral iron chelator 1,2-dimethyl-3-hydroxypyrid-4-one in patients with thalassemia. *Clin Pharmacol Ther* 1991; 50: 294–8.

Matte TD. Reducing blood lead levels: benefits and strategies. *J Am Med Assoc* 1999; 281: 2340–2.

Mays CW, Taylor GN, Wrenn ME. Status of chelation research: a review. In: *Actinides in Man and Animals: Proceedings of the Snowbird Actinide Workshop*. Wrenn ME (ed.) Salt Lake City: RD Press, 1981: 351–68.

Meggs WJ, Gerr F, Aly MH, Kierena T, Roberts DL, Shih R, Kim HC, Hoffman R. The treatment of lead poisoning from gunshot wounds with succimer (DMSA). *Clin Toxicol* 1994; 32: 377–85.

Mehta J, Singhal S, Revankar R, Walvalkar A, Chablani A, Mehta BC. Fatal systemic lupus erythematosus in patient taking oral iron chelator L1 [letter]. *Lancet* 1991; 337: 298.

Mehta J, Singhal S, Mehta BC. Future of oral iron chelator deferiprone (L1) [letter]. *Lancet* 1993; 341: 1480.

Meredith TJ, Jacobsen D, Haines JA, Berger J-C (eds). *Naloxone, Flumazenil and Dantrolene as Antidotes. IPCS/CEC Evaluation of Antidotes Series*, Volume 1. Cambridge: Cambridge University Press, 1993: 77.

Miranda M, Villagra R. Pregnancy and Wilson's disease: is penicillamine innocuous? [in Spanish]. *Rev Méd Chile* 1997; 125: 497–8.

Moel DI, Kumar K. Reversible nephrotoxic reactions to a combined 2,3-dimercapto-1-propanol and calcium disodium ethylenediaminetetraacetic acid regimen in asymptomatic children with elevated blood lead levels. *Pediatrics* 1982; 70: 259–62.

Moore DF, O'Callaghan CA, Berlyne G, Ogg CS, Alban Davies H, House IH, Henry JA. Acute arsenic poisoning: absence of polyneuropathy after treatment with 2,3-dimercapto-propanesulphonate (DMPS). *J Neurol Neurosurg Psychiat* 1994; 57: 2233–5.

Morgan JM. Chelation therapy in lead neuropathy. *South Med J* 1975; 68: 1001–6.

Mortensen ME, Walson PD. Chelation therapy for childhood lead poisoning. *Clin Pediatr* 1993; 32: 284–91.

Mückter H, Liebl B, Reichl F-X, Hunder G, Walther U, Fichtl B. Are we ready to replace dimercaprol (BAL) as an arsenic antidote? *Hum Exp Toxicol* 1997; 16: 460–5.

Muller-Eberhard U, Erlandson ME, Ginn HE, Smith CH. Effect of trisodium calcium diethylenetriaminepenta-acetate on bivalent cations in thalassamia major. *Blood* 1963; 22: 209–17.

Naganuma A, Anderson ME, Meister A. Cellular glutathione as a determinant of sensitivity to mercuric chloride toxicity: prevention of toxicity by giving glutathione monoester. *Biochem Pharmacol* 1990; 40: 693–7.

Netter P, Bannwarth B, Péré P, Nicolas A. Clinical pharmacokinetics of D-penicillamine. *Clin Pharmacokinet* 1987; 13: 317–33.

Nienhuis AW. Vitamin C and iron. *N Engl J Med* 1981; 304: 170–1.

Norman EH, Bordley WC. Lead toxicity intervention in children. *J R Soc Med* 1995; 88: 121–4.

Nwokolo CU, Pounder RE. D-Penicillamine does not increase urinary bismuth excretion in patients treated with tripotassium dicitrato bismuthate. *Br J Clin Pharmacol* 1990; 30: 648–50.

Ohlsson WTL. Penicillamine as lead-chelating substance in man. *Br Med J* 1962; ii: 1454–6.

CHAPTER 2

Olivieri NF, Buncic JR, Chew E, Gallant T, Harrison RV, Keenan N, Logan W, Mitchell D, Ricci G, Skarf B, Taylor M, Freedman MH. Visual and auditory neurotoxicity in patients receiving subcutaneous deferoxamine infusions. *N Engl J Med* 1986; 314: 869–73.

Olivieri NF, Koren G, Hermann C, Bentur Y, Chung D, Klein J, St Louis P, Freedman MH, McClelland RA, Templeton DM. Comparison of oral iron chelator L1 and desferrioxamine in iron-loaded patients. *Lancet* 1990; 336: 1275–9.

Olivieri NF, Brittenham GM, Matsui D, Berkovitch M, Blendis LM, Cameron RG, McClelland RA, Liu PP, Templeton DM, Koren G. Iron-chelation therapy with oral deferiprone in patients with thalassemia major. *N Engl J Med* 1995; 332: 918–22.

Ortega A, Domingo JL, Gómez M, Corbella J. Treatment of experimental acute uranium poisoning by chelating agents. *Pharmacol Toxicol* 1989; 64: 247–51.

Osterloh J, Becker CE. Pharmacokinetics of $CaNa_2EDTA$ and chelation of lead in renal failure. *Clin Pharmacol Ther* 1986; 40: 686–93.

Owen LN, Sultanbawa MUS. Olefinic acids. VII. The addition of thiols to propiolic and acetylenedicarboxylic acid. *J Chem Soc* 1949: 3109–13.

Palatnick W, Tenenbein M. Leukocytosis, hyperglycemia, vomiting, and positive X-rays are not indicators of severity of iron overdose in adults. *Am J Emerg Med* 1996; 14: 454–5.

Pall H, Blake DR, Winyard P, Lunec J, Williams A, Good PA, Kritzinger EE, Cornish A, Hider RC. Ocular toxicity of desferrioxamine – an example of copper promoted auto-oxidative damage? *Br J Ophthalmol* 1989; 73: 42–7.

Paredes SR, Kozicki PA, Batlle AM del C. S-Adenosyl-L-methionine: a counter to lead intoxication? *Comp Biochem Physiol* 1985; 82B: 751–7.

Perrett D. The metabolism and pharmacology of D-penicillamine in man. *J Rheumatol* 1981; 8 (Suppl 7): 41–50.

Pestaner JP, Ishak KG, Mullick FG, Centeno JA. Ferrous sulfate toxicity: a review of autopsy findings. *Biol Trace Elem Res* 1999; 69: 191–8.

Peters RA, Stocken LA, Thompson RHS. British anti-lewisite (BAL). *Nature* 1945; 156: 616–19.

Petersilge CL. Prolonged anuria following a single injection of a bismuth preparation. Possible response to therapy with BAL. *J Pediatr* 1947; 31: 580–3.

Petrunkin VE. Synthesis and properties of dimercapto derivatives of alkylsulphonic acids. 1: Synthesis of sodium 2,3-dimercaptopropylsulphonate (unithiol) and sodium 2-mercaptoethyl-sulphonate [in Russian]. *Ukrain Khim Zhurn* 1956; 22: 603–7.

Pfannkuch F, Bentley P, Schnebli HP. Future of oral iron chelator deferiprone (L1) [letter]. *Lancet* 1993; 341: 1480.

Pippard MJ, Callender ST, Finch CA. Ferrioxamine excretion in iron-loaded man. *Blood* 1982; 60: 288–94.

Pitt CG. Structure and activity relationships of iron chelating drugs. In: *Development of Iron Chelators for Clinical Use*. Martell AE, Anderson WF, Badman DG (eds). New York: Elsevier, 1981: 105–31.

Pitt CG, Bao Y, Thompson J, Wani MC, Rosencrantz H, Metterville J. Esters and lactones of phenolic amino carboxylic acids: prodrugs for iron chelation. *J Med Chem* 1986; 29: 1231–7.

Playford RJ, Matthews CH, Campbell MJ, Delves HT, Hla KK, Hodgson HJF, Calam J. Bismuth induced encephalopathy caused by tripotassium dicitrato bismuthate in a patient with chronic renal failure. *Gut* 1990; 31: 359–60.

Porter JB. Evaluation of new iron chelators for clinical use. *Acta Haematol* 1996; 95: 13–25.

Porter JB. Deferoxamine pharmacokinetics. *Semin Hematol* 2001; 38 (Suppl 1): 63–8.

Porter JB, Gyparaki M, Burke LC, Huehns ER, Sarpong P, Saez V, Hider RC. Iron mobilization from hepatocyte monolayer cultures by chelators: the importance of membrane permeability and iron-binding constant. *Blood* 1988; 72: 1497–503.

Porter JB, Huehns ER, Hider RC. Development of iron chelating drugs. *Baillière's Clin Haematol* 1989a; 2: 257–92.

Porter JB, Hoyes KP, Abeysinghe R, Huehns ER, Hider RC. Animal toxicology of iron chelator L1 [letter]. *Lancet* 1989b; ii: 156.

Portnyagina VA, Morgun MI. N-(Mercaptopropyl)-substituted monoamides and imides of phthalic acid [in Russian]. *Ukrain Khim Zhur* 1966; 32: 1081–4.

Propper RD, Shurin SB, Nathan DG. Reassessment of the use of desferrioxamine B in iron overload. *N Engl J Med* 1976; 294: 1421–3.

Proudfoot AT. Antidotes: benefits and risks. *Toxicol Lett* 1995; 82/83: 779–83.

Proudfoot AT, Simpson D, Dyson EH. Management of acute iron poisoning. *Med Toxicol Adverse Drug Exp* 1986; 1: 83–100.

Rabinowitz MB, Wetherill GW, Kopple JD. Kinetic analysis of lead metabolism in healthy humans. *J Clin Invest* 1976; 58: 260–70.

Reichl F-X, Hunder G, Liebl B, Fichtl B, Forth W. Effect of DMPS and various adsorbents on the arsenic excretion in guinea-pigs after injection with As_2O_3. *Arch Toxicol* 1995; 69: 712–17.

Richardson DR. The controversial role of deferiprone in the treatment of thalassemia. *J Lab Clin Med* 2001; 137: 324–9.

Rivera M, Zheng W, Aposhian HV, Fernando Q. Determination and metabolism of dithiol chelating agents. VIII. Metal complexes of *meso*-dimercaptosuccinic acid. *Toxicol Appl Pharmacol* 1989; 100: 96–106.

Rodgers SJ, Lee C-W, Ng CY, Raymond KN. Ferric iron sequestering agents. 15. Synthesis, solution chemistry, and electrochemistry of a new cationic analogue of enterobactin. *Inorg Chem* 1987; 26: 1622–5.

Rudge SR, Perrett D. The pharmacology and biochemical action of second-line agents. *Ballière's Clin Rheumatol* 1988; 2: 185–210.

Ruff HH, Bijur PE, Markowitz M, Ma Y-C, Rosen JF. Declining blood lead levels and cognitive changes in moderately lead-poisoned children. *J Am Med Assoc* 1993; 269: 1641–6.

Saenger P, Rosen JF, Markowitz M. Diagnostic significance of edetate disodium calcium testing in children with increased lead absorption. *Am J Dis Childh* 1982; 136: 312–15.

Saryan LA, Zenz C. Lead and its compounds. In: *Occupational Medicine*, 3rd edn. Zenz C, Dickerson OB, Horvath EP (eds). St Louis: Mosby, 1994: 506–41.

Schäfer SG, Forth W. Excretion of metals into the rat intestine. *Biol Trace Element Res* 1983; 5: 205–17.

Scheinberg IH. Wilson's disease. *J Rheumatol* 1981; 8 (Suppl 7): 90–3.

Schumacher HR, Osterman AL, Choi S-J, Weisz PB. Calcinosis at the site of leakage from extravasation of calcium disodium edetate chelator therapy in a child with lead poisoning. *Clin Orthopediatr Rel Res* 1987; 219: 221–5.

Schwarzenbach G, Ackermann H. Komplexone XII. Die Homologen der Äthylendiamintetraessigsäure und ihre Erdalkalikomplexe. *Helvet Chim Acta* 1948; 31: 1029–48.

Seward JP. Occupational lead exposure and management. *West J Med* 1996; 165: 222–4.

Shum S, Skarbovig J, Habersang R. Acute lethal arsenite poisoning in mice: effect of treatment with N-acetylcysteine, D-penicillamine and dimercaprol on survival time. *Vet Hum Toxicol* 1981: 23 (Suppl): 39–42.

Shum S, Whitehead J, Vaughn L, Shum S, Hale T. Chelation of organoarsenate with dimercaptosuccinic acid. *Vet Hum Toxicol* 1995: 37: 239–42.

Slater EC, de Vries S. Identification of the BAL-labile factor. *Nature* 1980; 288: 717–18.

Slikkerveer A, Jong HB, Helmich RB, de Wolff FA. Development of a therapeutic procedure for bismuth intoxication with chelating agents. *J Lab Clin Med* 1992; 119: 529–37.

Speyer JL, Green MD, Zeleniuch-Jacquotte A, Wernz JC, Rey M, Sanger J, Kramer E, Ferrans V, Hochster H, Meyers M, Blum RH, Feit F, Attubato M, Burrows W, Muggia FM. ICRF-187 Permits longer treatment with doxorubicin in women with breast cancer. *J Clin Oncol* 1992; 10: 117–27.

Stather JW, Stradling GN, Gray SA, Moody J, Hodgson A. Use of DTPA for increasing the rate of elimination of plutonium-238 and americium-241 from rodents after their inhalation as the nitrates. *Hum Toxicol* 1985; 4: 573–82.

Stevens W, van Peteghem C, Heyndrickx A, Barbier F. Eleven cases of thallium intoxication treated with Prussian Blue. *Int J Clin Pharmacol* 1974; 10: 1–22.

Stivelman J, Schulman G, Fosburg M, Lazarus JM, Hakim RM. Kinetics and efficacy of deferoxamine in iron-overloaded hemodialysis patients. *Kidney Int* 1989; 36: 1125–32.

Stohler HR, Frey JR. Chemotherapy of experimental schistosomiasis mansoni: influence of dimercaptosuccinic acid on the toxicity and antischistosomal activity of sodium antimony dimercaptosuccinate and other antimony compounds in mice. *Ann Trop Med Parasitol* 1964; 58: 431–8.

Stradling GN, Bulman RA. Recent research on decorporation therapy at National Radiological Protection Board. In: *Actinides in Man and Animals: Proceedings of the Snowbird Actinide Workshop*, Wrenn ME (ed.). Salt Lake City: RD Press, 1981: 369–79.

Summers MR, Jacobs A, Tudway D, Perera P, Ricketts C. Studies of desferrioxamine and ferrioxamine in normal and iron-loaded subjects. *Br J Haematol* 1979; 42: 547–55.

Sunderman FW. Efficacy of sodium diethyldithiocarbamate (dithiocarb) in acute nickel carbonyl poisoning. *Ann Clin Lab Sci* 1979; 9: 1–10.

Sunderman FW. Use of sodium diethyldithiocarbamate in the treatment of nickel carbonyl poisoning. *Ann Clin Lab Sci* 1990; 20: 12–21.

Tandon SK, Mathur AK. Chelation in metal intoxication. III. Lowering of nickel content in poisoned rat organs. *Acta Pharmacol Toxicol* 1976; 38: 401–8.

Tandon SK, Flora SJS. Singh S. Chelation in Metal Intoxication XXIV: Influence of various components of vitamin B complex on the therapeutic efficacy of disodium calcium versenate in lead intoxication. *Pharmacol Toxicol* 1987; 60: 62–5.

Tandon SK, Singh S, Jain VK. Efficacy of combined chelation in lead intoxication. *Chem Res Toxicol* 1994; 7: 585–9.

Taylor DM, Volf V. Oral chelation treatment of injected ^{241}Am or ^{239}Pu in rats. *Health Phys* 1980; 38: 147–58.

Tenenbein M. Benefits of parenteral deferoxamine for acute iron poisoning. *J Toxicol Clin Toxicol* 1996; 34: 485–9.

Tenenbein M, Kowalski S, Sienko A, Bowden DH, Adamson IYR. Pulmonary toxic effects of continuous desferrioxamine administration in acute iron poisoning. *Lancet* 1992; 339: 699–701.

Thomas DJ, Chisolm JJ. Lead, zinc and copper decorporation during calcium disodium ethylenedieamine tetraacetate treatment of lead-poisoned children. *J Pharmacol Exp Ther* 1986; 239: 829–35.

Thompson DF. Management of thallium poisoning. *Clin Toxicol* 1981; 18: 979–90.

Tolot F, Prost G, Neulat G. Insuffisance rénale aiguë au cours d'un saturnisme; rôle de l'EDTA. *Nouv Presse Med* 1978; 36: 3252–3.

Topham R, Goger M, Pearce K, Schultz P. The mobilization of ferritin iron by liver cytosol. A comparison of xanthine and NADH as reducing substrates. *Biochem J* 1989; 261: 137–43.

Truhaut R, Boudène C, Lutz M, Métivier H. On the comparative efficacy of desferrioxamine and DTPA as agents for the elimination of plutonium in poisoned rats [in French]. *Arch Mal Prof* 1966; 27: 669–76.

Ubios AM, Braun EM, Cabrini RL. Lethality due to uranium poisoning is prevented by ethane-1-hydroxy-1,1-biphosphonate (EHBP). *Hlth Phys* 1994; 66: 540–4.

Uysal Z, Akar N, Kemahli S, Dincer N, Arcasoy A. Desferrioxamine and urinary zinc excretion in β-thalassemia major. *Pediatr Hematol Oncol* 1993; 10: 257–60.

Vale JA, Meredith TJ. Antidotal therapy: pharmacokinetic aspects. In: *New Concepts and Developments in Toxicology*. Chambers PL, Gehring P, Sakai F (eds). Amsterdam: Elsevier, 1986: 329–38.

Vassallo S, Howland MA. Severe dichromate poisoning: survival after therapy with IV N-acetylcysteine and hemodialysis [abstract]. *Vet Hum Toxicol* 1988; 30: 347.

Vaziri ND, Upham T, Barton CH. Hemodialysis clearance of arsenic. *Clin Toxicol* 1980; 17: 451–6.

Walker EM, Stone A, Milligan LB, Gale GR, Atkins LM, Smith AB, Jones MM, Singh PK, Basinger MA. Mobilization of lead in mice by administration of monoalkyl esters of *meso*-2,3-dimercaptosuccinic acid. *Toxicology* 1992; 76: 79–87.

Walshe JM. Penicillamine, a new oral therapy for Wilson's disease. *Am J Med* 1956; 21: 487–95.

Walshe JM. Treatment of Wilson's disease with trientine (triethylene tetramine) dihydrochloride. *Lancet* 1982; i: 643–7.

Walshe JM. Unithiol in Wilson's disease. *Br Med J* 1985; 290: 673–4.

Wang S-C, Ting K-S, Wu C-C. Chelating therapy with Na-DMS in occupational lead and mercury intoxications. *Chinese Med J* 1965; 84: 437–9.

Wedeen RP, Batuman V, Landy E. The safety of the EDTA lead-mobilization test. *Environ Res* 1983; 30: 58–62.

Westlin WF. Deferoxamine as a chelating agent. *J Toxicol Clin Toxicol* 1971; 4: 597–602.

Williams A, Hoy T, Pugh A, Jacobs A. Pyridoxal complexes as potential chelating agents for oral therapy in transfusional iron overload. *J Pharm Pharmacol* 1982; 34: 730–2.

Xie J, Funakoshi T, Shimada H, Kojima S. Effects of chelating agents on testicular toxicity in mice caused by acute exposure to nickel. *Toxicology* 1995; 103: 147–55.

Yonaga T, Morita K. Comparison of the effect of N-(2,3-dimercaptopropyl) phthalamidic acid, DL-penicillamine, and dimercaprol on the excretion and tissue retention of mercury in mice. *Toxicol Appl Pharmacol* 1981; 57: 197–207.

Zalups RK, Barfuss DW. Participation of mercuric conjugates of cysteine, homocysteine and N-acetylcysteine in mechanisms involved in the renal tubular uptake of inorganic mercury. *J Am Soc Nephrol* 1998; 9: 551–61.

CHAPTER 2

Immunotherapy

Contents

3.1 ANTIVENINS

Antibodies have been used to inactivate protein poisons from animals and microbes *in vivo* for many years. Antivenins used to treat poisoning with snake venom are one example. This topic has been reviewed previously (Sullivan, 1986; Howland and Smilkstein, 1991). The term antivenin was used for the first antiserum for snake venom poisoning prepared for human use (Calmette, 1907 – see section 4.3.2). It has been retained in many parts of the world on the basis of historical precedent, and because it identifies a specific process, immunization, in its preparation. The term antivenom, on the other hand, is frequently used for any product that acts against venom, such as trypsin.

3.1.1 The treatment of snake bite

In Africa, snake bite causes hundreds of deaths annually and thousands of cases of permanent physical disability. In Nigeria, some 70 % of hospital beds are occupied by snake bite victims at times of the year when people are working outdoors (Theakston and Warrell, 2000). There are 50–70,000 deaths annually in India and Pakistan (Warrell, 1999). There are some 50,000 cases of snake bite every year in the USA, of which about 8,000 are inflicted by a venomous snake, with some 6,000 being treated with antivenin. Pit vipers (Crotalinae) are responsible for about 98 % of all bites and considerable morbidity. There were some 7–15 deaths per annum between 1960 and 1990 (Stolpe *et al.*, 1989; Johnson, 1991; Consroe *et al.*, 1995). In Australia, although cases of envenomation reported to poisons centres are dominated by spider bites and insect stings, snake bites affect 1,000–3,000 people per year with two or so deaths annually (White, 1998). Brown snakes (*Pseudonaja*) cause most deaths and bites, with tiger snakes (*Notechis*) and taipans (*Oxyuranus*) accounting for nearly all other fatalities. Up to 500 cases require antivenin treatment annually, most victims coming from the rural areas of the most populated states. All Australian venomous snakes are front-fanged elapids.

Snake envenomation is a medical emergency that requires urgent clinical judgement. As more people engage in outdoor activities there has been an increase in both the occurrence of snake bite and the need for treatment. Unfortunately, cost is an important factor influencing antivenin availability, especially in less developed countries (Theakston and Warrell, 2000). Treatment protocols, even for venomous bites, are controversial. The wider availability of snake venom detection kits in countries such as Australia has allowed specific antivenin, rather than polyvalent antivenin, to be used more frequently, but polyvalent antivenin is still used in some 50 % of cases. The use of adrenaline premedication before antivenin administration also remains controversial (Tibballs, 1994).

The amount of venom injected via a bite is very variable as it depends on the length of time since the snake has eaten, the size of the prey and the degree of aggression shown by the snake. Snake venoms are complex mixtures of proteins and small polypeptides with enzymatic activity (Russell, 1991). Venom composition within a species can show considerable geographical variation (Daltry *et al.*, 1996). Crotalid venoms produce changes in capillary walls that lead to fluid loss into tissues, particularly into the bitten area, but also into other organs. These phenomena are recognized clinically as oedema, bruising, hypoproteinaemia and haemoconcentration (Johnson, 1991). The arbitrary grouping of snake venoms into neurotoxins, haemotoxins and cardiotoxins is toxicologically misleading and can result in serious clinical errors. This is because a so-called neurotoxin can produce marked cardiovascular changes or direct haematological effects (Russell, 1991).

Poisonous species of snakes mainly fall into the following families or subfamilies: Viperidae, including the true vipers (Viperinae) such as Russell's viper and puff adder; the pit vipers (Crotalinae); and Elapidae, the elapids, which include the cobras, king cobras, kraits, coral snakes and sea snakes.

3.1.2 Crotalinae: pit vipers

The pit vipers consist of rattlesnakes and moccasins (copperheads and cottonmouths). The snakes are distinguishable by the pit located between each eye and nostril. The pit viper's head appears triangular as a result of the venom glands located in the temporal region. They have two sharp, canalized fangs that are long and movable and retract posteriorly.

The rattlesnakes are divided into two types. The genus *Crotalus* contains the more dangerous rattlesnakes, as well as a greater number of species, and is distributed over a far greater range. It is distinguished from the genus *Sistrurus* because it has small scales on the crown of the head whereas the latter has large plates. As the name implies, both possess rattles at the end of the tail, and together they account for about 65 % of all venomous snake bites in the USA every year. Most fatal bites result from the Eastern (*C. adamanteus*) or Western (*C. atrox*) diamondback rattlesnake. The Mojave rattlesnake (*C. scutulatus scutulatus*) has the most neurotoxic venom of all rattlesnakes but is fortunately responsible for only a few bites every year (Jansen *et al.*, 1992).

There are two species of moccasins: the cottonmouth (*Agkistrodon piscivorus*) and the copperhead (*A. contortrix*). Moccasins are distinguished by their facial pits, elliptical pupils, the absence of rattles and the presence of a single row of scales on the undersurface of the tail. They do, however, vibrate their tails like a rattlesnake. The cottonmouth is an aquatic snake that lives in swamps, lakes, ditches and rice fields. It is usually dark olive with dark cross-bands. When disturbed, the snake will often open its white mouth in a characteristically threatening manner. Copperheads have inverted Ys and hourglass configurations on their bodies. Their heads may be copper or brown. The average adult varies in length from 50 to 100 cm. They are often found on mountains, hillsides, rocks and sawdust piles but may also live within city limits and in suburban developments. When disturbed they can strike very quickly, but the majority of bites by copperheads do not result in death.

3.1.2.1 Crotalid poisoning: clinical features

These vary considerably depending on the species, the amount of venom injected and the premorbid state of the patient. The most diagnostic sign is rapid, progressive, painful swelling. Usually there is some swelling around the bite area within 5–10 min, often spreading to involve the entire hand or foot. Superficial lacerations produced by fangs usually do not result in envenomation. A common symptom following the bites of the Eastern diamondback rattlesnake and the Pacific rattlesnakes is tingling around the mouth, forehead and scalp. Bruising is common in most cases of moderate or severe rattlesnake poisoning and usually appears around the bite within 3–6 h. It tends to be severe following bites by Eastern and Western diamondbacks, the prairie and Pacific rattlesnakes, and less severe following copperhead bites. Vesicles may form in the area of the bite within the first 8 h, often becoming blood filled. It is difficult to determine the severity of envenomation during the first few hours after a crotalid snake bite, and estimates may need to be revised as poisoning progresses. A bite may appear minor at 1 h but prove serious or fatal at 3 h. In about 20 % of rattlesnake bites, the snake may not inject venom.

There may be swelling, pain, bruising, weakness, nausea, vomiting and alteration of temperature, pulse and blood pressure. Paraesthesiae, fasciculations, haemo-concentration, platelet loss, petechiae and shock can also occur. Severe envenomation may be accompanied by low blood pressure, which usually occurs 30 min or more after the bite, facial numbness and generalized fasciculations due to neurotoxin (Gold and Barish, 1992). If a bite is close to a vein, local swelling may be minimal, but patients may develop coagulopathy and haemorrhage. Particularly after bites by the Mojave rattlesnake, respiratory distress may occur, and muscular weakness may be seen in severe cases. If oedema and erythema or systemic effects have not occurred within 4 h of the bite, it is safe to assume that the patient does not have pit viper envenomation (White and Weber, 1991).

Most of the grading systems for crotalid bites are poor, as they depend upon a few key clinical features, and these are often stipulated for a specific time. It is more practical, however, to grade them as minimal, moderate or severe based on all clinical findings and laboratory data (Table 3.1; Johnson, 1991). The grading may need to be changed as the course of poisoning or treatment progresses. Bites by the Mojave rattlesnake, for example, may be graded as minimal, but the consequences of giving too little antivenin may be a poor outcome or even death. The grading of poisoning after crotalid envenomation is often determined by the most severe clinical feature.

After a crotalid snake bite, the bitten part and preferably the whole patient should be immediately immobilized to limit the spread of venom (Burgess *et al.*, 1992; Gold and Barish, 1992). If the snake was killed it should be brought to hospital for identification. If a live snake is brought to hospital it should be placed in a refrigerator in its container for at least 30 min. This allows for safer identification. Wound excision, cryotherapy and the use of ligatures have been tried and may increase morbidity after pit viper envenomation (Burgess *et al.*, 1992). Suction, using an extractor applied to the fang punctures, may be of value in the first 30–60 min. The wound should be cleaned.

CHAPTER 3

TABLE 3.1
Assessment of the severity of crotalid envenomation

Mild poisoning	Moderate poisoning	Severe poisoning
Local swelling	Local swelling	Marked swelling
Erythema	Erythema	Marked erythema
Bruising	Bruising	Marked bruising
No systemic features	Mild systemic manifestations	Marked systemic manifestations: hypotension, tachycardia, respiratory compromise, neurological changes
No laboratory abnormalities	Some laboratory abnormalities	Coagulopathy: abnormal prothrombin time, abnormal partial thromboplastin time, abnormal platelet count, abnormal fibrinogen

Broad-spectrum antibiotic treatment is generally recommended. The critical therapy for moderate to severe envenomation is appropriate antivenin.

3.1.2.2 Crotalid antivenins

Polyvalent Crotalinae antivenin (Wyeth) contains globulins that neutralize the systemic toxicity of venoms of crotalids native to North, Central and South America, including rattlesnakes (*Crotalus, Sistrurus*), cottonmouth (*Agkistrodon piscivorus*) and copperhead (*A. contortrix*) moccasins, species of *Bothrops* including *B. atrox* (Fer-de-lance*)*, the tropical rattlesnake (*C. durissus terrificus* and similar species), the cantil *(A. bilineatus*) and bushmaster (*Lachesis mutus*) of Central and South America, *A. hayls, Trimeresurus flavoviridis* and *T. purpureomaculatus*. The antivenin is not effective against the venoms of coral snakes and should never be used in the management of poisoning by these snakes.

Antivenin should not be routinely administered to every patient suffering from pit viper bite. It is unnecessary in most cases of copperhead bites, unless the bite is considered moderate to severe, or possibly when the victim is a small child. Envenomation from cottonmouths usually requires lower antivenin doses (Russell, 1991). Although antivenin appears to be effective in neutralizing the lethality of the venom, it is less effective in protecting against local tissue damage (Kelly *et al.*, 1991).

Before starting antivenin therapy, careful inquiry must be made about any history of allergy. An intradermal sensitivity test should be performed before antivenin is given therapeutically, regardless of the history. This is done by injection of 0.02 mL of 0.9 % (w/v) sodium chloride-diluted antiserum at a site distant from the bite. The injection site is then observed for at least 10 min for the development of redness, hives, pruritus or other adverse effects. A syringe containing 0.5 mL of 1:1,000 adrenaline must be available for treating allergic reactions whenever antivenin is administered. In general, the shorter the interval between injection and reaction, the greater the degree of sensitivity. However, a negative skin test does not indicate whether serum sickness will occur after administration of full doses of the antivenin. If an immediate hypersensitivity reaction occurs, it usually happens within 30 min of administration of the antivenin (Table 3.2).

Antivenin-induced serum sickness is generally dose related. If a hypersensitivity reaction occurs, administration of the antivenin should be immediately discontinued and the patient given an oral antihistamine if the reaction is mild or i.m. adrenaline if

TABLE 3.2

Crotalid antivenin hypersensitivity reactions

Immediate reaction (within minutes)	Delayed (5–24 days) serum sickness
Apprehension	Malaise
Itch or urticaria	Fever
Swelling of face, tongue or throat	Urticaria
Dyspnoea	Lymphadenopathy
Cyanosis	Arthralgia
Nausea	Nausea
Vomiting	Vomiting
Cardiovascular collapse	Peripheral neuropathy (arms)
	Meningism

the reaction is moderate to severe. If infusion of the antivenin is restarted, administration should be at a slower rate. Steroids are commonly given to treat serum sickness reactions, although their value remains to be established.

Antivenin must not be injected into a finger or toe. For i.v. infusion, a 1+1 to 1+9 dilution of reconstituted antivenin in 0.9 % (w/v) sodium chloride or 5 % (w/v) D-glucose is prepared. To avoid foaming, dilutions of antivenin should be mixed not by shaking, but by gentle swirling. An initial 5–10 mL of diluted antivenin should be infused over 3–5 min with careful observation of the patient; if there are no indications of any immediate systemic reaction (Table 3.2), the infusion should be continued at the maximum safe rate of i.v. fluid administration. The rate of administration should be based on the severity of the case and the patient's tolerance to the antivenin. Pregnancy is not a contraindication to administration of antivenin.

The greatest danger from snake bites occur within the first day or two after the bite, and therefore the entire initial dose of antivenin should be given as soon as possible and preferably within 4 h of the bite. Antivenin is less effective when given after 8 h and is of questionable value beyond 12 h. However, in severe envenomation, antivenin may be given even 24 h after the time of the bite and has been shown to reverse coagulation deficits even at 30 h. The recommended doses for children and adults are given in Table 3.3.

Bites by large snakes may need relatively high doses, particularly in children or small adults. The dose of antivenin given to children is based not on body weight, but on the clinical response to the initial dose and continuing assessment of the patient in respect to the severity of poisoning. If swelling continues to progress, systemic features of envenomation increase in severity or new manifestations appear, such as low blood pressure or reduced haematocrit, an additional 10–50 mL (contents of 1–5 vials) should be administered.

Details of some further crotalid antivenins are given in Table 3.4. Broadly speaking, these antivenins should be used in the same way as described for polyvalent crotalid antivenin, although local advice on their use should be sought if possible.

3.1.2.3 F_{ab} antibody fragments and other approaches

A preparation is now being investigated that consists of fragments of antibodies raised in sheep and specific for crotalid venom (F_{ab}AV, Therapeutic Antibodies). The production of these fragments is very similar to the method of generating antidigoxin antibody fragments (section 3.2.1). It should provide a less immunogenic alternative than the antivenin produced from horse serum. Use of the product in three patients was associated with rapid and complete reversal of neurotoxicity (Clark *et al.*, 1997). It has

TABLE 3.3
Crotalid polyvalent antivenin dosage recommendations

Degree of envenomation	Antivenin dose
Nil	None
Minimal	20–40 mL (2–4 vials)
Moderate	50–90 mL (5–9 vials)
Severe	100–150 mL or more (10+ vials)

TABLE 3.4
Some further Crotalid snake bite antivenins (see also Warrell, 1999)

Antivenin	Origin	Effective against
Sharp-nosed pit viper	National Institute of Preventive Medicine, Taiwan	*Agkistrodon acutus* (= *Deinagkistrodon acutus*)
Malayan pit viper	Thai Red Cross, Bangkok	*Calloselasma rhodostoma* (= *Agkistrodon rhodostoma*)
Green pit viper	Thai Red Cross, Bangkok	*Trimermesurus poperum*
Trimermesurus bivalent	National Institute of Preventive Medicine, Taiwan	*Trimermesurus mucrosquamatus* (Chinese habu), *T. gramineus* (= *T. stejnegeri* – Chinese bamboo viper)
Polyvalent	Perum Bio Pharma (Pasteur Institute), Bandung, Indonesia	*Calloselasma rhodostoma*, also *Bungarus fasciatus* (banded krait), *Naja naja sputatrix* (= *N. sumatrana* – Sumatran spitting cobra)
	Costa Rica	*Crotalus durissus terrificus* (tropical rattlesnake, cascabel), *Bothropsatrox* (Fer-de-lance), *Lachesis mutus* (bushmaster)

recently been approved by the Food and Drug Administration of the USA (FDA), but costs £6,000 per treatment (Theakston and Warrell, 2000).

Molecular and DNA immunization techniques are also being used to generate venom toxin-specific antibodies as the source material for developing improved antivenins (Harrison *et al.*, 2000). It is thought that, by generating a bank of antibodies, each specific to a distinct venom toxin, more rational antivenins than those resulting from conventional, whole-venom immunization can be prepared. Moreover, it is thought that antivenins prepared in this way are less likely to induce anaphylaxis and allergic reactions, such as often occur when conventional equine and ovine antivenins are given to humans.

3.1.3 Elapidae (including cobras and coral snakes)

3.1.3.1 Diagnosis of envenomation by elapids

Elapidae envenomations differ significantly from those of pit vipers. They may be little or no pain or swelling immediately after the bite. Occasionally there is a delay of 1–6 h before the onset of systemic symptoms (Table 3.5). Clinical features of poisoning include difficulty in speaking and swallowing and intense salivation. Loss of deep reflexes and respiratory depression occur later as a result of the neurotoxin component. In contrast to crotalid bites, severe poisoning can be present without indications of a substantial local tissue reaction. The earliest signs may be euphoria or drowsiness, followed by nausea and vomiting, salivation and paralysis. Systemic features of poisoning usually occur within 6 h of the bite, although they may be delayed for up to 18 h. Once systemic poisoning becomes manifest, progression is often rapid. Paralysis has occurred within

TABLE 3.5

Diagnosis of Elapidae envenomation

Local effects	Systemic effects
Little or no pain	Anxiety
Little/no early swelling	Diplopia
Scratch marks	Drowsiness
Small degree of erythema	Dysphagia
	Dyspnoea
	Headache
	Lethargy
	Motor paralysis/weakness
	Respiratory depression
	Salivation
	Fits
	Nausea and vomiting

2–3 h after a bite and has involved the cranial motor nerves. Death from respiratory paralysis has occurred within 4 h of a bite. Children are prone to fits after coral snake bites. The mechanism for this is unclear because the toxins do not cross the blood–brain barrier, but hypoxia may be a factor. Cardiac failure has also been noted. With vigorous supportive therapy and close observation, patients with complete neuromuscular paralysis have recovered, but death may result from either cardiac or respiratory failure.

3.1.3.2 Treatment of coral snake bite

Coral snakes (in North America the Arizona coral snake, *Micuroides euryxanthus;* Eastern coral snake, *Micrurus fulvius fulvius;* Texas coral snake, *M. fulvius tenere*) bite, chew and hang on to the area attacked in order to envenomate. Hence flat surfaces are not usually bitten and death rarely results (Norris and Dart, 1989). Coral snake bites probably result in envenomation in less than 40 % of cases. However, there is no reliable method of predicting those bitten individuals that have been injected with venom.

Coral snakes may be completely black, completely white or partially pigmented but are usually not seen because they are shy and nocturnal. The small size of the fangs makes it difficult for a coral snake bite to penetrate clothing. Most bites occur on the hands as a result of direct handling of the snakes. The most deleterious components of the venom appear to be various neurotoxic, low-formula-weight polypeptides that cause a curare-like post-synaptic block at the neuromuscular junction by binding competitively to the acetylcholine receptor. This is delayed in onset and extremely prolonged. Unlike pit viper venoms, coral snake venom lacks proteolytic enzymes, which explains the relative paucity of local signs and symptoms following the bite. There may be very mild swelling and pain or paraesthesiae at the bite site, but often only fang marks are seen.

Suspected coral snake bites should receive prompt evaluation, and if there is evidence of a break in the skin the patient should be hospitalized for observation for at least 24 h. The bite site should be cleaned. As the venom is very rapidly absorbed by the venous system, there is no point in bandage occlusion. Although acetylcholinesterase

(AChE) inhibitors might have a theoretical use in reversing neuromuscular blockade, no studies have been performed in man.

Hospital management is based on the use of specific 'Wyeth North American coral snake antivenin' or multivalent coral snake antivenin (Costa Rica). It is important before giving the antivenin to be sure that the victim has indeed been bitten by a coral snake, as the Wyeth antivenin is made from horse serum and has the same potential adverse effects as crotalid antivenin (Gold and Barish, 1992). For this reason, skin testing and enquiry about a history of allergy is essential (see Crotalid antivenin test, section 3.1.2.2). If fang marks are present, even in the absence of other clinical features of poisoning, it is important to begin antivenin therapy. Once systemic poisoning becomes manifest, it may be difficult to reverse them or slow their progression even with the use of antivenin.

After a negative skin test, the reconstituted antivenin should be diluted in 0.9 % (w/v) sodium chloride. There are no studies on appropriate dosage (Norris and Dart, 1989). Some suggest that 50–60 mL (contents of 5–6 vials) be given to patients if pain or neurological features of toxicity are evident. Doses up to 80–100 mL (contents of 8– 10 vials) should be given if bulbar signs of paralysis are present. Bites from large snakes may need relatively high doses, particularly in children or small adults. The dose given to children is not based on body weight. The need for additional doses is based on the clinical response to the initial dose and on the severity of poisoning. If necessary, additional antivenin may be administered, usually in doses of 10–50 mL. Some patients may need 100 mL or more. It should be noted that the Wyeth antivenin is not effective in bites by the Arizona coral snake (*Micruroides*). However, the venom from this snake is relatively non-toxic and there has not been a report of a fatality.

3.1.3.3 Treatment of snake bite in South-East Asia

The diagnosis and treatment of snake bite in the Indian subcontinent, Myanmar, Thailand, Lao PDR, Cambodia, Vietnam, Malaysia, Singapore, Brunei, the Philippines and parts of Indonesia are the subjects of a recent WHO publication (Warrell, 1999). Some antivenins used in this area, the Middle East and in Africa are listed in Table 3.6.

3.1.3.4 Treatment of snake bite in Australia

Australia's venomous snakes fall into five groups based on clinical features of poisoning and the specific antivenin required (White, 1998). Group 1 consists of the brown snakes, the most common cause of bites and deaths. Group 2 contains the tiger snakes, copperheads, the rough-scaled snake and the broad-headed snakes. These snakes should be considered potentially deadly as it has recently been established that their bite can cause massive coagulopathy. The third group consists of the mulga and black snakes, the fourth group the taipans and the last group the death adders.

Australian snakes do cause some local effects around the bite, but these are more important for their diagnostic utility than for the morbidity caused, which is usually minor. However, the systemic effects are of major importance. Of these, four predominate, though not all species cause all four. Neurotoxic paralysis is rarely lethal given modern intensive care facilities. Rhabdomyolysis is still occasionally fatal, most often through development of secondary renal failure or hyperkalaemia. Coagulopathy

TABLE 3.6

Some further snake bite antivenins (see also Warrell, 1999)

Antivenin	Origin	Effective against
Cobra	Knoll AG, Germany	*Naja naja sputatrix* (= *N. sumatrana* – Sumatran spitting cobra)
	Thai Red Cross, Bangkok	*Naja kaouthia* (monocellate cobra)
	Myanmar, Yangon, Burma	*Naja kaouthia*
Philippine cobra	Biological Production Service, Philippines Department of Health	*Naja philippinensis*
King cobra (hamadryad)	Thai Red Cross, Bangkok	*Ophiophagus hannah*
Banded krait	Thai Red Cross, Bangkok	*Bungarus fasciatus*
Russell's viper	Thai Red Cross, Bangkok	*Vipera russelli* (= *Daboia russelli*)
	Myanmar, Yangon, Burma	*Vipera russelli*
Elapid bivalent	National Institute of Preventive Medicine, Taiwan	*Bungarus multicinctus* (Chinese krait) and *Naja atra* (Chinese cobra)
Bivalent	Serum Institute of India, Pune	*Echis carinatus*, *Vipera russelli*
Echis bivalent	South African Institute for Medical Research	*Echis carinatus*, *E. coloratus*
Polyvalent	National Institute of Health, Pakistan	*Bungarus caeruleus* (common krait), *Echis carinatus*, *Naja naja* (common spectacled Indian cobra), *Vipera lebetina* (=*Macrovipera lebetina*), *V. russelli*
	State Serum and Vaccine Institute, Tehran, Iran	*Naja oxiana* (north Indian or oxus cobra), *Vipera lebetina*, *Echis carinatus* and/or *E. sochureki* (saw-scaled or carpet vipers), *Pseudocerastes persicus*
	Haffkine Bio-Pharmaceuticals, Mumbai, India	*Bungarus caeruleus*, *Echis carinatus*, *Naja naja*, *Vipera russelli*
	Serum Institute of India, Pune	*Bungarus caeruleus*, *Echis carinatus*, *Naja naja*, *Vipera russelli*
	Central Research Institute, Kasauli, India	*Bungarus caeruleus*, *Echis carinatus*, *Naja naja*, *Vipera russelli*
	South African Institute for Medical Research	African night adders (*Causus*), cobras (*Naja*), mambas (*Dendroaspis*) and puff adders (*Bitis*)

is probably the leading cause of deaths at present. Primary or secondary renal failure remains an important problem.

Complete defibrination may be seen as soon as 20 min after a brown snake bite. However venoms targeting extravascular sites, such as neurotoxins and myotoxins, may take longer to reach effective concentrations and cause clinically detectable effects. Thus, myolysis or paralysis is often not obvious for 2–6 h post bite. Whatever the dynamics of individual components, the clinician may be faced with a complex multisystem disorder as evidenced by a taipan bite with complete paralysis, coagulopathy, secondary haemorrhage and anaemia, rhabdomyolysis, acute renal failure and secondary pneumonia (White, 1995).

The hospital management of snake bite revolves around early recognition of the diagnosis and prompt effective response. It is vital to look for paralysis. The first sign is usually ptosis, followed by ophthalmoplegia, then fixed dilated pupils and dysarthria, after which early intubation may be needed. Myolysis may mimic paralysis, with muscle weakness, but this is invariably accompanied by myoglobinuria, unless there is acute renal failure. Coagulopathy may be silent or obvious. Investigations are always useful in ascertaining the type and extent of systemic envenomation, especially snake venom detection, coagulation tests and creatine phosphokinase assay. Classic defibrination results, as seen in brown snake bite, show a very low fibrinogen, with fibrin degradation products being grossly elevated. The prothrombin time (international normalized ratio, INR) is also prolonged. In contrast, in anticoagulation as caused by mulga snakes and their relatives, there will be prolongation of the INR but concentrations of fibrinogen and its degradation products are unaffected.

All current Australian Commonwealth Serum Laboratories (CSL) snake antivenins are F(ab)$_2$ equine liquid products. There is a dominance of use of brown snake and tiger snake antivenin, but in 31 % of cases polyvalent antivenin is used (White, 1998). Snake venom detection kits use enzyme-linked immunosorbent assays (ELISAs) and can detect the type of snake involved, allowing use of specific antivenin (Table 3.7). A result can be obtained in 25 min, based on bite site or urine. Blood is less reliable. Sometimes the bite is too severe to wait for a result. There are many other clues to the type of snake involved, including geographic location, physical description of the snake and local and systemic effects, particularly the presence or absence of paralysis, coagulopathy or myolysis (White, 1998). Using a combination of all the available information, it is often possible to guess the type of snake most likely to be involved, thus allowing the use of specific antivenom. Later venom detection can verify the validity of diagnosis.

3.1.3.5 Viperidae: European adder

The adder, *Vipera berus*, is found throughout Western Europe and is the only naturally occurring poisonous snake in the UK. Bites usually result from trying to pick up the snake in the summer months, as they hibernate in winter (Hawley, 1988). Probably less than 50 % of bites are associated with venom injection.

The bite usually comprises two puncture marks about a centimetre apart on the extremity of a limb. It may go unnoticed until swelling develops, but often there is immediate pain. Swelling at the site often occurs within an hour and indicates that injection of venom has occurred. Rarely, systemic poisoning may occur in the absence of a local reaction. Vomiting, abdominal pain and diarrhoea may occur within a few

TABLE 3.7

Poisonous snakes of Australia

Group	Latin name	Common name	Type of antivenin
1	*Pseudonaja textilis*	Eastern brown snake	CSL brown snake antivenin
	P. nuchalis	Western brown snake or Gwardar	
	P. affinis	Dugite	
	P. inframacula	Peninsula brown snake	
	P. guttata	Speckled brown snake	
	P. ingrami	Ingram's brown snake	
2	*Notechis scutatus*	Common tiger snake	Monovalent CSL tiger snake antivenin
	N. ater	Black tiger snake	
	N. occidentalis	Western tiger snake	
	Austrelaps superbus	Lowland copperhead	
	A. ramsayi	Highland copperhead	
	A. labialis	Pygmy copperhead	
	Tropidechis carinatus	Rough-scaled snake	
	Hoplocephalus bungaroides	Broad-headed snake	
	H. bitorquatus	Pale-headed snake	
	H. stephensi	Stephen's banded snake	
	Rhinoplocephalus nigrescens	Eastern small-eyed snake	
3	*Pseudechis australis*	Mulga or king brown snake	CSL black snake antivenin
	P. butleri	Butler's mulga snake	
	P. colletii	Collett's snake	
	P. guttatus	Spotted or blue-bellied black snake	
	P. porphyriacus	Red-bellied black snake	
4	*Oxyuranus scutellatus*	Common taipan	CSL taipan antivenin
	O. microlepidotus	Inland taipan	
5	*Acanthophis antarcticus*	Common death adder	CSL death adder antivenin
	A. pyrrhus	Desert death adder	
	A. praelongus	Northern death adder	

■ CHAPTER 3 ■

minutes, and hypotension and loss of consciousness can also occur at an early stage (Cederholm and Lennmarken, 1987). Gastrointestinal symptoms may continue for 2 days, and over this time the limb swells further and becomes haemorrhagic, blood loss often being sufficient to cause anaemia. Hypotension may persist for up to 36 h after the bite and this, together with development of bleeding, oliguria, a neutrophil leucocytosis and non-specific ECG changes, such as T-wave inversion, indicate severe systemic poisoning (Moore, 1988).

The bite should not be cut or sucked, but cleaned and covered with a dry dressing. If hospital is more than 30 min away a bandage or light ligature should be placed around a limb proximal to the bite to impede venous return. Every victim should be referred to hospital and observed for at least 24 h. The heart rate and blood pressure should be recorded hourly and a careful note made of urine output and volumes of fluid lost through vomiting or diarrhoea. The extent of swelling should be recorded, and the white cell count, plasma urea and electrolytes should be measured daily. A coagulation screen is recommended if bleeding occurs. Death from adder bites is extremely rare. Adults usually take slightly longer to recover than children.

The only generally available antivenin is Zagreb antivenin, although clinical trials of a viper-specific $F(ab')_2$ antibody fragment (Viperfav) have started (de Haro et al., 1996; Scherrmann et al., 1996). European adder (Zagreb) antivenin can be used for bites by the long-nosed viper, Vipera berus, and by V. aspis. The principal indications for the use of Zagreb antivenin are:

- persistent or recurrent hypotension;
- bleeding;
- ECG changes such as T-wave inversion;
- white blood count 20,000 per mm^3 or greater;
- in adults, swelling extending up the limb within 2 h of the bite (to reduce disability from the local effects of the poison).

The benefits of antivenin have to be weighed against the risk of hypersensitivity reaction to the serum. Therefore, a history of asthma or other allergies is a relative contraindication. However, it is remarkably safe. The s.c. injection of a small dose as a test of hypersensitivity may give misleading results and is not recommended. A small amount (0.5 mL) of 1:1,000 adrenaline (0.5 mg) must be drawn into the syringe before giving antivenin. Two ampoules (total of 4 mL) of European viper venom antiserum should be added to 100 mL of 0.9 % (w/v) sodium chloride and infused at a rate of 15 mL/min. Immediate reactions to the antivenin can be controlled by temporarily stopping the infusion and oral administration of antihistamines or i.m. injection of the adrenaline. In severely affected patients, in whom swelling continues, the dose of antivenin may need to be repeated.

3.1.4 Spiders

3.1.4.1 Black widow spider

The black widow spider (Lactrodectus mactans) is one of the most potent envenomators of humans, and its bites cause a massive transmitter release from nerve terminals, with resultant pain and cramping of large muscles. One high-molecular-weight neurotoxin, 'α-latrotoxin', activates cation channels in the presynaptic membrane after binding to a specific receptor (Clark et al., 1992). Although both male and female spiders are venomous, only the females have fangs large and strong enough to penetrate human skin. The black widow spider is easily recognized by the jet-black body with a red hourglass mark on the underside of the abdomen. Black widows stay close by webs placed on or close to the ground and in secluded, dimly lit areas that have access to flying insects. Other common preferred sites are abandoned rodent burrows, nests, sheds and garages.

Most bites are a pinprick or painless and occur on the extremities, and generalized pain in the back or abdomen is the most frequent presenting complaint of patients. Two tiny red marks are occasionally identifiable at the site of the bite. The middle of the site may be white, with surrounding erythema and a reddish blue border (Allen,

1992). Pain usually progresses from the bite up the limb and will finally localize in the abdomen and back. The abdominal muscles become rigid and severe cramps develop. In addition, nausea, vomiting, urine retention, insomnia, tremors, speech defects, sweating and a small rise in body temperature may be noted within 1 h. The symptoms may appear within a few hours or a few minutes of the bite. Other clinical features may include headache, eyelid oedema, skin rash, conjunctivitis and an increase in blood pressure. Severely poisoned patients may lapse into coma. Respiratory muscle paralysis and cardiovascular collapse may also occur (Clark *et al.*, 1992).

If pain is intense, ice can be placed over the wound. Therapy is mainly supportive and should include stabilization of vital signs if necessary, with attention being paid to end-organ damage resulting from acetylcholine release. Supplemental oxygen, i.v. access and cardiac monitoring are indicated in symptomatic young and elderly patients. As with any break in the skin, tetanus prophylaxis should be updated if necessary. Although calcium salts have been recommended for abdominal pain, there is limited evidence that they are of value. In the acute phase, oral diazepam may help with muscle cramps as well as with the symptoms of less severe poisoning.

Antivenin against the black widow spider is of horse origin (Pasteur Merieux, MSD) and is recommended for patients who have heart disease or respiratory distress, for pregnant patients who show features of poisoning and for those younger than 16 and older than 65 years of age who show signs of envenomation or serious poisoning (Allen, 1992; Clark *et al.*, 1992). Patients with allergies to horse serum products can be given the infusion, albeit with caution. One vial of antivenin can be added to 15–100 mL of 5 % (w/v) D-glucose or 0.9 % (w/v) sodium chloride solution and then infused over 20–30 min. The normal dose is 1–2 vials, and prompt resolution of features of poisoning is characteristic within 1 h. Although treatment with antivenin may be beneficial in individuals, its efficacy is unproven.

3.1.4.2 Funnel web spiders

These spiders occur in Australia. They are irritable and possess a venom that is potentially deadly to humans. The toxic component, atraxotoxin, is a neurotoxin that acts directly on nerve membranes, causing widespread release of neurotransmitters. Therefore, acetylcholine is released at motor end plates and acetylcholine, adrenaline and noradrenaline through the autonomic nervous system. Clinical features include neuromuscular paralysis and hypertension. Funnel web spider antivenin (CSL Australia) covers the funnel web spider (*Atrax robustus*) and *Hadronyche* and *Missulena* species and should be used for any patient developing more than a local bite reaction.

3.1.4.3 Brown recluse spider

The brown recluse spider (*Loxosceles reclusa*) is also called the Arizona brown spider and tends to be found in central and south-eastern USA. Adults are 7–30 mm in length and vary in colour from yellow to dark brown. The violin-shaped dark markings immediately behind the eyes are the most conspicuous recognition characteristic (Madrigal *et al.*, 1972). Unlike black widow spiders, both sexes are equal in size and danger. Brown recluse spiders have six eyes in three pairs. As most other spiders have eight eyes, this feature eliminates many spiders suspected of being a brown recluse. They are usually nocturnal and live in warm, dry areas, such as undisturbed cellars or abandoned buildings. The largest populations are found in indoor areas. They will bite only if molested or otherwise threatened. Human victims are often bitten while putting on clothing in which the spider is accidentally trapped and traumatized (Madrigal *et al.*, 1972; Magrina and Masterson, 1981).

The venom of the brown recluse spider is complex and composed of at least eight different proteins (Arnold, 1976). These induce injury to arteries and veins, which become occluded with thrombus composed of white cells and platelets. Capillary stasis ensues followed by tissue infarction (Alario *et al.*, 1987; Allen, 1992). Membrane damage along with other activities of brown recluse spider venom results in a chain reaction with release of inflammatory mediators such as leukotrienes and prostaglandins.

The clinical response to envenomation varies from a mild local stinging reaction to severe systemic involvement and death (Gendron, 1990). Because the bite frequently occurs at night, the spider is crushed, hence the origin of the bite is rarely positively identified. Only after 2–80 h as pain, varying from mild to severe, begins at the site of the bite does the victim notice transient erythema, followed by a blister with an irregular area of ischaemia. A zone of haemorrhage with a surrounding halo is seen, which, over several days, turns dark in colour and tender to touch (Arnold, 1976). Within 7 days, the central area is depressed, sharply demarcated and dark, and between 7 and 14 days a scar falls off, leaving a wound that heals by secondary intention (Alario *et al.*, 1987). The two features of colour and configuration help differentiate these bites from other venomous spider bites. Others tend not to be necrotic (Alario *et al.*, 1987).

Although the skin lesions are painful and disfiguring, death is usually related to circulatory or renal failure. In nearly all fatalities, haemoglobininuria and acute renal failure have been preterminal events (Madrigal *et al.*, 1972). In severe cases, systemic features occur 24–72 h post bite and include a morbilliform rash, urticaria, fever, nausea and vomiting and haemolysis (Vorse *et al.*, 1972; Eichner, 1984). The systemic symptoms are not directly proportional to the severity of the skin lesions. Next come haemorrhage, ecchymoses, haemoglobinuria and renal failure.

Symptomatic support with red cell transfusions is important in treatment (Eichner, 1984). Maintenance of good hydration and monitoring of renal function help ensure that haemoglobinuria does not cause renal failure. Systemic steroids (1–2 mg/kg daily, 4 days), although not of proven efficacy, may be given in the acute phase (4–5 days) in an attempt to stop red cell destruction (Gendron, 1990). There are no controlled human studies evaluating other treatment options for brown recluse bites, including local excision, polymorphonuclear inhibitors and, most recently, hyperbaric oxygen. Most skin lesions can be managed by good wound care, elevation, ice packs and mobilization. Although bites can become infected, prophylactic antibiotics are controversial and probably not indicated (Gendron, 1990).

More recently, a goat-derived specific antivenin to the brown recluse spider was developed and tested in the field. This is the Brazilian Butanan Institute (*Titus phonentria*, *Loxosceles* spider) antivenin. When administered within 24 h of the bite, it prevented or markedly attenuated toxicity. The product is not yet readily available commercially.

3.1.4.4 Red back spider

The red back spider (*Latrodectus hasselti*) is often found in urban habitats in Australia and, although not aggressive, the sheer volume of encounters with humans ensures several thousands bites annually. CSL red back spider antivenin is the most commonly used antivenin in Australia. It is reported as being efficacious in 94 % of cases, with one ampoule being used in 75 % of cases, two ampoules in 18 % and three or more in 6 %. Clinical experience suggests that only 20 % of red back spider bites require antivenin therapy. Premedication with adrenaline was used in 45 % of cases and the incidence of adverse reactions was low (White, 1998).

3.1.5 Scorpions

Scorpions are found throughout the tropics, arid deserts and semiburied grasslands. They frequently concentrate in areas of human habitation to take advantage of shelter, water and prey. There are some 30 species of scorpions found in the New World; of these, about seven are of medical importance. The scorpion is characterized by a long, segmented tail, which ends in a bulbous sack and a conspicuous sting. They may be black with yellow in colour, and can vary from 1.5 to 20 cm in length. They are nocturnal and during the day remain hidden under stones and other objects. When indoors, they hide in shoes and stored materials. The sting response is commonest in circumstances in which scorpions become trapped in clothing or sleeping bags. If movement persists multiple stings may result. The most deadly scorpion is *Centruroides sculpturatus*.

There are two distinct types of scorpion venom. One has local effects but is relatively harmless. The other contains a neurotoxin that causes dramatic and sometimes fatal reactions. The venom of the North American scorpion (*Centruroides*) is the most toxic. The venom simulates the clinical features of strychnine poisoning by acting on both smooth and striated muscle, causing increased excitability and muscle contraction, trembling and, finally, paralysis. Sodium channels are disturbed with resulting prolongation of the action potential as well as spontaneous nerve repolarization. Stimulation of the autonomic system results in a massive outpouring of adrenaline, and sympathetic overdrive manifestations may include tachycardia, hypertension and seizures as well as sweating and piloerection. The venom of non-lethal scorpions causes local reactions such as burning, swelling, and discoloration at the site of the skin lesion. Rarely, anaphylaxis occurs.

The poisonous varieties that possess very potent neurotoxins may produce no local swelling or discoloration. The sharp pain first produced by the sting is quickly followed by paraesthesiae in the bite area, which extends very rapidly. This may be followed by numbness or drowsiness. Local muscle contractions may begin in close proximity to the sting site and may advance to more central effects. Excessive peripheral neuromuscular activity may manifest as simple restlessness from apprehension or pain, but may progress to uncontrollable spasm. Stings by more toxic American scorpions produce additional symptoms of skin flushing, parasympathetic activity, hyperirritability and hyperactivity, hypertension and muscle weakness.

Local pain and paraesthesiae both at the site and peripherally are best treated with local compresses and oral analgesia. More severe symptoms may require intensive support. Tachyarrhythmias may be treated with propranolol. If hypertension is a concern, an α-blocker should be used (Gueron *et al.*, 1992). Other treatments, such as antihistamines, calcium, steroids and sympathetic drugs, have been shown to be of little value. Systemic toxicity, or a painless sting from a lethal species in an individual thought to be at risk, is best treated with antivenin.

One prospective, randomized, controlled trial found no benefit in routine administration of scorpion antivenin after scorpion sting, irrespective of the severity of poisoning as assessed clinically, even though the antivenin dose used was twice that normally employed (Abroug *et al.*, 1999). However, no very seriously poisoned patients were included (Burdett *et al.*, 2000), and the efficacy of the antivenin used was questioned (Possani, 2000). Whatever the benefit of antivenin, meticulous supportive care is critical to a good outcome if serious poisoning occurs (Elatrous *et al.*, 1999; Gueron and Ilia, 1999).

3.1.5.1 *North African scorpion antivenin*

North African scorpion antivenin (Twyford Pharmaceuticals) covers *Androctonus australis, A. aeneas, A. crassicauda, Buthacus arenicola, B. occitanus, Leiurus quinquestriatus, Buthus, Buthiscus* and *Buthotus* species.

3.1.5.2 **Centruroides** *antivenin*

Since the early 1960s *Centruroides* scorpion antivenin (Myn Laboratories, Mexico City) has been made by lyophilizing microfiltered hypersensitized goat serum. The rapid and safe resolution of the severe symptoms of *Centruroides* envenomation following antivenin therapy has led some to recommend its use in unselected patients. Others, seeking to avoid any potential risks associated with the administration of the foreign protein, have pronounced against its use. The fact that the antivenin has not been subjected to FDA controls has also been cited as a cause for caution. When making a decision about the use of antivenin, consideration must be given to the benefits of immediate symptom resolution, cost savings by patient discharge from the emergency room and the avoidance of sedation, paralysis and intubation. Antivenin is usually administered to severely poisoned patients, but particularly the very young, the old or those individuals with hypertension. There is less justification for the use of the antivenin in mildly affected children or adults (Bond, 1992; Bush, 1999).

3.1.5.3 *SAIMR scorpion antivenin*

SAIMR (South African Institute of Medical Research) scorpion antivenin covers *Parabuthus granulatus, P. transvaalicus* and other *Parabuthus* species.

3.1.6 Stonefish

This specific antivenin (CSL, Australia) works against envenomation by *Synanceja trechynis* and *S. verrucosa*.

3.2 USE OF F_{ab} ANTIBODY FRAGMENTS TO TREAT POISONING WITH LOW-FORMULA-MASS COMPOUNDS

The aim of immunotoxicotherapy is to sequester, extract or redistribute and eliminate toxins by giving antibodies or antibody fragments that possess specific active binding sites for the poison in question. For immunotoxicotherapy to be possible and cost-effective, the toxin must be able to stimulate the production of antibodies and carry a high risk either of causing death through acute toxicity (e.g. tricyclic antidepressants) or of having long-term effects due to accumulation in tissues (e.g. polychlorinated biphenyl compounds) (Bismuth *et al.*, 1997).

The ability to prepare antisera to low-formula-mass drugs and other poisons suggested that 'immunotherapy' might be used similarly to inactivate such compounds *in vivo* and facilitate their excretion. However, the ability to manufacture an antibody with the necessary affinity for the poison and to administer it in the quantities needed to reverse toxicity fully have so far limited the practical development of this approach to treating severe poisoning with digoxin and other digitalis glycosides, colchicine and tricyclic antidepressants (Scherrmann, 1994). Stoichiometric neutralization with antibodies is effective against toxins present in microgram quantities, such as cardiac glycosides. Fortunately, for some toxins taken in doses that are 100–1,000 times higher, such as tricyclic antidepressants and colchicine, partial neutralization is effective as the cost of full stoichiometric neutralization would be prohibitive (Schaumann *et al.*,

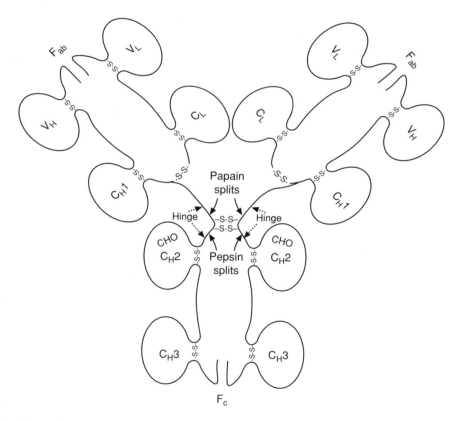

Figure 3.1: Schematic diagram of the human immunoglobin (IgG) molecule. The molecule is composed of two 'heavy' and two 'light' polypeptide chains and has two antigen binding sites (F_{ab}) and a complement-fixing site (F_c). V_L and V_H denote light- and heavy-chain variable regions, respectively, and C_H1, C_H2 and C_H3 and 'constant' regions on the 'heavy' chain; C_L is a 'constant' region of the 'light' chain. Reproduced from Kabat (1982) with the permission of the American Society for Pharmacology and Therapeutics

1986). Most antibodies are polyclonal and have broad specificity, which permits successful treatment of poisoning with closely related compounds (Bismuth *et al.*, 1997).

In recent years there have been dramatic innovations in the safety and efficacy of immunotherapy, highlighted by the successes seen in digitalis and colchicine poisoning. It should be emphasized, however, that immunotherapy is only an adjunct to the intensive supportive care of poisoned patients. The limitations of immunotherapy are its high costs and restriction, at present, to drugs having toxic doses in the low milligram range.

3.2.1 Antidigoxin F_{ab} antibody fragments

Mortality is high in severe digoxin poisoning. The development of antidigoxin antibodies for use in measuring plasma concentrations of this drug, and the subsequent use of the antibodies to abolish digoxin toxicity in animals, were important advances (Schmidt and Butler, 1971). Unfortunately, whole antibodies are themselves immunogenic by virtue of the presence of the F_c fragment (Figure 3.1), and they are also too large to be readily excreted in urine. Moreover, degradation of the circulating antibody–digoxin complexes could eventually release large quantities of digoxin back into the circulation (Butler *et al.*, 1977a).

The use of digoxin-specific F_{ab} antibody fragments derived from antibodies raised in sheep has overcome these problems (Smith *et al.*, 1976, 1982). Papain digestion cleaves the IgG molecule into three fragments: a crystallizable fraction (F_c), which is unwanted, and two F_{ab} fragments. These fragments include the digoxin binding sites (Figure 3.1). F_{ab} fragments lack immunogenicity and are small enough (relative formula mass *c.* 50,000) to diffuse into the interstitial space and then be readily excreted in the urine. The fragmentation of antibodies limits the risk of anaphylaxis but reduces the stability of the toxin–antibody complex. The plasma half-life of F_{ab} antibody fragments in the baboon is 9–13 h and that of the parent IgG antibody is 61 h; the total V_D of F_{ab} antibody fragments in the baboon is 8.7 times greater than that of IgG (Smith *et al.*, 1979). The affinity constant for digoxin is high (10^{10}), and greater than that of digoxin for its receptor (Na^+,K^+-activated ATPase), implicated in the development of digoxin toxicity. The affinity constant of the antibody fragment for digitoxin is also high (10^9). Administered i.v., the fragments bind to circulating glycoside, forming relatively stable complexes that are unable to bind to tissue digitalis receptors. F_{ab} fragments cannot cross membranes and hence stay in the extracellular compartment. In animals, F_{ab} antibody fragments reverse digoxin effects much more quickly than does IgG. There is a suggestion that reversal of inotropy lags behind reversal of electrical arrhythmic effects (Ochs *et al.*, 1978).

The antibody fragments were first used in man in 1976, and many patients have now been treated with them (Smith, 1985; Schaumann *et al.*, 1986; Sullivan, 1986; Stolshek *et al.*, 1988; Antman *et al.*, 1990; Howland and Smilkstein, 1991). Digibind (GlaxoWellcome) is generally available in North America and in the UK, and Digitalis Antidot BM (Boehringer Mannheim GmbH) has been released in Europe (Smolarz *et al.*, 1985). Both show some cross-reaction with digitoxin (Hess *et al.*, 1983; Smolarz *et al.*, 1985; Wenger *et al.*, 1985) and lanatoside C (Hess *et al.*, 1979). Digibind has been shown to reverse β-methyldigoxin- and β-acetyldigoxin-induced arrhythmias in guinea pigs (data on file, GlaxoWellcome, 1995). Unfortunately, both preparations are very expensive. A new preparation is under development (Therapeutic Antibodies) but is not licensed yet. Antidigoxin antibody fragments should be stored in a refrigerator (2–8 °C) or in a freezer (–20 °C or below). Their efficacy is not impaired by brief freezing and thawing before use (Baud *et al.*, 1992). Indications for use of F_{ab} fragments for digoxin poisoning are shown in Table 3.8.

Sixty-three patients with severe digitalis toxicity, i.e. with life-threatening arrhythmias or hyperkalaemia, or both, were given the Wellcome preparation i.v. over 15–30 min. They ranged in age from a few days to 85 years and included 28 who had taken massive overdoses. Fifty-three of the 56 patients suitable for analysis recovered completely (Wenger *et al.*, 1985). Digibind can reverse ventricular arrhythmias within 2 min, with persistence of ventricular extrasystoles for a further 15 min, and in general rhythm and conduction disturbances settle within 30 min (Smith *et al.*, 1982). In a trial of Digitalis Antidote BM, 32 of 34 patients were successfully treated (Smolarz *et al.*, 1985). Of 29 children and adolescents (aged up to 18 years) with severe digoxin poisoning treated with Digibind (GlaxoWellcome), digoxin toxicity was resolved in 27; three patients required additional F_{ab} treatment (Woolf *et al.*, 1992). In no series could deaths be attributed to failure to reverse toxicity.

In some cases, the rate of reversal of toxicity has been dramatic: gastrointestinal features of toxicity disappeared almost immediately, and hyperkalaemia was corrected within 30–60 min of ending the infusion (Spiegel and Marchlinski, 1985). Arrhythmias were corrected equally quickly in some patients (Spiegel and Marchlinski, 1985), but more slowly (up to 13 h; mean 3.2 h) in others (Smolarz *et al.*, 1985). Even digitoxin-induced thrombocytopenia was considerably improved within hours (Hess *et al.*, 1983).

Reported values for the elimination half-life of digoxin after the administration of F_{ab} antibody fragments are conflicting. Claimed elimination half-lives are 16–20 h (Wenger *et al.*, 1985) or 20–30 h compared with 160 h for spontaneous elimination (Smolarz *et al.*, 1985). During the first 12 h after infusion of F_{ab} fragments all of the free digoxin in serum is bound to the fragments and therefore rendered inactive (Smith *et al.*, 1976). Treatment with F_{ab} fragments increases the renal clearance of digoxin by 20–30 % (Butler *et al.*, 1977b). Thus, F_{ab} fragments for digoxin have both toxicokinetic and toxicodynamic actions. Conventional serum immunoassays of glycoside concentration are no longer useful when the patient has been treated with F_{ab} fragments (Gibb *et al.*, 1983; Gibb and Adams, 1985; Hursting *et al.*, 1987; Sinclair *et al.*, 1989).

The dose of F_{ab} fragments required is governed by the need for equimolar neutralization of the body load of digoxin or other cardiac glycoside (Smith *et al.*, 1982). The body burden of digoxin can be estimated in two ways. The first is from information on the amount acutely ingested, multiplied by 0.8 to take account of digoxin bioavailability (80 %) (Figure 3.2). The second is from the plasma concentration in the quasi-steady state, which in practice is the plasma (or serum) digoxin concentration 4–6 h or more post dose. The plasma digoxin concentration (µg/L) is multiplied by

CHAPTER 3

TABLE 3.8

Indications for use of F_{ab} antibody fragments in digoxin poisoning (Smith *et al.*, 1982)

Cardiovascular shock
Heart rhythm disturbances including any degree of heart block or ventricular arrhythmias
History of large ingested dose, confirmed by very high plasma digoxin concentrations
Hyperkalaemia (serum potassium 5 mmol/L or more)
Use early if patient over 55 years of age or has pre-existing cardiovascular disease

---

Estimation of body burden

Digoxin
1   If the dose (mg) ingested is known, multiply by 0.8 (oral bioavailability of digoxin 80 %)
2   If the dose ingested is not known, the digoxin body burden (mg) is calculated thus:

[Plasma digoxin concentration[a] (µg/L) $\times$ 5 (L/kg) $\times$ body weight (kg)]/1000

Digitoxin
1   If the dose (mg) ingested is known, use this figure directly (oral bioavailability of digitoxin 100 %)
2   If the dose ingested is not known, the digitoxin body burden (mg) is calculated thus:

[Plasma digitoxin concentration[a,b] (µg/L) $\times$ 0.5 (L/kg) $\times$ body weight (kg)]/1000

Calculation of dose of F_{ab} fragments

As 80 mg F_{ab} fragments will sequester approximately 1 mg of digoxin or digitoxin, the dose of F_{ab} fragments (mg) is calculated from:

Estimated digoxin body burden (mg) $\times$ 80

The number of vials of F_{ab} fragments used [Digibind (GlaxoWellcome) vials each contain 38 mg F_{ab} fragments] should be rounded up to the nearest whole vial.

Notes

[a]Normally, blood for therapeutic monitoring of cardiac glycosides is taken at least 6 h post dose to allow time for absorption and tissue distribution to be completed. However, after massive acute oral overdosage these processes may not be complete even at 6 h. Moreover, the time of ingestion may not be known accurately. In these circumstances it may not be appropriate to delay taking blood for plasma glycoside assay if the clinical condition of the patient and any accompanying history suggests that use of F_{ab} fragments may be indicated. If the blood is taken before absorption/distribution is complete, use of the resulting plasma digoxin concentration in the above equation may lead to overestimation of the digoxin body burden and thus of the F_{ab} fragment dose required. However, in a life-threatening situation this is preferable to undue delay.
[b]Plasma digitoxin assays are not widely available, but digitoxin cross-reacts on digoxin assay kits and thus a plasma 'digitoxin' result can be obtained.

Figure 3.2: Estimation of dose of F_{ab} fragments required for digoxin and digitoxin poisoning

---

$0.005 \times$ body weight (kg) to obtain an estimate of total body burden in milligrams (Figure 3.2). The plasma concentration factor is derived from the V_D (5 L/kg body weight) divided by 1,000 to reduce the body load estimate to milligrams. The approximate formula mass ratio of F_{ab} and digoxin is 80. Hence, the approximate dose of F_{ab} fragments (mg) required is 80 times the digoxin body burden (mg). There is no correction for per cent absorbed dose in digitoxin poisoning (bioavailability of digitoxin 100 % – Baud *et al.*, 1992). However, the plasma concentration factor is 10-fold smaller in digitoxin poisoning than in digoxin poisoning (Figure 3.2) (digitoxin V_D 0.5 L/kg). If neither the dose ingested nor the plasma digoxin concentration is known, it is conventional practice in an adult to infuse the contents of 10 vials of Digibind (GlaxoWellcome), i.e. 380 mg F_{ab} fragments.

The fragments are given i.v. diluted to at least 250 mL by plasma protein solution (except in infants, in whom the volume infused can be reduced) over 15–30 min. A longer duration of infusion diminishes the efficacy of the antidote (Smith *et al.*, 1982). Factors limiting the efficacy of F_{ab} fragments are the dose given, the duration of the infusion and any delay in administration. In one case, where the dose given was insufficient, the patient died from recurrence of ventricular fibrillation (Smith *et al.*, 1991). Administration at too slow a rate (over 4 h) in one case resulted in reduced efficacy (Smolarz *et al.*, 1985). Rapid infusion of F_{ab} fragments seems necessary for them to 'catch' the glycoside in the extracellular compartment.

The gastrointestinal tract, kidney, liver, spleen and lymph nodes are among the potential sites of catabolism of F_{ab} antibody fragments. Circulating F_{ab} fragments are filtered through the glomeruli and rapidly and extensively reabsorbed in the proximal tubules. However, some 60–70 % of F_{ab} total body clearance is non-renal (Scherrmann, 1994). The elimination half-life of F_{ab} fragments in humans is about 12 h (Thanh-Barthet *et al.*, 1993).

Infusion of F_{ab} fragments is generally well tolerated. A case of erythema at the injection site and a case of urticaria have been reported. No delayed hypersensitivity reactions have been reported. The risk of anaphylaxis on repeated administration of F_{ab} fragments has not been evaluated. However, adverse effects attributable to F_{ab} treatment, notably hypokalaemia and exacerbation of congestive cardiac failure, have been recorded (Smolarz *et al.*, 1985; Wenger *et al.*, 1985; Smith, 1991), and there is concern that renal function could be impaired in some patients. A recent study has shown that F_{ab} fragments reduce glomerular filtration rate in the rabbit (Timsina and Hewick, 1992).

Digoxin-specific F_{ab} antibody fragments have also been used to reverse toxicity from cardiac glycosides present in plants such as *Digitalis purpurea* (purple foxglove) and *Nerium oleander* (oleander) (Eddleston and Warrell, 1999). *In vitro* trials have been undertaken of their possible use in treating poisoning due to the rodenticide scilliroside, one of the cardiac glycosides present in the bulb of red squill [sea onion, the red variety of *Urginea (Scilla) maritima*], and proscillaridin, a drug derived from scilliroside that has been used to treat cardiac failure in patients with poor renal function (Sabouraud *et al.*, 1990). Digidot (Boehringer Mannheim) antibody fragments were used. The affinity constants for the fragments for scilliroside and proscillaridin were, respectively, 80- and 500-fold weaker than for digoxin. Nevertheless, it was thought that sufficient binding to give clinical benefit might be achieved in treating poisoned patients.

Yew (*Taxus baccata* and other *Taxus* species) contains toxic alkaloids (taxanes) in almost all parts of the plant. Although these alkaloids are arrhythmogenic, they are structurally unrelated to the cardiac glycosides found in *Digitalis purpurea* for example, and it is unlikely that digoxin-specific F_{ab} fragments have any role in treating poisoning with *Taxus* species (Cummins *et al.*, 1990).

3.2.2 Other potential applications of F_{ab} antibody fragments

The possibility of using antiparaquat F_{ab} antibody fragments to remove paraquat from lung cells has been investigated (section 8.3). Antibodies from IgG- and IgM-secreting cell lines show high affinity for paraquat. After i.v. injection of 0.1 mg/kg paraquat, the plasma paraquat concentration in rats pretreated with antiparaquat antibodies was increased and the amount excreted in the urine was significantly decreased compared with controls (Nagao *et al.*, 1989). However, use of antiparaquat antibodies could not prevent paraquat from accumulating in tissues and is therefore unlikely to be of therapeutic benefit in man (Nagao *et al.*, 1989).

Infusion of anticolchicine, antidesipramine and antiphencyclidine F_{ab} antibody fragments causes redistribution of these drugs into plasma in animals (Owens and Mayersohn, 1986; Hursting *et al.*, 1989; Sabouraud *et al.*, 1992a,b).

Until recently, there was no successful specific therapy for colchicine poisoning, which is associated with a mortality of 90 % at doses of 0.8 mg/kg or more. Anticolchicine antibodies were prepared many years ago in rabbits (Wolff *et al.*, 1980). More recently, anticolchicine antibody F_{ab} fragments infused over 7 h have been used to treat a patient poisoned with colchicine (Scherrmann *et al.*, 1992). A very successful example of the use of immunotoxicotherapy in colchicine poisoning using goat colchicine-specific F_{ab} fragments was reported by Baud *et al.* (1995). Despite cardiogenic shock, bone marrow aplasia, sepsis, alopecia and transient peripheral neuropathy, the patient survived with no permanent physical sequelae. Substantial amounts of colchicine were removed from peripheral sites and redistributed into the extracellular space by F_{ab} infusion. The urinary colchicine excretion rate increased sixfold.

Tricyclic antidepressants (TCAs) are the commonest cause of death by intentional overdose of tablets in the USA. High-affinity TCA-specific monoclonal F_{ab} fragments have been prepared (Bowles *et al.*, 1988). Monoclonal F_{ab} or sheep polyclonal F_{ab} fragments rapidly reverse the cardiovascular toxicity of TCAs in rats, prolonging survival (Pentel and Keyler, 1995; Pentel *et al.*, 1995). The therapeutic effect occurs within minutes and is evident with F_{ab} doses that are 10–30 % of the stoichiometric dose. At the higher end of this dose range, cardiovascular deterioration or death has occurred, and thus strategies for reducing the required dose are desirable. As an example, combining TCA-specific F_{ab} with sodium bicarbonate is more effective than either treatment alone (Brunn *et al.*, 1992; Pentel *et al.*, 1995).

Similarly, antidesipramine antibody F_{ab} fragments administered in quantities equivalent to approximately 10 %, 20 % and 30 % of the desipramine dose caused dose-dependent amelioration in signs of toxicity (QRS interval, heart rate) in rats poisoned with desipramine (Brunn *et al.*, 1992; Dart *et al.*, 1996). There have been early anecdotal reports of the clinical value of this approach, but no reports of controlled studies have been published as yet.

3.3 IMMUNIZATION AGAINST BEE (*Hymenoptera*) STING

For most people, a bee sting is merely unpleasant and is followed by the development of small hives and itching that may persist for several hours. All traces of the sting usually disappear within a few hours. About 10 % of people who are stung develop a large local reaction consisting of extensive and persistent swelling at the sting site. The pathogenesis involves IgE-mediated late-phase and cell-mediated hypersensitivity reactions (Graft, 1989).

Systemic allergic reactions to insect stings may present in a variety of ways. In most severe episodes there is cardiovascular collapse or bronchospasm (Reisman and

Livingston, 1989). These reactions may first be indicated by cough, chest tightness, itching around the eyes, massive urticaria, sneezing, wheezing, tachycardia, hypotension and pallor. Some patients have a delayed serum sickness syndrome with symptoms including fever, headache and polyarthritis.

Local bites should be treated with oral antihistamines. If the swelling becomes extremely extensive and painful, steroid therapy is indicated (prednisolone 20–40 mg orally daily, for several days). When confronted with a patient with a severe reaction, adrenaline 1:1,000 in a dose of 0.3–0.5 mL for adults (0.2–0.3 mL for a child) should be given by deep s.c. injection, and the site massaged vigorously to enhance the rate of absorption. Patients should be observed closely because their response will determine whether or not the dose should be repeated. Patients at risk are taught how to self-inject.

Venom immunotherapy is indicated in individuals who have had an acute allergic reaction following an insect sting and have positive skin test reactions (Reisman and Livingston, 1989; Valentine *et al.*, 1990). The regimen begins with weekly injections of 0.01 μg of the appropriate venom and advances rapidly to 100 μg. The maintenance dose of 100 μg is given every 4 weeks for a year, after which the interval is lengthened to 6–8 weeks (Valentine *et al.*, 1990). It has been suggested that all patients who have had the more severe features of anaphylaxis, such as respiratory distress, hypotension or upper airway oedema, should receive venom immunotherapy regardless of age or the time interval since the sting reaction. Patients without systemic symptoms should not be given venom immunotherapy. Patients with large local reactions are not considered candidates for this form of therapy. Venom immunotherapy is 97 % effective in reducing the risk of anaphylaxis from stings in adults with previous systemic reactions. These reactions are potentially life-threatening in adults and children. A novel F_{ab}-based antivenin for the treatment of mass bee attacks (both *Apis mellifera scutellata* and *A. m. mellifera*) has recently been developed (Jones *et al.*, 1999).

REFERENCES

Abroug F, ElAtrous S, Nouira S, Haguiga H, Touzi N, Bouchoucha S. Serotherapy in scorpion envenomation: a randomised controlled trial. *Lancet* 1999; 354: 906–9.

Alario A, Price G, Stahl R, Bancroft P. Cutaneous necrosis following a spider bite: a case report and review. *Pediatrics* 1987; 79: 618–21.

Allen C. Arachnid envenomations. *Emerg Med Clin North Am* 1992; 10: 269–98.

Antman EM, Wenger TL, Butler VP, Haber E, Smith TW. Treatment of 150 cases of life-threatening digitalis intoxication with digoxin-specific Fab antibody fragments: final report of a multicenter study. *Circulation* 1990; 81: 1744–52.

Arnold RE. Brown recluse spider bites: five cases with a review of the literature. *J Am Coll Emerg Physicians* 1976; 5: 262–4.

Baud FJ, Brouard A, Haddad P. Fragments Fab d'anticorps spécifiques anti-digitaliques. In: *Les Antidotes*. Baud F, Barriot P, Riou B (eds). Paris: Masson, 1992: 127–38.

Baud FJ, Sabouraud A, Vicaut E, Taboulet P, Lang J, Bismuth C, Rouzioux JM, Scherrmann JM. Treatment of severe colchicine overdose with colchicine-specific Fab fragments. *N Engl J Med* 1995; 332: 642–5.

Bismuth C, Borron SW, Baud FJ, Taboulet P, Scherrmann JM. Immunotoxicotherapy: successes, disappointments and hopes. *Hum Exp Toxicol* 1997; 16: 602–8.

Bond GR. Antivenin administration for *Centruroides* scorpion sting: risks and benefits. *Ann Emerg Med* 1992; 21: 788–91.

CHAPTER 3

Bowles M, Johnston SC, Schoof DD, Pentel PR, Pond SM. Large scale production and purification of paraquat and desipramine monoclonal antibodies and their Fab fragments. *Int J Immunopharmacol* 1988; 10: 537–45.

Brunn GJ, Keyler DE, Pond SM, Pentel PR. Reversal of desipramine toxicity in rats using drug-specific antibody Fab' fragment: effects on hypotension and interaction with sodium bicarbonate. *J Pharmacol Exp Ther* 1992; 260: 1392–9.

Burdett T, McIntosh H, Murphy K, Parry R, Slater F. Antivenom for scorpion sting [letter]. *Lancet* 2000; 355: 66–72.

Burgess JL, Dart RC, Egen NB, Mayersohn M. Effects of constriction bands on rattlesnake venom absorption: a pharmacokinetic study. *Ann Emerg Med* 1992; 21: 1086–93.

Bush SP. Envenomation by the scorpion (*Centruroides limbatus*) outside its natural range and recognition of medically important scorpions. *Wilderness Environ Med* 1999; 10: 161–4.

Butler VP, Smith TW, Schmidt DH, Haber E. Immunological reversal of the effects of digoxin. *Fed Proc* 1977a; 36: 2235–41.

Butler VP, Schmidt DH, Smith TW, Haber E, Raynor BD, Demartini P. Effects of sheep digoxin-specific antibodies and their Fab fragments on digoxin pharmacokinetics in dogs. *J Clin Invest* 1977b; 59: 345–59.

Calmette A. *Les Venins, les Animaux Venimeux et la Sérothérapie Antivenimeuse*. Paris: Masson, 1907 (English translation: Austen EE. London: Bale, Sons and Danielsson, 1908).

Cederholm I, Lennmarken C. *Vipera berus* bites in children – experience of early antivenom treatment. *Acta Paediatr Scand* 1987; 76: 682–4.

Clark RF, Wethern-Kestner S, Vance MV, Gerkin R. Clinical presentation and treatment of black widow spider envenomation: a review of 163 cases. *Ann Emerg Med* 1992; 21: 782–7.

Clark RF, Williams SR, Nordt SP, Boyer-Hassen LV. Successful treatment of crotalid-induced neurotoxicity with a new polyspecific crotalid Fab antivenom. *Ann Emerg Med* 1997; 30: 54–7.

Consroe P, Egen NB, Russell FE, Gerrish K, Smith DC, Sidki A, Landon JT. Comparison of a new ovine antigen binding fragment (Fab) antivenin for United States Crotalidae with the commercial antivenin for protection against venom-induced lethality in mice. *Am J Trop Med Hyg* 1995; 53: 507–10.

Cummins RO, Haulman J, Quan L, Graves JR, Peterson D, Horan S. Near-fatal yew berry intoxication treated with external cardiac pacing and digoxin-specific FAB antibody fragments. *Ann Emerg Med* 1990; 19: 38–43.

Daltry JC, Wüster W, Thorpe RS. Diet and snake venom evolution. *Nature* 1996; 379: 537–9.

Dart RC, Sidki A, Sullivan JB, Egen NB, Garcia RA. Ovine desipramine antibody fragments reverse desipramine cardiovascular toxicity in the rat. *Ann Emerg Med* 1996; 27: 309–15.

Eddleston M, Warrell DA. Management of acute yellow oleander poisoning. *Q J Med* 1999; 92: 483–5.

Eichner ER. Spider bite hemolytic anaemia: positive Coombs' test, erythrophagocytosis, and leukoerythroblastic smear. *Am J Clin Pathol* 1984; 81: 683–7.

Elatrous S, Nouira S, Besbes-Ouanes L, Boussarsar M, Boukef R, Marghli S, Abroug F. Dobutamine in severe scorpion envenomation: effects on standard haemodynamics, right ventricular performance, and tissue oxygenation. *Chest* 1999; 116: 748–53.

Gendron BP. *Loxosceles reclusa* envenomation. *Am J Emerg Med* 1990; 8: 51–4.

Gibb I, Adams PC. Digoxin assay modifications to eliminate interference following immunotherapy for toxicity [abstract]. *Ann Biol Clin* 1985; 43: 696.

Gibb I, Adams PC, Parnham AJ, Jennings K. Plasma digoxin: assay anomalies in Fab-treated patients. *Br J Clin Pharmacol* 1983; 16: 445–7.

Gold BS, Barish RA. Venomous snakebites: current concepts in diagnosis, treatment, and management. *Emerg Med Clin North Am* 1992; 10: 249–67.

Graft DF. Stinging insect allergy: how management has changed. *Postgrad Med J* 1989; 85: 173–80.

Gueron M, Ilia R. Is antivenom the most successful therapy in scorpion victims? [letter]. *Toxicon* 1999; 37: 1655–7.

Gueron M, Ilia R, Sofer S. The cardiovascular system after scorpion envenomation. A review. *Clin Toxicol* 1992; 30: 245–8.

de Haro L, Lang J, Bedry R, Guelon D, Harry P, Marchel Mazet F, Jouglard J. Results of the tolerance study of an european F(ab')$_2$ antivenom (Viperfav®) given as an intravenous infusion to patients posoned by European vipers. *Proceedings of the XVII International Congress of the EAPCCT*, Marseilles, 1996: 92.

Harrison RA, Moura-ds-Silva AM, Laing GD, Wu Y, Richards A, Broadhead A, Bianco AE, Theakston RDG. Antibody from mice immunized with DNA encoding the carboxyl-disintegrin and cysteine-rich domain (JD9) of the haemorrhagic metalloprotease, Jararhagin, inhibits the main lethal component of viper venom. *Clin Exp Immunol* 2000; 121: 358–63.

Hawley A. Adder bites in Aldershot. *J R Army Med Corps* 1988; 134: 135–7.

Hess T, Stucki P, Barandun S, Scholtysik G, Riesen W. Treatment of a case of lanatoside C intoxication with digoxin-specific F(ab')$_2$ antibody fragments. *Am Heart J* 1979; 98: 767–71.

Hess T, Riesen W, Scholtysik G, Stucki P. Digitoxin intoxication with severe thrombocytopenia: reversal by digoxin-specific antibodies. *Eur J Clin Invest* 1983; 13: 159–63.

Howland MA, Smilkstein MJ. Primer on immunology with applications to toxicology. In: *Contemporary Management in Critical Care*, Vol. 1 (Part 3): *Critical Care Toxicology*. Hoffman RS, Goldfrank LR (eds). New York: Churchill Livingstone, 1991: 109–46.

Hursting MJ, Raisys VA, Opheim KE, Bell JL, Trobaugh GB, Smith TW. Determination of free digoxin concentrations in serum for monitoring Fab treatment of digoxin overdose. *Clin Chem* 1987; 33: 1652–5.

Hursting MJ, Opheim KE, Raisys VA, Kenny MA, Metzger G. Tricyclic antidepressant-specific Fab fragments alter the distribution and elimination of desipramine in the rabbit: a model for overdose treatment. *J Toxicol Clin Toxicol* 1989; 27: 53–66.

Jansen PW, Perkin RM, Van Stralen D. Mojave rattlesnake envenomation: prolonged neurotoxicity and rhabdomyolysis. *Ann Emerg Med* 1992; 21: 322–5.

Johnson CA. Management of snakebite. *Am Fam Physician* 1991; 44: 174–80.

Jones RGA, Corteling RL, To HP, Bhogal G, Landon J. A novel Fab-based antivenom for the treatment of mass bee attacks. *Am J Trop Med Hyg* 1999; 61: 361–6.

Kabat EA. Antibody diversity versus antibody complementarity. *Pharmacol Rev* 1982; 34: 23–38.

Kelly JJ, Sadeghani K, Gottlieb SF, Ownby CL, van Meter KW, Torbati D. Reduction of rattlesnake-venom-induced myonecrosis in mice by hyperbaric oxygen therapy. *J Emerg Med* 1991; 9: 1–7.

Madrigal GC, Ercolani RL, Wenzl JE. Toxicity from a bite of the brown spider (*Loxosceles reclusus*): skin necrosis, hemolytic anemia, and hemoglobinuria in a nine-year-old child. *Clin Pediatr* 1972; 11: 641–4.

Magrina JF, Masterson BJ. *Loxosceles reclusa* spider bite: a consideration in the differential diagnosis of chronic, nonmalignant ulcers of the vulva. *Am J Obstet Gynecol* 1981; 140: 341–3.

Moore RS. Second-degree heart block associated with envenomation by *Vipera berus*. *Arch Emerg Med* 1988; 5: 116–18.

Nagao M, Takatori T, Wu B, Terazawa K, Gotouda H, Akabane H. Immunotherapy for the treatment of acute paraquat poisoning. *Hum Toxicol* 1989; 8: 121–3.

Norris RL, Dart RC. Apparent coral snake envenomation in a patient without visible fang marks. *Am J Emerg Med* 1989; 7: 402–5.

Ochs HR, Vatner SF, Smith TW. Reversal of inotropic effects of digoxin by specific antibodies and their Fab fragments in the conscious dog. *J Pharmacol Exp Ther* 1978; 207: 64–71.

Owens SM, Mayersohn M. Phencyclidine-specific Fab fragments alter phencyclidine disposition in dogs. *Drug Metab Dispos* 1986; 14: 52–8.

Pentel PR, Keyler DE. Drug-specific antibodies as antidotes for tricyclic antidepressant overdose. *Toxicol Lett* 1995; 82/3: 801–6.

Pentel PR, Scarlett W, Ross CA, Landon J, Sidki A, Keyler DE. Reduction of desipramine cardiotoxicity and prolongation of survival in rats with the use of polyclonal drug-specific antibody Fab fragments. *Ann Emerg Med* 1995; 26: 334–41.

CHAPTER 3

Possani LD. Antivenom for scorpion sting [letter]. *Lancet* 2000; 355: 67.

Reisman RE, Livingston A. Late-onset allergic reactions, including serum sickness, after insect stings. *J Allergy Clin Immunol* 1989; 84: 331–7.

Russell FE. Snake venom poisoning. *Vet Hum Toxicol* 1991; 33: 584–6.

Sabouraud A, Urtizberea M, Cano N, Garnier R, Scherrmann JM. Specific anti-digoxin Fab fragments: an available antidote for proscillaridin and scilliroside poisoning. *Hum Exp Toxicol* 1990; 9: 191–3.

Sabouraud AE, Urtizberea M, Benmoussa K, Cano NJ, Scherrmann JM. Fab-bound colchicine appears to adopt Fab fragment disposition in rats. *J Pharm Pharmacol* 1992a; 44: 1015–19.

Sabouraud AE, Urtizberea M, Cano NJ, Grandgeorge M, Rouzioux J-M, Scherrmann JM. Colchicine-specific Fab fragments alter colchicine disposition in rabbits. *J Pharmacol Exp Ther* 1992b; 260: 1214–19.

Schaumann W, Kaufmann B, Neubert P, Smolarz A. Kinetics of the Fab fragments of digoxin antibodies and of bound digoxin in patients with severe digoxin intoxication. *Eur J Clin Pharmacol* 1986; 30: 527–33.

Scherrmann JM. Antibody treatment of toxin poisoning – recent advances. *Clin Toxicol* 1994; 32: 363–75.

Scherrmann JM, Sabouraud A, Urtizberea M, Rouzioux J, Lang J, Baud F, Bismuth C. Clinical use of colchicine specific Fab fragments in colchicine poisoning [abstract]. *Vet Hum Toxicol* 1992; 34: 334.

Scherrmann JM, Lang J, Pepin-Covatta S, Lutsch C. Recent advances on the immunoreactivity of a new purified equine F(ab')$_2$ preparation (Viperfav®) against European viper venom. *Proceedings of the XVII International Congress of the EAPCCT*, Marseilles, 1996: 90.

Schmidt DH, Butler VP. Reversal of digoxin toxicity with specific antibodies. *J Clin Invest* 1971; 50: 1738–44.

Sinclair AJ, Hewick DS, Johnston PC, Stevenson IH, Lemon M. Kinetics of digoxin and anti-digoxin antibody fragments during treatment of digoxin toxicity. *Br J Clin Pharmacol* 1989; 28: 352–6.

Smith TW. New advances in the assessment and treatment of digitalis toxicity. *J Clin Pharmacol* 1985; 25: 522–8.

Smith TW. Review of clinical experience with digoxin immune Fab (ovine). *Am J Emerg Med* 1991; 9 (Suppl 1): 1–6 (discussion 33–4).

Smith TW, Haber E, Yeatmen L, Butler VP. Reversal of advanced digoxin intoxication with F$_{ab}$ fragments of digoxin-specific antibodies. *N Engl J Med* 1976; 294: 797–800.

Smith TW, Lloyd BL, Spicer N, Haber E. Immunogenicity and kinetics of distribution and elimination of sheep digoxin-specific IgG and Fab fragments in the rabbit and baboon. *Clin Exp Immunol* 1979; 36: 384–96.

Smith TW, Butler VP, Haber E, Fozzard H, Marcus FI, Bremner F, Schulman IC, Phillips A. Treatment of life-threatening digitalis intoxication with digoxin-specific F$_{ab}$ antibody fragments. Experience in 26 cases. *N Engl J Med* 1982; 307: 1357–62.

Smolarz A, Roesch E, Lenz E, Neubert H, Abshagen P. Digoxin specific antibody (Fab) fragments in 34 cases of severe digitalis intoxication. *Clin Toxicol* 1985; 23: 327–40.

Spiegel A, Marchlinski FE. Time course for reversal of digoxin toxicity with digoxin-specific antibody fragments. *Am Heart J* 1985; 109: 1397–9.

Stolpe MR, Norris RL, Chisholm CD, Hartshorne MF, Okerberg C, Ehler WJ, Posch J. Preliminary observations on the effects of hyperbaric oxygen therapy on Western diamondback rattlesnake (*Crotalus atrox*) venom poisoning in the rabbit model. *Ann Emerg Med* 1989; 18: 871–4.

Stolshek BS, Osterhout SK, Dunham G. The role of digoxin-specific antibodies in the treatment of digitalis poisoning. *Med Toxicol Adverse Drug Exp* 1988; 3: 167–71.

Sullivan JB. Immunotherapy in the poisoned patient. Overview of present applications and future trends. *Med Toxicol Adverse Drug Exp* 1986; 1: 47–60.

Thanh-Barthet CV, Urtizberea M, Sabouraud AE, Cano NJ, Scherrmann JM. Development of a sensitive radioimmunoassay for Fab fragments: application to Fab parmacokinetics in humans. *Pharm Res* 1993; 10: 692–6.

Theakston RDG, Warrell DA. Crisis in snake venom supply for Africa [letter]. *Lancet* 2000; 356: 2104.

Tibballs J. Premedication for snake antivenom. *Med J Aust* 1994; 160: 4–7.

Timsina MP, Hewick DS. Digoxin-specific Fab fragments impair renal function in the rabbit. *J Pharm Pharmacol* 1992; 44: 867–9.

Valentine MD, Schuberth KC, Kagey-Sobotka A, Graft DF, Kwiterovich KA, Szklo M, Lichtenstein LM. The value of immunotherapy with venom in children with allergy to insect stings. *N Engl J Med* 1990; 323: 1601–3.

Vorse H, Seccareccio P, Woodruff K, Humphrey GB. Disseminated intravascular coagulopathy following fatal brown spider bite (necrotic arachnidism). *J Pediatr* 1972; 80: 1035–7.

Warrell DA (ed.). WHO/SEARO guidelines for the clinical management of snake bites in the Southeast Asian region. *SE Asian J Tropical Med Public Hlth* 1999; 30 (Suppl 1).

Wenger TL, Butler VP, Haber E, Smith TW. Treatment of 63 severely digitalis-toxic patients with digoxin-specific antibody fragments. *J Am Coll Cardiol* 1985; 5 (Suppl): 118A–23A.

White J. Clinical toxicology of snakebite in Australia and New Guinea. In: *Handbook of Clinical Toxicology of Animal Venoms and Poisons*. Meier J, White J (eds). Boca Raton: CRC Press, 1995: 595–617.

White J. Envenoming and antivenom use in Australia. *Toxicon* 1998; 36: 1483–92.

White RR, Weber RA. Poisonous snakebite in central Texas: possible indicators for antivenin treatment. *Ann Surg* 1991; 213: 466–72.

Wolff J, Capraro H-G, Brossi A, Hope Cook G. Colchicine binding to antibodies. *J Biol Chem* 1980; 255: 7144–8.

Woolf AD, Wenger T, Smith TW, Lovejoy FH. The use of digoxin-specific Fab fragments for severe digitalis intoxication in children. *N Engl J Med* 1992; 326: 1739–44.

■ CHAPTER 3 ■

Metabolic Antidotes

Contents

4.1 ACETIC ACID

Acetic acid (in the form of vinegar) inhibits nematocyst discharge after contact with *Chironex fleckeri*, the deadly north Australian box jellyfish. Vinegar application has become accepted first aid not only for box jellyfish stings, but also for stings by other jellyfish (Fenner *et al.*, 1993). However, in the case of stings by a newly differentiated species of *Physalia* found in Australian waters that can cause severe envenomation, vinegar was found to cause discharge of up to 30 % of nematocysts, and vinegar is therefore not recommended for the treatment of such stings as it may actually increase envenomation. Stings from the single-tentacled *Physalia utriculus* (the 'bluebottle') are not severe (tentacles with unfired nematocysts rarely adhere to the victim's skin), and vinegar dousing is not required. Vinegar treatment is therefore an unnecessary step in the first aid management of any *Physalia* sting but remains essential first aid for all cubozoan (box) jellyfish stings (Fenner *et al.*, 1993).

4.2 ALCOHOL DEHYDROGENASE INHIBITORS

Serious toxicity due to ethylene glycol (1,2-ethanediol) and to methanol is the result of hepatic metabolism to glycolate and thence to oxalate (Figure 4.1) and to formaldehyde and thence to formate respectively (Figure 4.2). The initial steps are catalysed by alcohol dehydrogenase (ADH, alcohol:NAD$^+$ oxidoreductase, EC 1.1.1.1), and it is possible to minimize production of these toxic metabolites by giving the ADH inhibitors ethanol or fomepizole (4-methylpyrazole) (Kowalczyk *et al.*, 1998; Jacobsen, 1999). Sodium bicarbonate should be used to correct significant metabolic acidosis (Table 1.2), and haemodialysis may be needed to remove unchanged toxin and any toxic metabolites already formed, especially if renal function is impaired. Haemodialysis incorporating bicarbonate buffer and ethanol in the dialysate is commonly used where acidosis is a clinical problem. If haemodialysis is not available, peritoneal dialysis removes unchanged toxin and metabolites, albeit less effectively.

CHAPTER 4

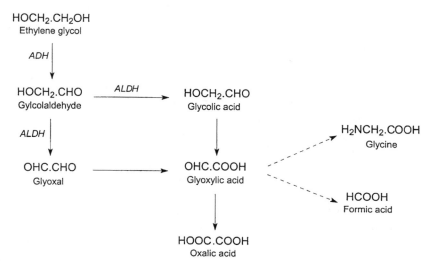

Figure 4.1: Mammalian metabolism of ethylene glycol (ADH, alcohol dehydrogenase; ALDH, aldehyde dehydrogenase)

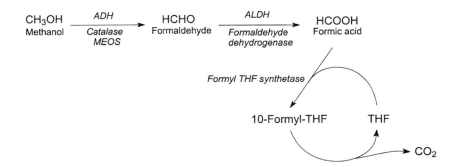

Figure 4.2: Mammalian metabolism of methanol (ADH, alcohol dehydrogenase; ALDH, aldehyde dehydrogenase; MEOS, microsomal ethanol oxidizing system; THF, tetrahydrofolate)

Methanol is often added in relatively small amounts (5–10 % v/v) to denature ethanol intended for industrial or domestic use, for example as a fuel ('methylated spirit', 'meths'). Ingestion of such mixtures rarely results in serious methanol poisoning as relatively large amounts of antidote (ethanol) will have been co-ingested.

2-Chloroethanol (ethylene chlorohydrin) is also metabolized to a toxic metabolite (chloroacetaldehyde) by ADH. Chloroacetaldehyde is detoxified by reaction with reduced glutathione (GSH). Administration of ethanol and also methionine was associated with survival in a 21-month-old girl who had ingested film cements containing 2-chloroethanol (Kvistad *et al.*, 1983). A further compound that is activated *in vivo* by ADH is 1,3-difluoro-2-propanol, the major ingredient of the pesticide Gliftor, and thus ethanol or fomepizole might be of use in treating poisoning with this agent (Feldwick *et al.*, 1998). Recent case reports suggest that ethanol or fomepizole may also be useful in diethylene glycol $[O(CH_2CH_2OH)_2]$ and triethylene glycol $[HO(CH_2)_2O-(CH_2)_2O(CH_2)_2OH]$ poisoning (Vassiliadis *et al.*, 1999; Brophy *et al.*, 2000).

4.2.1 Ethanol

Ethanol is readily available and blocks ADH by competitive inhibition. Ethanol should be given if (i) the history suggests that a potentially toxic amount of ethylene glycol or methanol has been ingested or (ii) features compatible with serious toxicity (significant metabolic acidosis, drowsiness, visual disturbances) are present *and* hyperglycaemia is absent (it is important to exclude the common medical differential diagnosis of diabetic ketoacidosis) (Barceloux *et al.*, 1999). The results of biochemical investigations (osmolality, anion gap) may provide additional useful information in the differential diagnosis of metabolic acidosis due to either diabetic ketoacidosis or toxic alcohols.

The aim of antidotal therapy is to maintain blood ethanol concentrations of 1–1.5 g/L until the blood ethylene glycol and/or methanol concentration is < 0.2 g/L. Oral ethanol may be given if the patient is conscious – 100–150 mL of whisky or brandy [40 % (v/v) or 320 g/L ethanol] is a suitable loading dose for an adult and will need to be supplemented with an i.v. infusion or further oral doses of at least 7 g/h. A suitable paediatric dose of 95 % (v/v) ethanol is 0.8–1.0 mL/kg, diluted in orange juice (Litovitz, 1986).

If the patient is drowsy or severely poisoned, ethanol should be given i.v., ideally with a glucose infusion. The dose is 1 g/kg initially, and the infusion should be continued at a rate of 66 mg kg^{-1} h^{-1} using a 10 % (v/v) ethanol solution in 5 % (w/v) D-glucose or 0.9 % (w/v) sodium chloride. Thereafter, the maintenance infusion rate is adjusted on the basis of plasma ethanol concentration. Regular consumers of alcohol and patients undergoing dialysis require higher ethanol dosage (Table 4.1). Massive ethylene glycol ingestion can be treated in this way using an ethanol-enriched, bicarbonate-based dialysate (Nzerue *et al.*, 1999).

The dose of ethanol required is difficult to predict because the initial rate of ethanol metabolism is very variable between patients. Secondly, ethanol metabolism is saturable, the plasma ethanol concentration at which saturation is achieved also varying between patients (Holford, 1987). It is thus important that blood ethanol concentrations are measured frequently. Adverse effects of ethanol at the doses used may include nausea and vomiting, drowsiness, confusion and, particularly in children, hypoglycaemia. The blood glucose concentration should thus also be monitored regularly. If the patient requires haemodialysis, the dose of ethanol will have to be increased by up to 100 mg kg^{-1} h^{-1}. Alternatively, ethanol (1–2 g per litre of dialysate) may be added to peritoneal dialysis or to haemodialysis fluid (Chow *et al.*, 1997).

If the patient (i) is prescribed or has co-ingested metronidazole, (ii) has gastrointestinal ulceration, (iii) is a child aged under 5 years or (iv) has severe hepatic disease, use of fomepizole, if available, rather than ethanol might be preferable.

TABLE 4.1
Suggested dose of ethanol for maintenance treatment (oral or i.v.) of methanol or ethylene glycol poisoning

Patient	Amount of ethanol needed (mg kg^{-1} h^{-1})	5 % (v/v) Ethanol[a] (mL kg^{-1} h^{-1})[b]	10 % (v/v) Ethanol[a] (mL kg^{-1} h^{-1})[b]
Non-drinker or child	66	1.65	0.83
Average adult	110	2.76	1.38
Chronic drinker	154	3.90	1.95

Notes
a   5 % (v/v) ethanol = 40 g/L; 10 % (v/v) ethanol = 80 g/L.
b   Prepared in 5 % (w/v) D-glucose or 0.9 % (w/v) sodium chloride.

4.2.2 Fomepizole

Fomepizole [4-methylpyrazole (4-MP); Antizol, Orphan Medical; CAS 5547-65-6; Figure 4.3) is a potent competitive ADH inhibitor and has advantages over ethanol in that it has a longer duration of action and has no central depressant or other toxic effects at the doses used clinically (Baud *et al.*, 1988; McMartin and Heath, 1989; Harry *et al.*, 1994, 1998; Borron *et al.*, 1999; Goldfarb, 1999). On the other hand, it is much more expensive than ethanol and availability is limited. Fomepizole is sometimes used for treatment of ethylene glycol and methanol poisoning, on occasions avoiding the need for haemodialysis. Elimination is largely by metabolism, with only some 1 % of a dose being excreted unchanged in urine (Jacobsen *et al.*, 1989). 4-Hydroxymethylpyrazole

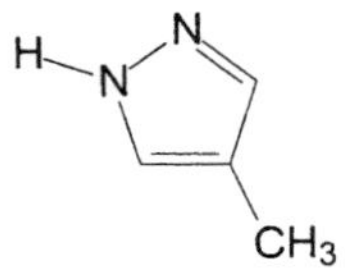

Figure 4.3: Structural formula of fomepizole

and 4-carboxypyrazole are major urinary metabolites (McMartin *et al.*, 1987). An *N*-glucuronide is also formed. Fomepizole is easily removed by dialysis, and this must be taken into account when it is used clinically (Jacobsen *et al.*, 1996a; Brent *et al.*, 1999). Fomepizole also inhibits ethanol metabolism and vice versa (Jacobsen *et al.*, 1996b), and has been suggested at a dose of 2.5–10 mg/kg for use in treating severe disulfiram–ethanol reactions in alcoholics (Lindros *et al.*, 1981) and for alleviation of acute acetaldehyde toxicity in hypersensitive individuals (Inoue *et al.*, 1985).

Indications for giving fomepizole rather than ethanol to treat methanol/ethylene glycol poisoning are: (i) ingestion of more than one poison and/or decreased level of consciousness and (ii) lack of adequate intensive care staffing or laboratory support to monitor ethanol administration adequately. The only absolute contraindication to use of fomepizole is if the patient is prescribed or has co-ingested disulfiram because of the risk of an Antabuse-type reaction.

In treating ethylene glycol or methanol poisoning, the loading dose of fomepizole is 15 mg/kg i.v., followed by 10 mg/kg i.v. 12-hourly for four doses, and then 15 mg/kg i.v. 12-hourly until the plasma concentration of ethylene glycol and/or methanol is less than 0.2 g/L. If ethanol is also being given at a dose of 1 g kg^{-1} h^{-1}, the rate of fomepizole elimination is reduced by 50 %.

An oral preparation of fomepizole (100 mg in 20 mL) is available is some countries and, although logic suggests that this is probably the most effective way to give the antidote in the early stages of methanol or ethylene glycol poisoning, in many countries fomepizole is given exclusively i.v. The oral dose is 15 mg/kg as a loading dose, followed by 5 mg/kg 12 h later and then 10 mg/kg every 12 h until the ethylene glycol or methanol is no longer detectable in plasma (Baud *et al.*, 1992). At doses between 10 and 100 mg/kg fomepizole demonstrates zero-order kinetics.

Adverse reactions to fomepizole include headache, nausea and dizziness (McMartin *et al.*, 1987; Jacobsen *et al.*, 1988). Rash, eosinophilia, anaemia, leucopenia and thrombocytopenia have also been reported (Baud *et al.*, 1986/7). A hepatitic reaction and cholestasis have been described, as has renal failure. However, provided a dose of less than 20 mg/kg is given for no more than 5 days, then, by analogy with pyrazole (Wilson and Bottiglieri, 1962), adverse effects are thought to be unlikely. In clinical trials in adults there were no adverse effects of fomepizole at doses of either 7 mg/kg i.v. or 10–1,000 mg orally (Jacobsen *et al.*, 1990).

4.3 CALCIUM SALTS

Calcium gluconate (calcium D-gluconate; CAS 299-28-5; Figure 4.4) gel (2.5 % w/w) is used topically to treat hydrofluoric acid burns. Insoluble calcium fluoride is formed, thus preventing further skin penetration of the poison. The gel should be applied to the affected area for at least 30 min. If pain persists, 10 % (w/v) calcium gluconate

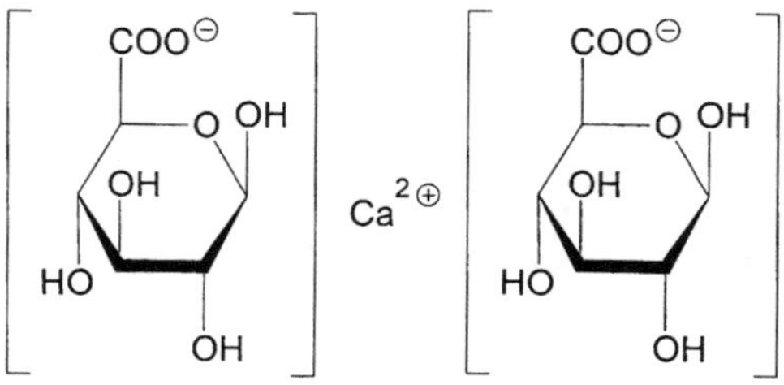

Figure 4.4: Molecular formula of calcium gluconate

should be injected (0.5-mL depots) under the site of the injury to achieve intradermal and subcutaneous penetration. Intra-arterial or i.v. infusion of calcium gluconate [10 mL 10 % (w/v) calcium gluconate diluted with 40 mL 5 % (w/v) D-glucose] has also been suggested to treat hydrofluoric acid burns on the arms or legs (Velvart, 1983; Vance *et al.*, 1986; Caravati, 1988; Graudins *et al.*, 1997; Ryan *et al.*, 1997). Oral calcium gluconate administration has been suggested for treating poisoning due to the ingestion of fluoride salts (Lheureux *et al.*, 1990).

Calcium gluconate given i.v. has also been used to raise extracellular calcium concentrations after overdosage with calcium channel blockers such as nifedipine or verapamil, although its efficacy remains unproven (Jaeger *et al.*, 2000). Calcium gluconate has also been claimed to have a role in severe poisoning with β-blockers such as atenolol (Pertoldi *et al.*, 1998). Calcium chloride can be used for these same purposes and has the advantage that it contains more calcium (w/w) than calcium gluconate. Calcium chloride is preferable to calcium gluconate in patients with hepatic impairment. A dose of 0.2–0.5 mL/kg of a 10 % (w/v) solution of the gluconate (maximum 10 mL) is given i.v. over 5–10 min. If necessary, the dose may be repeated in 10–15 min. It should never be coadministered with a sodium bicarbonate infusion as insoluble calcium carbonate will be formed *in vitro*. A similar regimen (0.1–0.2 mL gluconate per kilogram) has been used to reverse hypocalcaemia in severe poisoning with ethylene glycol or oxalates, although only symptomatic hypocalcaemia should be corrected as excessive administration can lead to increased calcium oxalate deposition in the kidneys and hence potentiate renal damage.

Finally, calcium gluconate may reverse the neuromuscular paralysis associated with hyperkalaemia and hypermagnesaemia as well as muscle spasm occurring after *Lactrodectus mactans* (black widow spider) envenomation (section 3.1.2.1), although it appears ineffective in relieving pain associated with such bites (Clark *et al.*, 1992). It also protects against the cardiotoxicity associated with drug-induced hyperkalaemia (except that associated with digoxin and related glycosides), and can stabilize the situation until the hyperkalaemia can be corrected either by haemodialysis or by i.v. infusion of D-glucose and insulin.

4.4 COPPER SALTS

Copper salts are used in veterinary medicine to treat chronic molybdenum poisoning in ruminants (Underwood, 1977). Copper sulphate is a topical antidote to yellow phosphorus. Yellow phosphorus is sometimes picked up by people on beaches as the contents of old munitions dumps are washed ashore.

■ CHAPTER 4 ■

4.5 IODATES

Potassium iodate is used to enhance elimination of radioactive iodine. It has been considered for distribution to civilians at time of nuclear threat and acts by competitive displacement of radioactive iodine from the thyroid. In overdosage it has been associated with retinopathy (Singalavanija *et al.*, 2000).

4.6 IOPANOIC ACID

Iopanoic acid (Telepaque; CAS 96-83-8; Figure 4.5) is an iodinated radiocontrast agent and is a potent inhibitor of the conversion of thyroxine to tri-iodothyronine. Iopanoic acid (125 mg/d orally, 5 days) has been used to treat a boy aged 2.5 years who had ingested an unknown amount of thyroxine and who was showing only limited response to propylthiouracil (75 mg/d) and propranolol (15 mg 6-hourly) (Brown *et al.*, 1998). In general, however, thyroxine overdoses are not sinister and seldom even require symptomatic treatment with β-adrenoceptor blockers (section 5.2).

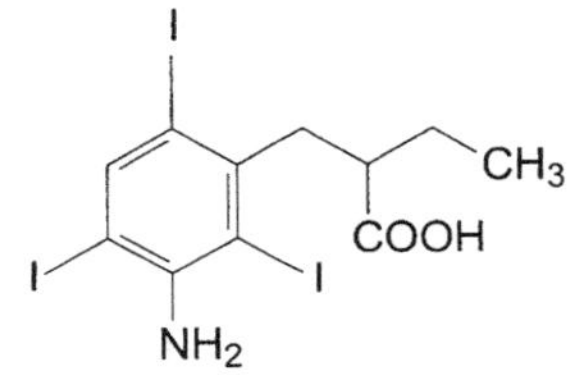

Figure 4.5: Structural formula of iopanoic acid

4.7 LEUCOVORIN

Folate antagonists such as methotrexate, pyrimethamine and trimethoprim inhibit dihydrofolate reductase (EC 1.5.1.3) and prevent the formation of tetrahydrofolate, which is required for nucleoprotein synthesis and erythropoiesis. Mild poisoning with folate antagonists often requires nothing more than monitoring of the full blood count. Significant or potentially significant poisoning with folate antagonists can be treated with the 5-formyl tetrahydrofolate derivative leucovorin (folinic acid; Figure 4.6). The pharmaceutical formulation of leucovorin is a mixture of the 6-S and 6-R stereoisomers

Leucovorin	
CAS registry number	58-05-9
Relative formula mass	473.4
pK_a	3.1, 4.8, 10.4
Oral absorption (6-S isoform) (%)	90
Presystemic metabolism (6-S isoform)	High
Plasma half-life (6-S isoform) (min)	32
Volume of distribution (6-S isoform) (L)	17.5
Plasma protein binding (%)	54

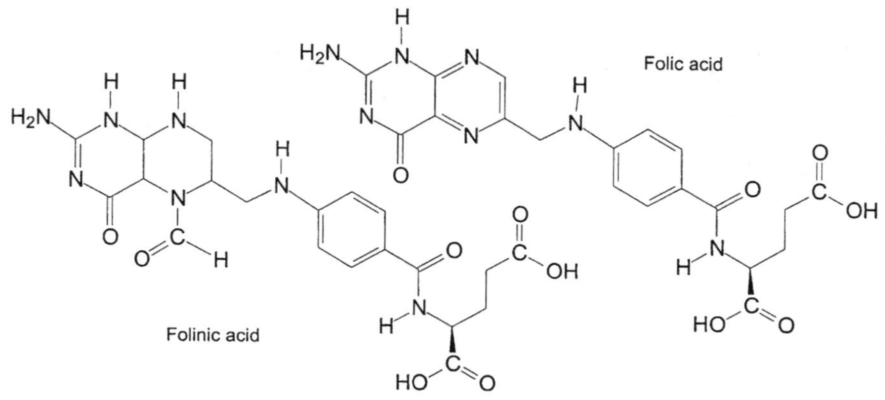

Figure 4.6: Structural formulae of leucovorin (folinic acid) and folic acid

of 5-formyltetrahydrofolate. Leucovorin should be given, preferably within 1 h of the overdose, if there is evidence to suggest marrow depression, although administration of the antidote should not await the development of overt bone marrow depression. The initial i.v. leucovorin dose is equal to the amount of folate antagonist ingested, if known. Otherwise 100 mg/m^2 body surface area should be given. Further (oral) doses (15 mg for an adult) should be given 6-hourly after methotrexate until the blood methotrexate concentration is < 23 µg/L (50 nmol/L), and daily after trimethoprim, for 5–7 days. Allergic reactions should be treated with conventional antihistamine therapy.

It has been suggested that leucovorin administration (1 mg/kg orally or i.v., 6-hourly) may enhance methanol and formate metabolism via the folate-dependent one-carbon cycle pool (Figure 4.2), but this is of little practical value in acute methanol poisoning as unchanged methanol and metabolites are readily excreted in urine or removed by dialysis. However, successful treatment of serious acute formic acid poisoning with leucovorin together with supportive measures including urinary alkalinization has been described previously (Moore *et al.*, 1994); seven doses of leucovorin (1 mg/kg i.v. 4-hourly) were given.

4.8 MAGNESIUM SALTS

Many poisons cause prolongation of the QT interval in the heart with risk of *torsade de pointes* arrhythmia (Figure 4.7). An infusion of magnesium ions is sometimes effective in stopping associated ventricular tachycardia or ventricular fibrillation, especially if hypokalaemia has occurred (hypomagnesaemia is often also present in such cases). The usual dose (magnesium sulphate) is 8 mmol Mg^{2+} i.v. over 10 min for an adult, repeated once if necessary (British National Formulary, 2000a).

Barium compounds can cause neuromuscular blockade and hypokalaemia. Patients with barium poisoning may present with headache, paraesthesiae, peripheral weakness, paralysis, diarrhoea and arrhythmias or other ECG abnormalities. Magnesium ion infusions are effective in treating tachycardia associated with barium poisoning. The same dose as used to treat arrhythmias associated with the long QT syndrome is used (see above).

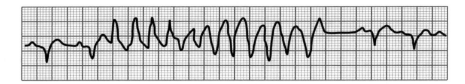

Figure 4.7: *Torsade de pointes* arrhythmia, treated successfully with intravenous magnesium sulphate

The magnesium ion is thought to have an antioxidant effect *in vivo*. Dietary magnesium restriction enhances paraquat toxicity in rats, but attempts to use magnesium salts to treat paraquat poisoning in man have shown no clear effect (section 8.3). Magnesium sulphate (1 g/h i.v. for 4 h, then 1 g i.v. every 4–6 h up to a maximum of 5 days) was used to treat 25 patients poisoned with aluminium phosphide (Chugh *et al.*, 1997). Mortality was 25 % as opposed to 40 % in an untreated group, suggesting possible benefit from the treatment.

4.9 NICOTINAMIDE

Nicotinamide [niacinamide; vitamin B_3 (this latter term is also used to refer to nicotinic acid); CAS 98-92-0; Figure 4.8] is used for the management of intoxication with pyriminil (*N*-3-pyridylmethyl-*N'*-(4-nitrophenyl)urea, PNU), a yellow–green powder used as a rodenticide. Insulin-dependent diabetes mellitus and a severe peripheral neuropathy developed in a fit 25-year-old man several days after ingesting PNU (Prosser and Karam, 1978). After 10 months, a glucose tolerance test was abnormal and nerve conduction studies showed sensory and motor neuropathy. At least 15 other cases of PNU-induced diabetes in humans have been reported. Its mechanism of action may be by interference with nicotinamide metabolism in the pancreas, where it destroys β-cells (Kallman *et al.*, 1992), CNS and heart. Nicotinamide is the suggested antidote. The dosage regimen for an adult is 500 mg i.v. or 200 mg i.m., followed by 200 mg i.v. or i.m. every 2 h to a total of 3 g/d (Flomenbaum, 1998). Subsequent dosage is 100 mg orally three times daily for 2 weeks. Vigilance to the later development of diabetes is required. Neurological deficit may progress despite later nicotinamide administration (LeWitt, 1980).

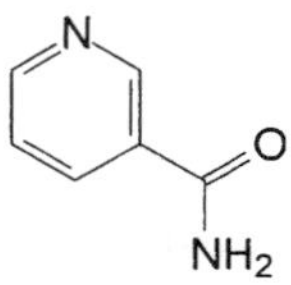

Figure 4.8: Structural formula of nicotinamide

4.10 PHYTOMENADIONE (VITAMIN K_1)

Phytomenadione (vitamin K_1; phytononadione; phylloquinone; 2-methyl-3-phytyl-1,4-naphthoquinone; Konakion, Roche; Figure 4.9) is a fat-soluble compound that is required for the hepatic synthesis of blood coagulation factors II (prothrombin), VII

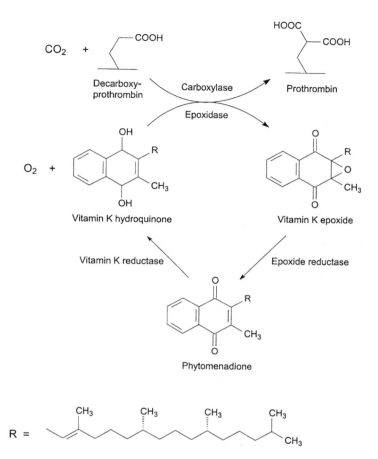

Figure 4.9: The phytomenadione (vitamin K$_1$)–phytomenadione epoxide cycle

(proconvertin), IX (Christmas) and X (Stuart-Prower) (Stenflo and Suttie, 1977). Excess vitamin K is rapidly metabolized. In adequate doses phytomenadione reverses the inhibitory effects of coumarin and indandione anticoagulants on the synthesis of these factors. It is probable that a phytomenadione concentration of 0.5 mg/L is needed to drive clotting factor synthesis in most clinical situations (10 mg should be given slowly i.v. to an adult in most cases) (Park *et al.*, 1984). Phytomenadione will not reverse either low-molecular-weight heparin or conventional heparin-induced bleeding which necessitates the use of protamine sulphate injections (section 5.22). Phytomenadione, unlike vitamin K$_3$ (menadione), is effective in treating poisoning with 'superwarfarins' such as brodifacoum, and oral treatment with phytomenadione may need to be continued for several months (Corke, 1997; Bruno *et al.*, 2000).

Phytomenadione dosage (2–10 mg i.v. or i.m.) is repeated every 4–8 h based on serial prothrombin time or international normalized ratio (INR) measurements. If the patient has a metal heart valve and anticoagulation therefore cannot be wholly reversed, use of DE-Fix or fresh-frozen plasma is recommended, rather than phytomenadione. Some clinicians use 1–2 mg of phytomenadione in such patients but risk over-reversal of

Phytomenadione

CAS registry number	84-80-0
Relative formula mass	450.7
pK_a	Not ionizable
Oral absorption (range) (%)	10–63
Plasma half-life (h) (mean, range)	2.2 (1.2–3.5)
Volume of distribution (L)	3.5
Plasma protein binding	Extensive

anticoagulation. The infusion rate should not exceed 1 mg/min to minimize the risk of side-effects due to histamine release (flushing, sweating, bronchoconstriction, chest tightness). Dilution of the phytomenadione solution in 20 mL 0.9 % (w/v) sodium chloride with infusion over 15 min reduces this risk (Park *et al.*, 1984; Choonara *et al.*, 1985). In severe poisoning with warfarin or similar compounds phytomenadione doses of up to 50 mg i.v. may be needed initially (Bjornsson and Blaschke, 1978). Injection i.m. is best avoided in the presence of haemorrhage because of the risk of haematoma formation at the injection site and because an oily mixture is extremely painful on injection. The onset of action is delayed until the activated clotting factor concentrations in blood reach an effective amount, usually after 4–6 h. The maximum effect occurs about 24 h post dose. Severe haemorrhage may require infusion of fresh-frozen plasma, DE-fix or fresh whole blood, in addition to i.v. phytomenadione. Close observation is required to detect falls in blood pressure, development of tachycardia and more obvious signs of bleeding such as blood in the mouth.

4.11 POTASSIUM SALTS

An infusion of a potassium salt (normally potassium chloride) has been shown to correct the potassium-displacing capacity of absorbed soluble barium salts (Berning, 1975). To prevent the risk of sudden cardiac death, no more than 20 mmol K^+ should be infused per hour into an adult.

In thallium poisoning, the administration of potassium chloride i.v. has been suggested in order to enhance the excretion of thallium into the gut, but the effect is small and the procedure potentially dangerous. However, sufficient potassium should be administered to keep the serum potassium between 4.5 and 5.0 mmol/L. Oral potassium supplements should be avoided if Prussian Blue is being given because potassium ions may interfere with the exchange between potassium and thallium ions in the gut.

Potassium permanganate (1 % w/v) solution can be used topically in conjunction with sodium bicarbonate to treat yellow phosphorus burns.

4.12 PYRIDOXINE (VITAMIN B$_6$)

Pyridoxine (vitamin B$_6$; Figure 4.10) is sometimes given prophylactically to patients being treated with the antitubercular drug isoniazid in order to prevent the development of peripheral neuropathy. Isoniazid is thought to react with pyridoxal 5-phosphate, the

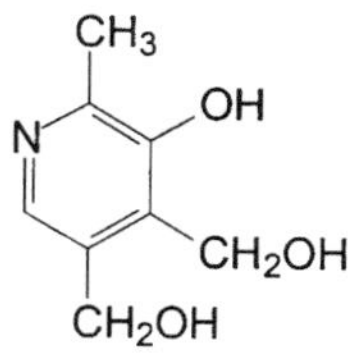

Figure 4.10: Structural formula of pyridoxine (vitamin B$_6$)

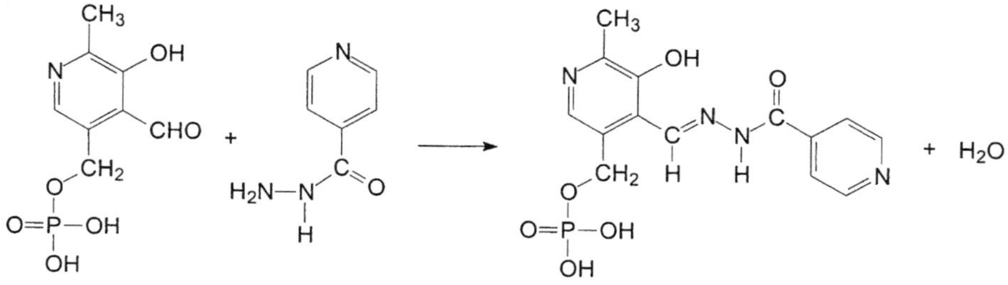

Figure 4.11: Reaction of pyridoxal 5-phosphate with isoniazid to form a hydrazone

biologically active form of the vitamin, to form a hydrazone (Figure 4.11). The hydrazone is a very strong inhibitor of pyridoxal phosphate kinase, and thus tissue depletion of this essential cofactor may occur unless supplemental pyridoxine is given. Pyridoxal 5-phosphate itself has been advocated in the treatment of cyanide poisoning (Keniston *et al.*, 1987), but has not found application in this role (section 6.2.1).

In acute overdosage, isoniazid may induce convulsions, which are thought to be caused by inhibition of pyridoxal 5-phosphatase leading to γ-aminobutyric acid (GABA) deficiency in the brain. Pyridoxine is used to prevent or control isoniazid-induced convulsions and the consequent lactic acidosis, and also shorten the period of coma (Wason *et al.*, 1981).

Pyridoxine may also reduce the hepatic, renal and CNS toxicity resulting from monomethylhydrazine inhibition of pyridoxine metabolism in *Gyrometria* (false morrel) poisoning. In addition, pyridoxine has been advocated for treating poisoning with cycloserine and hydrazine, and it has been suggested that it may enhance the detoxification of the toxic metabolites of ethylene glycol. Pyridoxine (1 g i.v.) had no

Pyridoxine (hydrochloride)

CAS registry number	58-56-0
Relative formula mass (free base)	205.6 (169.2)
pK$_a$	5.0, 9.0
Oral absorption	High
Presystemic metabolism	Negligible
Plasma half-life (days)	15–20
Plasma protein binding	Nil for non-phosphorylated forms

CHAPTER 4

effect on either level of consciousness or rate of metabolism of ethanol after acute self-poisoning with ethanol (Mardel *et al.*, 1994).

In acute isoniazid poisoning, a single i.v. infusion (gram for gram equivalent basis, up to 10 g) in 5 % (w/v) D-glucose over 30–60 min is used. If the amount of isoniazid ingested is unknown, give 5 g pyridoxine to an adult (Yarborough and Wood, 1983). One dose is usually enough to reverse isoniazid-induced convulsions, which usually settle within 30 min of administration of the antidote. Benzodiazepines can be given concurrently, but usually smaller doses are needed. In a child give 70 mg/kg by infusion as above. For monomethylhydrazine toxicity the dose is 25 mg/kg i.v. This may be increased up to 300 mg kg^{-1} d^{-1} if necessary. Pyridoxine (10–25 mg/d) should be given concurrently with D-penicillamine (section 2.2.6).

Pyridoxine is metabolized to pyridoxal 5-phosphate, the active form of the vitamin and a cofactor in more than 100 enzymic reactions. It is relatively safe in therapeutic doses. At such doses, more than 50 % is eliminated by metabolism to a 4-pyridolic acid. However, 0.5–2 g/d over several years may lead to progressive sensory neuropathy, although there is considerable inter-individual variation in susceptibility (Schaumberg *et al.*, 1983; Bendich and Cohen, 1990). Pyridoxine should be stored in the dark.

4.13 REDOX REAGENTS

Methaemoglobin (oxidized haemoglobin) may be formed after exposure to oxidizing agents such as aniline, chlorates, dapsone, ferricyanide, nitrates, nitrites, nitrobenzene, primaquine, sulphonamides and some local anaesthetics (Table 4.2). The diagnosis should be suspected in any patient who has cyanosis unresponsive to oxygen administration (Stambach *et al.*, 1997). Patients with more than 30 % methaemo-globinaemia and who are breathless require treatment. Methylthioninium chloride is the preferred treatment (section 4.1.3.2).

TABLE 4.2
Some agents causing methaemoglobinaemia

Toxin	Use
Acetanilide, phenacetin	Analgesics
Aniline derivatives	Dyes
Benzocaine, prilocaine	Local anaesthetics
Chlorates	Weedkiller
Dapsone	Treatment of dermatitis herpetiformis
Methylthioninium chloride	Treatment of methaemoglobinaemia
Nitrates	Cardiovascular drugs, munitions
Nitrites	Cardiovascular and recreational drugs, treatment of cyanide poisoning
Nitrobenzene and derivatives	Synthetic chemistry
Nitroglycerine	Cardiovascular drug, munitions
Nitrous oxide	Inhalational anaesthetic, propellant gas, 'injected oxygen'
Nitrotoluene and derivatives	Munitions, synthetic chemistry
Primaquine	Antimalarial drug
Quinine	Antimalarial drug

4.13.1 Ascorbic acid (vitamin C)

Ascorbic acid (CAS 50-81-7; Figure 4.12) promotes conversion of methaemoglobin to haemoglobin and should be used instead of methylthioninium chloride in poisoning with oxidizing agents and other chemicals causing methaemoglobinaemia in patients with glucose-6-phosphate dehydrogenase (G6PDH) deficiency. The dose is 1 g i.v. or 200 mg by mouth three times daily. The possible contribution of ascorbate in enhancing iron excretion in iron-overloaded patients treated with DFO, for example, has been discussed above (section 2.3.2). Ascorbate protects against the toxicity of sodium metavanadate in mice, possibly by reducing V^{5+} to the less toxic V^{4+} (Domingo *et al.*, 1986).

Ascorbate (10 mg/kg daily) has also been used to remove the odour of garlic from the breath in selenium and in tellurium poisoning (Hunter, 1978). In sodium selenate poisoning, use of ascorbic acid (1 g i.m. and then 4 g/d orally) together with dimercaprol (initially 150 mg 6-hourly i.v.) has been reported to be effective (Civil and McDonald, 1978 – section 2.2.4).

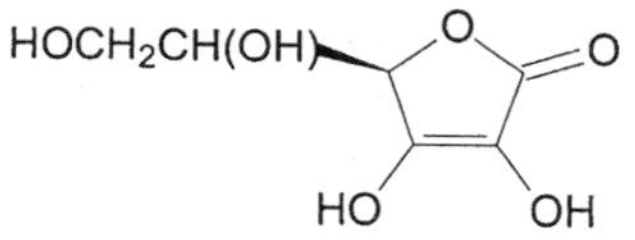

Figure 4.12: Structural formula of ascorbic acid

4.13.2 Methylthioninium chloride (methylene blue) and tolonium chloride

The transport of oxygen in the blood in man and animals at atmospheric pressure is dependent on haemoglobin, and for transport to occur the constituent iron of haemoglobin must be in a reduced state (ferrohaemoglobin, Fe^{2+}). A physiologically normal subject is exposed to endogenous oxidizing substances that oxidize about 3 % of his or her haemoglobin to methaemoglobin (Fe^{3+}) each day. This is normally easily converted back to haemoglobin by an endogenous NADH-dependent reductase (diaphorase), so that in normal adults only about 1 % of the total haemoglobin is in the oxidized form (1 % methaemoglobinaemia).

This endogenous methaemoglobin reductase system has limited capacity, and exposure to several oxidizing agents (Table 4.2) can induce pathological methaemoglobinaemia. This impairs the oxygen-carrying capacity of the blood, causing hypoxia. The diagnosis of methaemoglobinaemia clinically rests on four key elements: clinical history, including circumstances of poisoning; the clinical features of methaemoglobinaemia, i.e. blue coloration or central cyanosis, breathlessness and tiredness; direct measurement of the blood methaemoglobin; and the confirmatory test of failure of the hypoxia to correct after the administration of oxygen at a high flow rate via a face mask. There is a rough correlation between clinical features of poisoning and blood methaemoglobin concentration (Table 4.3). Classically, the blood is said to look chocolate brown, although this seems not to be a universal finding.

At low concentrations methylthioninium chloride (methylene blue; tetra-methylthionine chloride; Swiss blue; Figure 4.13) either acts as an electron acceptor

TABLE 4.3

Interpretation of blood methaemoglobin concentrations

Methaemoglobin (% of total haemoglobin)	Clinical features
0–15 %	Nil
16–20 %	Cyanosis
21–45 %	Dyspnoea, syncope
46–55 %	CNS depression
56–70 %	Coma, convulsions, cardiac failure, arrhythmias
> 70 %	Possible death

for an NADPH-dependent methaemoglobin reductase or is reduced by a further enzyme. A colourless product that rapidly and non-enzymically reduces methaemoglobin to haemoglobin within the red blood cell is formed (Figure 4.14). At high concentrations, methylthioninium may catalyse the oxidation of ferrous iron in haemoglobin to ferric iron, hence forming methaemoglobin, but the evidence for this is conflicting (Smith, 1969). Tolonium chloride (toluidine blue O; CAS 92-31-9; Figure 4.13) acts similarly to methylthioninium chloride but is very rarely used in clinical practice.

The effect of i.v. methylthioninium chloride in reversing chemically induced methaemoglobinaemia was observed by accident in a chemist who had been exposed to 4-bromoaniline and who presented with an intense cyanosis (Williams and Challis, 1933). Steele and Spink (1933) also reported rapid reversal of severe methaemoglobinaemia by i.v. methylthioninium chloride in patients poisoned with substances thought to be aniline or a related compound and acetanilide. Subsequent animal and clinical studies confirmed that the drug was effective in reversing methaemoglobinaemia due to a wide range of poisons (Table 4.2), although the efficiency with which methaemoglobin is reduced varies between different poisons. Even with hydroxylamine, which generates a methaemoglobinaemia that is particularly difficult to reverse with methylthioninium chloride, some efficacy has been demonstrated in animal studies (Smith, 1969). The continued action of methylthioninium chloride in reducing methaemoglobin in the presence of an oxidizing agent depends upon a continued supply of NADPH, and it is possible that these observed differences in efficiency between different poisons reflect further actions of the compounds in question in interrupting the supply of NADPH.

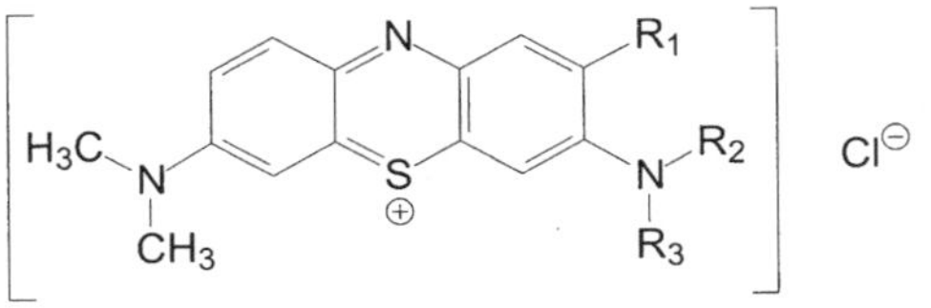

	R_1	R_2	R_3
Methylthioninium chloride	H	CH_3	CH_3
Tolonium chloride	CH_3	H	H

Figure 4.13: Structural formulae of methylthioninium chloride and of tolonium chloride

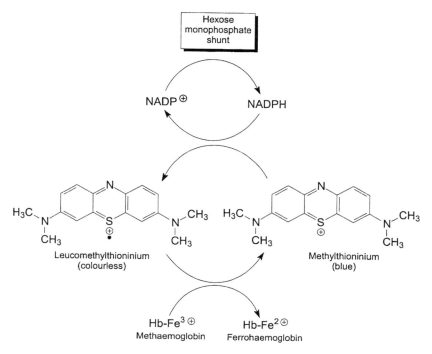

Figure 4.14: *In vivo* reduction of methaemoglobin by methylthioninium chloride

Methylthioninium chloride is given as a 1 % (w/v) aqueous solution at doses of 1–2 mg/kg i.v. over 5 min. The dose may be repeated at hourly intervals depending on the blood methaemoglobin concentration and clinical response (Mansouri, 1985). Doses higher than 7 mg/kg i.v. over 5 min may produce nausea, vomiting, abdominal/chest pain, dizziness, sweating, confusion, haemolysis and cyanosis as a result of methaemoglobin formation (Finch, 1948; Mansouri, 1985).

Methylthioninium chloride is given only if a patient shows features of poisoning such as breathlessness, and usually only once methaemoglobinaemia exceeds 40 %. Oxygen should be given to increase the amount of oxygen delivered to tissue dissolved in blood as opposed to carried by haemoglobin. Methylthioninium chloride acts within 1 h of administration. Arterial blood gases and methaemoglobin concentration should be monitored regularly. The drug should not be given s.c. as necrotic ulcers have been reported at injection sites (Perry and Meinhard, 1974). The frequency of methylthioninium chloride administration will often depend on the cause of the

Methylthioninium chloride	
CAS registry number	61-73-4
Relative formula mass	373.9
pK_a	3.8
Oral absorption (%)	53–97
Presystemic metabolism	Negligible

methaemoglobinaemia. A dapsone overdose, for example, may necessitate methylthioninium chloride administration for much longer than after ingestion of nitrites because of the long half-life of dapsone.

Methylthioninium chloride should not be used if methaemoglobinaemia is not present, as it may then itself induce methaemoglobinaemia. Anaphylactic reactions to the drug are recognized. The methylthioninium ion is eliminated largely by renal excretion, and thus methylthioninium chloride should be used cautiously in patients with renal dysfunction. The methylthioninium ion can be excreted in its unchanged blue form or its leuco (colourless) form (DiSanto and Wagner, 1972). Renal excretion starts from *c.* 30 min post injection and can continue for up to 3–5 days (Nadler *et al.*, 1934). Methylthioninium chloride may cause haemolysis if administered to G6PDH-deficient patients (Beutler, 1969) and ascorbic acid or exchange transfusion should be considered as an alternative treatment for methaemoglobinaemia in such patients.

4.14 RIBOFLAVIN (VITAMIN B₂)

Riboflavin (vitamin B$_2$; CAS 83-88-5; Figure 4.15) has been reported to provide some protection against the toxicity of boric acid in laboratory animals (Roe *et al.*, 1972). However, supportive care alone has been used thus far to treat borate poisoning in man. Riboflavin has also been reported to be of value in activating the NADPH-dependent methaemoglobin reductase system, and can be used to treat congenital methaemoglobinaemia (Hirano *et al.*, 1981). It is particularly useful in patients with methaemoglobinaemia who cannot tolerate methylthioninium chloride or ascorbate (section 4.13). Oral dosage (20–120 mg/d, divided doses) has been used (Donovan, 1990). Riboflavin administration is not associated with adverse reactions.

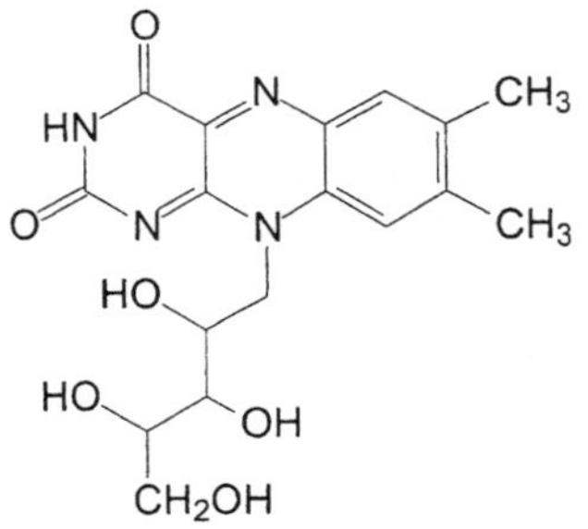

Figure 4.15: Structural formula of riboflavin (vitamin B$_2$)

4.15 SODIUM SALTS

Oral sodium chloride precipitates silver as silver chloride. Sodium chloride may also be used to enhance the urinary excretion of bromide ion in acutely poisoned patients who do not require haemodialysis. Administration of 0.9 % (w/v) sodium chloride i.v. decreased the plasma half-life of bromide from 332 h to 65 h in one patient (Wieth and Funder, 1963). Antidotal uses of sodium nitrite and sodium thiosulphate are discussed in sections 6.2.3.1 and 6.2.5 respectively.

Sodium bicarbonate given i.v. or orally has a non-specific role in correcting acidosis in severe poisoning with compounds such as ethylene glycol, iron, methanol and some other compounds (Table 1.2). It tends to be reserved for more seriously poisoned patients (blood pH < 7.2) as there is a theoretical risk that exogenous bicarbonate could worsen intracellular acidosis. Sodium bicarbonate in combination with other agents has also been suggested for use in poisoning with OP insecticides (section 5.9.1).

Sodium bicarbonate given i.v. is valuable in treating severe poisoning with strong acids such as salicylates and chlorophenoxy herbicides, and some weaker acids (chlorpropamide, barbitone, phenobarbitone) (Wax and Hoffman, 1991). Here sodium bicarbonate administration acts not only by correcting acidosis, but also by promoting diffusion of the poison from tissues into plasma and hence promoting metabolism or excretion in urine or in bile (Flanagan *et al.*, 1990; Wax and Hoffman, 1991 – Figures 4.16 and 4.17).

The dose used to promote an alkaline diuresis is 1 L of 1.26 % (w/v) sodium bicarbonate infused i.v. over 2 h, repeated as necessary. Urine pH should be closely monitored to ensure that it remains between 7 and 8 so that effective renal elimination can occur. The blood pH should not exceed 7.55. When giving sodium bicarbonate by infusion it is important to monitor serum potassium and ensure adequate potassium replacement – an effective alkaline diuresis cannot occur without renal potassium loss.

Sodium bicarbonate finds extensive use in the prophylaxis of arrhythmias in tricyclic antidepressant poisoning. It should be given whenever the QRS complex on the ECG is widened (> 110 ms for example), even in the absence of acidosis (Figure 4.18). It is also effective in stopping ventricular arrhythmias and is first-line therapy. Its prophylactic and antiarrhythmic action is most probably due to sodium channel blockade (Frommer *et al.*, 1987; McCabe *et al.*, 1998; Love *et al.*, 2000), although an effect on blood pH and thus on drug or metabolite ionization and therefore tissue (especially CNS) penetration may also be important (Wax and Hoffman, 1991; Newton *et al.*, 1994;

■ CHAPTER 4 ■

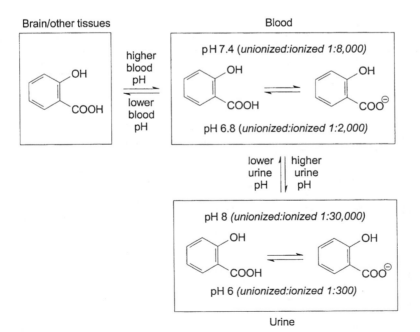

Figure 4.16: Effect of changes in blood and urine pH on the ionization of salicylate

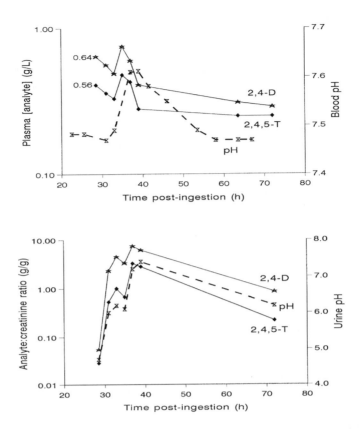

Figure 4.17: Effect of i.v. sodium bicarbonate given some 32 h post ingestion on blood and urine pH and on plasma concentrations and urinary excretion of 2,4-dichlorophenoxyacetic acid (2,4-D) and 2,4,5-trichlorophenoxyacetic acid (2,4,5-T) (Flanagan *et al.*, 1990)

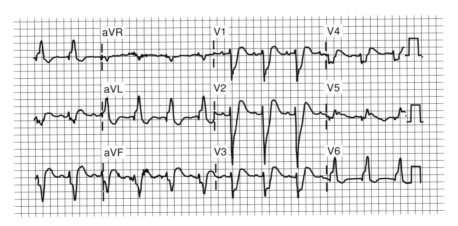

Figure 4.18: Significant QRS prolongation on an ECG (QRS 200 ms), an indication for the use of i.v. sodium bicarbonate in tricyclic antidepressant poisoning

Mackway-Jones and Thomas, 1999). In rats, the effect of sodium bicarbonate in tricyclic antidepressant poisoning is in addition to the effect of adrenaline (Knudsen and Abrahamsson, 1997). There is recent evidence that sodium bicarbonate may be of value in treating ventricular tachycardia associated with acebutolol overdosage (Donovan *et al.*, 1999) and hypotension due to verapamil (Tanen *et al.*, 2000). However, i.v. administration was ineffective in treating experimental propranolol poisoning in dogs (Love *et al.*, 2000).

The dose of sodium bicarbonate used for the prophylaxis and treatment of cardiac arrhythmias is normally 1–2 mmol/kg 8.4 % (w/v) sodium bicarbonate i.v. infused over 15 min. Repeat bolus doses may be used as necessary. Care should be taken not to exceed a blood pH of 7.55. If multiple doses of 8.4 % (w/v) sodium bicarbonate are anticipated, patients may benefit from insertion of a central line as peripheral sodium bicarbonate administration causes venous damage.

Sodium bicarbonate should not be given orally after ingestion of strong acids, as it gives rise to a severe exothermic reaction with the risk of increasing tissue injury. Oral sodium bicarbonate could be given after ingestion of ferrous salts such as ferrous sulphate as it forms insoluble ferrous carbonate and thus should minimize further iron absorption. However, in practice it is rarely used in this way. Sodium bicarbonate is used topically in conjunction with potassium permanganate (section 4.11) to treat yellow phosphorus burns.

4.16 SULPHYDRYL DONORS

Administration of sulphydryl donors, notably D,L-methionine (racemethionine) or NAC (acetylcysteine; *N*-acetyl-L-cysteine; *N*-acetyl-3-mercaptoalanine; L-α-acetamido-mercaptopropionic acid; mercapturic acid; Mucomyst; Parvolex, Evans), has achieved great prominence as either of these compounds can protect against paracetamol (acetaminophen) cytotoxicity if given with 12 h or so of ingestion (Prescott *et al.*, 1979; Meredith *et al.*, 1995; Vale and Proudfoot, 1995). NAC especially may protect against the cytotoxicity of some other compounds (Anonymous, 1991; Flanagan and Meredith, 1991; Holdiness, 1991).

4.16.1 Treatment of paracetamol poisoning

The cytotoxicity of paracetamol is probably mediated by a reactive metabolite, *N*-acetyl-4-quinoneimine (NAPQI), a strong electrophile and oxidizing agent formed in the liver and in the kidney by oxidative metabolism. Cells in which NAPQI is formed are normally protected by intracellular GSH (Figure 4.19). However, if mitochondrial and cytosolic GSH become depleted (to 20–30 % of normal), covalent binding of NAPQI to nucleophilic cell macromolecules and other reactions followed eventually by cell death may ensue. Disturbed calcium homeostasis due to oxidation of intracellular thiol-containing enzymes, in particular Ca^{2+} translocases, may be important in this process (Reed, 1990).

4.16.1.1 Mechanism of action of sulphydryl compounds

In animals, prior administration of high doses of inhibitors of oxidative metabolism such as cimetidine can reduce NAPQI formation and thus the frequency and severity

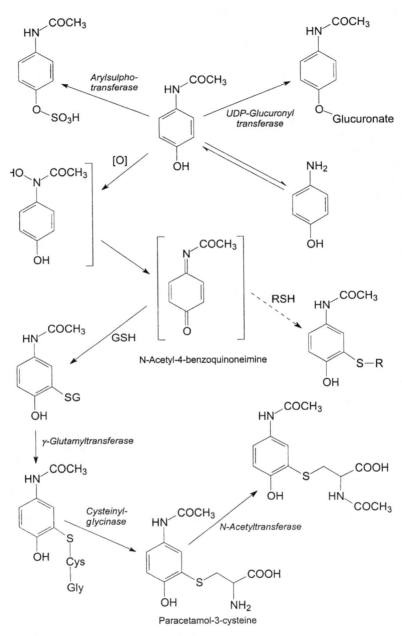

Figure 4.19: Summary of paracetamol metabolism (GSH, reduced glutathione; RSH, cell macromolecule)

of hepatotoxicity. However, such an approach is impractical for the treatment of poisoning in man because the agent concerned would have to be given before the paracetamol overdose (Kaufenberg and Shepherd, 1998). The use of other sulphur compounds to prevent the development of hepatorenal damage has been investigated. However, cysteine is unstable in solution. In one study, dimercaprol and D-penicillamine were found to provide little or no protection against paracetamol-induced hepatorenal toxicity in humans at the doses used (Prescott, 1983). Cysteamine (mercaptamine, 2-mercaptoethanolamine), an effective protective agent when used in paracetamol poisoning up to 10 h post ingestion, has unacceptable side-effects including nausea, vomiting, drowsiness and cardiotoxicity at the doses used (Prescott, 1983).

Carbocysteine (S-carboxymethyl-L-cysteine) has shown similar activity to NAC in protecting against paracetamol poisoning in animals (Ioannides *et al.*, 1983). However, this compound does not contain a free sulphydryl moiety, and clinical data on its use are lacking. Although NAC can act as a precursor of inorganic sulphate (Lin and Levy, 1981), NAC and L-methionine are more likely to act by repleting intracellular GSH (Miners *et al.*, 1984; Burgunder *et al.*, 1989). Clearly, both L-methionine and NAC require conversion to cysteine prior to incorporation in GSH, NAC being deacetylated and L-methionine undergoing sequential metabolism by five enzymes (Kretzschmar and Klinger, 1990; Figure 4.20). However, L-cysteine synthesis from L-methionine is not possible in individuals with homocystinuria, and there is thus a theoretical argument against the use of methionine to treat paracetamol poisoning in such cases (Meredith *et al.*, 1995).

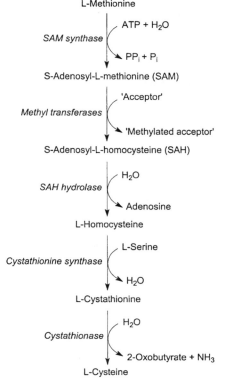

Figure 4.20: Hepatic L-cysteine synthesis from L-methionine: the cystathionine pathway

Pretreatment of mice with buthionine sulphoximine, a specific inhibitor of GSH synthesis, removed the protective effect of NAC and of methionine against paracetamol toxicity (Miners *et al.*, 1984). The exertion of a general cytoprotective effect by NAC via other mechanisms including reduction of NAPQI, oxidized thiol enzymes and other cell constituents is also a possible mechanism of action in humans; NAC may even be conjugated directly with NAPQI (Figure 4.21). Other mechanisms by which NAC could exert a cytoprotective effect include inhibition of neutrophil accumulation (Mitchell,

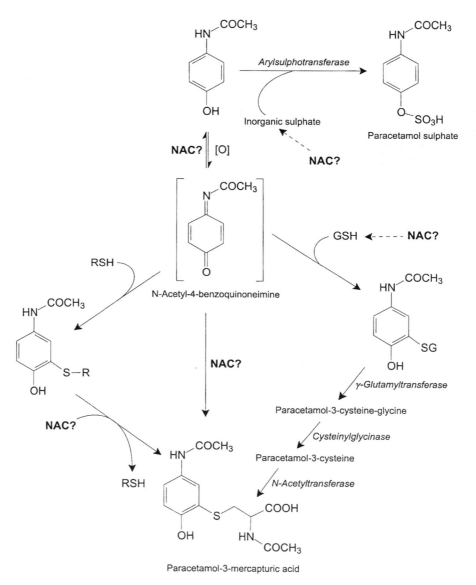

Figure 4.21: Some possible modes of action of *N*-acetylcysteine in preventing or ameliorating paracetamol-induced hepatorenal damage

1988) and restoration of the ability of proteolytic enzymes to dispose of arylated protein (Bruno *et al.*, 1988). However, direct interaction with NAPQI seems less likely as it appears that covalent binding, GSH depletion, etc. occur relatively soon after the overdose yet NAC or methionine can prevent progression to overt hepatocellular damage if given in time.

4.16.1.2 Antidotal treatment

NAC or methionine should be given if the plasma paracetamol concentration is above a line joining 200 mg/L (1.32 mmol/L) at 4 h post ingestion and 30 mg/L (0.20 mmol/L) at 15 h post ingestion on a semilogarithmic plot (Prescott, 1983; Figure 4.22). In the USA, a treatment line is used that is 25 % lower than the above, a factor which should be borne in mind when comparing studies between different centres (Meredith *et al.*, 1995). A plasma paracetamol measurement performed before 4 h post ingestion can be misleading because absorption may be incomplete. Treatment should not await a paracetamol measurement if the patient presents more than 8 h after ingesting a paracetamol dose of more than 150 mg/kg as the efficacy of NAC diminishes if it is given more than 10 h post ingestion (Prescott *et al.*, 1979). The time after ingestion, the occurrence of coma or vomiting and the risk of adverse reactions to i.v. NAC should also be considered when taking the decision to give an antidote.

	N-*Acetylcysteine*	D,L-*Methionine*
CAS registry number	616-91-1	59-51-8
Relative formula mass	163.2	149.2
pK_a	3.2; 9.65; 11.2	2.3, 9.2
Oral absorption	Extensive	High
Presystemic metabolism (%)	90–95	–
Plasma half-life (h) (mean, range)	2.6 (0.5–6.6)	–
Volume of distribution (L/kg)	0.5	–
Plasma protein binding (%)	> 80	–

Further considerations that may complicate the interpretation of plasma paracetamol concentrations are that the time of ingestion may be difficult to determine precisely and concomitant ingestion of opioids or anticholinergic drugs may delay gastric emptying. Some patients ingest several paracetamol overdoses in succession before being admitted to hospital, and in such cases antidotal therapy should be considered irrespective of the plasma paracetamol concentration (Vale and Proudfoot, 1995), especially if an adult is thought to have ingested more than 150 mg/kg over 24 h (75 mg/kg in 'high-risk' patients – Dargan *et al.*, 2001).

Some 20–40 % of patients with paracetamol concentrations above the 200 mg/L 'treatment line' after a single overdose (Figure 4.22) will escape serious hepatorenal damage even if untreated; such damage occurs only rarely in patients with concentrations below this line. However, there are several groups that may be at special risk. In particular, chronic alcohol abusers may be at risk of hepatic toxicity from high

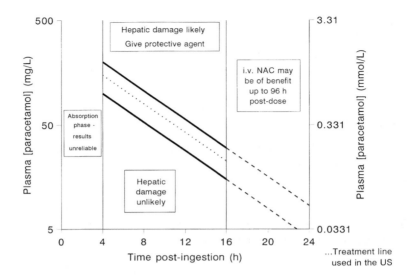

Figure 4.22: Nomogram relating time post ingestion and plasma paracetamol concentration to the suggested requirement for antidotal therapy. The lower 'treatment line' should be used for alcoholics, AIDS patients, patients with eating disorders and patients prescribed enzyme-inducing drugs such as anticonvulsants and isoniazid (see text)

therapeutic paracetamol dosage as hepatic GSH may be low initially (Seeff *et al.*, 1986; Lauterberg and Velez, 1988), although this view has been challenged (Prescott, 2000). For the same reason, individuals who are infected with human immunodeficiency virus (HIV) and those with eating disorders may be particularly susceptible to paracetamol-induced hepatotoxicity (Henry, 1990; Vale and Proudfoot, 1995). Patients may also be at greater risk because of other factors, for example those taking anticonvulsants or other enzyme inducers such as isoniazid may form NAPQI more readily, thus depleting endogenous GSH more quickly (Pirotte, 1984; Bray *et al.*, 1992; Crippin, 1993). Those considered at special risk (enzyme induction or GSH depletion) should be treated according to a 'high-risk' line that joins 100 mg/L paracetamol at 4 h to 15 mg/L at 15 h (British National Formulary, 2000b).

The incorporation of methionine into tablets containing paracetamol has been suggested as a means of protecting against hepatorenal toxicity following paracetamol overdosage (McLean and Day, 1975). This has been recommended for patients who are at special risk of self-poisoning, but concern has been voiced about possible carcinogenicity, cardiovascular toxicity and risk in pregnancy due to production of excess homocysteine (Jones *et al.*, 1997a). However, methionine loading at the amount ingested when taking combination paracetamol–methionine tablets may not in fact raise plasma homocysteine concentrations markedly, hence cardiovascular toxicity may be a theoretical rather than a real problem (McAuley *et al.*, 1999), although there may still be risk in pregnancy. Adding methionine to paracetamol preparations might be especially valuable in less developed countries where overdose treatment facilities are sparse (Krenzelock, 1997).

Although young children seem to be less susceptible than adults to the hepatorenal toxicity of paracetamol, those thought to be at risk of hepatorenal damage on the basis of a plasma paracetamol measurement should be treated in the same way as adults. No adverse sequelae were reported when two pregnant paracetamol overdose patients were treated with oral or i.v. NAC, one at 36 and one at 32 weeks (Byer *et al.*, 1982; Rosevear and Hope, 1989). In a study of 60 pregnant patients who had ingested an overdose of paracetamol, 24 were thought to be at risk of developing hepatorenal damage on the basis of plasma paracetamol concentrations and were given oral NAC (Riggs *et al.*, 1989). There was a significant correlation between time to loading dose of NAC and outcome, with an increase in the incidence of spontaneous abortion or fetal death when treatment was delayed. This suggests that treatment should be given to all such patients as soon as possible after the overdose. Administration i.v. would result in protection being achieved more quickly and reliably than with oral dosing.

NAC administered both orally and i.v. has been used to treat paracetamol poisoning, whereas methionine is normally given orally. The dosage regimens advocated were derived empirically, and it is therefore difficult to compare the relative efficacy of treatments, particularly as patients show great variation in the severity of hepatorenal damage sustained after paracetamol overdosage, even if similar amounts have been ingested. Some reports suggest possible benefit from i.v. NAC (20-h regimen) when commenced up to 24 h (Harrison *et al.*, 1990), and possibly even up to 36 h (Parker *et al.*, 1990), after the overdose, while some protection up to 24 h seems apparent with the 72-h oral NAC regimen (Smilkstein *et al.*, 1988).

NAC given i.v. to patients with paracetamol-induced fulminant hepatic failure appears to improve survival (Keays *et al.*, 1991). The mechanism underlying this observation is a matter of much interest (Proudfoot, 1995; Jones, 1998). Although once felt to be due to improved tissue microperfusion, and hence oxygen delivery (Harrison *et al.*, 1991), this view has recently been challenged using end-tidal carbon dioxide measurements, a sensitive measure of oxygen kinetics (Walsh *et al.*, 1998). NAC may act by protecting protein thiols against oxidation, by haemodynamic effects on regional blood flow to critical organs, by free radical scavenging or by interfering with the production of cytokines.

There have been many attempts to find compounds effective in the later stages of paracetamol poisoning when the efficacy of NAC or methionine is reduced or absent. Recent work has suggested that activated Kupffer cells and compounds secreted by these cells, such as cytokines (chemokines), may play a role in the progression of paracetamol-induced liver injury (McClain *et al.*, 1999; Hogaboam *et al.*, 2000). Some studies suggested that inhibition of tumour necrosis factor α (TNF-α) is effective in preventing hepatic necrosis after exposure to certain hepatotoxins, but studies in mice showed no protective effect after exposure to paracetamol (Simpson *et al.*, 2000). The possible use of ELR-containing CXC chemokines (chemokines are low-molecular-weight, 8–12 kDa, basic proteins that have been classified into four distinct families, CXC, CC, C and CX3C, based on the position of their first two conserved cysteine residues), i.e. CXC chemokines containing the amino acid sequence Glu–Leu–Arg, to induce hepatocyte proliferation and liver regeneration after paracetamol poisoning has been discussed (Hogaboam *et al.*, 1999a,b, 2001).

4.16.1.3 *Clinical use of* N-*acetylcysteine and methionine*

Both methionine and NAC are effective in treating paracetamol poisoning in humans, although both are less effective if given more than 10–12 h post ingestion (Prescott *et al.*, 1979). Methionine is safe and oral therapy (4 × 2.5 g over 12 h; child < 6 years, 4 × 1 g) has been used widely (Vale *et al.*, 1981). Oral NAC (140 mg/kg then 17 × 70 mg/kg 4-hourly) is also effective if given within 10 h (Smilkstein *et al.*, 1988). Note that the dose of methionine in a 70-kg adult (10 g over 12 h) is much less than the dose of NAC (93 g over 72 h) yet efficacy appears similar. However, oral therapy is difficult if the patient is unconscious, and efficacy may be reduced if the patient vomits or is given oral activated charcoal.

NAC given i.v. is used extensively to treat paracetamol poisoning in the UK and in Australia (Buckley *et al.*, 1999a). An initial dose of 150 mg/kg is infused in 200 mL of 5 % (w/v) D-glucose over 15 min, followed by 50 mg/kg in 500 mL of 5 % D-glucose over 4 h and 100 mg/kg in 1 L of 5 % D-glucose over the next 16 h, i.e. 300 mg/kg NAC (21 g in a 70-kg adult) over 20 h (Prescott *et al.*, 1979, 1983). The quantity of i.v. fluid used in children should take into account age and weight, but fluid overload remains a potential risk in patients under 10 kg body weight. Decision trees have been developed to guide management (Dargan *et al.*, 2001; see Appendix 3).

NAC treatment may need to be prolonged (50 mg/kg i.v. over 8 h repeated as necessary) in patients presenting more than 12 h post ingestion. In the presence of evidence of hepatic damage, prolonged NAC administration is continued until the prothrombin time, the most sensitive marker of such damage, begins to improve. In general, antidotal therapy commenced before the result of a plasma paracetamol measurement becomes available should be withdrawn in patients subsequently found not to be at risk using the standard nomogram (Figure 4.22). However, if the patient presents to hospital 16 or so hours post ingestion, commonly available paracetamol assays may not have sufficient sensitivity to measure the plasma paracetamol accurately. In such circumstances, antidotal treatment should be continued notwithstanding.

Smilkstein *et al.* (1991) reported that in 179 patients i.v. NAC dosage over 52 h [an initial dose of 140 mg/kg followed by 12 × 70 mg/kg doses – hourly, i.e. a total dose of 980 mg/kg (68.6 g in a 70-kg adult)] was more effective than the 20-h protocol in preventing hepatotoxicity in patients presenting 16–24 h post ingestion. The efficacy of this regimen appears to be similar to that of the 72-h oral NAC regimen (Perry and Shannon, 1998). The use of a lower NAC dosage in the early stages of the infusion should reduce the risk of adverse reactions while still giving adequate cytoprotection.

NAC is given orally as a 5 % (w/v) solution in a soft drink or, if given intragastrically, in water. NAC preparations suitable for oral use are available in other countries. If the patient vomits within 1 h of a dose, the dose should be repeated. In the absence of FDA approval for the use of methionine or i.v. NAC to treat paracetamol poisoning, oral NAC has been employed extensively in the USA. One argument used in favour of oral therapy is that NAC and metabolites absorbed from the intestine pass directly to the liver via the portal circulation. However, this argument takes no account of the fact that the kidney is also at risk.

In six volunteers activated charcoal had no significant effect on oral NAC absorption (Renzi *et al.*, 1985) but was associated with a mean reduction in NAC bioavailability of 40 % in a second study in 19 subjects (Ekins *et al.*, 1987). Vomiting is a contraindication to oral therapy (charcoal, methionine or NAC), although it may itself be associated with the use of oral NAC. On the other hand, prompt administration of activated charcoal to paracetamol overdose patients presenting within 1–2 h of the ingestion may reduce the need for i.v. NAC (Buckley *et al.*, 1999b).

4.16.1.4 *Pharmacokinetics and metabolism* of N-acetylcysteine

Study of the pharmacokinetics of NAC is complicated because of the variety of forms (free, protein-bound in either reduced or oxidized form, mixed disulphides with other thiols, including protein thiols) in which NAC can be present. Thus, NAC is deacetylated to give cysteine, cystine, methionine, GSH and other products; mixed disulphides (N,N'-diacetylcystine, N-acetylcysteine-cysteine, etc.) also occur (Olsson *et al.*, 1988). NAC absorption occurs rapidly after oral administration of doses of 100–200 mg, although bioavailability is less than 12 % (Burgunder *et al.*, 1989; Borgström and Kågedal, 1990). This is thought to be because of extensive deacetylation, most probably in the intestinal mucosa (Sjödin *et al.*, 1989). After i.v. administration, plasma half-lives of 2–6 h have been reported; 20–30 % of the dose is excreted unchanged in urine (Borgström *et al.*, 1986; Prescott *et al.*, 1989). NAC does not accumulate in plasma on chronic dosing (Borgström and Kågedal, 1990), although NAC clearance is impaired in the presence of chronic liver disease (Jones *et al.*, 1997b).

In plasma, most of a dose of NAC is present as disulphides. In one study, oral NAC increased free cysteine in plasma although total cysteine and free and total glutathione concentrations remained unchanged (Burgunder *et al.*, 1989). Plasma total NAC concentrations soon after the start of an infusion (20-h i.v. regimen) range from 300 to 900 mg/L, whereas concentrations of only 11–90 mg/L are maintained towards the end (Prescott *et al.*, 1989). The latter concentrations are similar to those attained following oral NAC administration (Burgunder *et al.*, 1989).

4.16.1.5 *Adverse reactions to* N-acetylcysteine

When used to treat paracetamol poisoning, oral NAC is rarely accompanied by serious adverse reactions although, after repeated oral doses, nausea/vomiting and diarrhoea have been reported in up to 50 % and 35 % of patients respectively. Headache, rash, hypotension and respiratory distress occur (Miller and Rumack, 1983). Urticaria has also been reported (Charley *et al.*, 1987). Hepatotoxicity following combined oral and rectal administration of NAC in high doses (106 g in 3 days) to treat meconium ileus equivalent in a 3-year-old boy with cystic fibrosis has also been observed (Bailey and Andres, 1987).

NAC given i.v. may be accompanied by anaphylactoid reactions such as flushing, rash/pruritus, angioedema, bronchospasm, nausea/vomiting, hypotension, tachycardia and respiratory distress. These reactions occur 15–60 min into the infusion in some 5 % of patients (Dawson *et al.*, 1989). Asthmatics are at special risk – respiratory arrest during the early stages of an infusion in a previously healthy 17-year-old girl with mild asthma has been reported (Reynard *et al.*, 1992). These toxic reactions appear to be due to histamine release by NAC rather than any other component of the infusion (Bateman *et al.*, 1984) and occur at the time of peak plasma concentration, i.e. within 1 h of starting the infusion when plasma total NAC concentrations exceed 300 mg/L (Prescott *et al.*, 1989). Flushing may also be caused, at least in part, by vasodilatation due to the hyperosmolarity of the NAC infusion (Jones *et al.*, 1994).

Following accidental NAC overdosage the adverse effects observed are similar but of greater severity (Mant *et al.*, 1984). In a recent study, the ratio of the measured to intended NAC concentrations (median, range) in 198 infusion bags (66 patients, three bags each) used in treating paracetamol poisoning were: bag 1 – 1.07 (0.61–3.58), bag

CHAPTER 4

2 – 1.34 (0.46–2.90) and bag 3 – 1.36 (0.56–2.93). Over twice the intended NAC dose was given to four patients while one received only 60 % of that intended. Overall, only about 25 % of patients had a NAC dose within 10 % of that intended (Ferner *et al.*, 1999). It was thought that volumetric errors in preparing the dilutions rather than miscalculation were responsible for most errors.

Treatment of NAC toxicity is normally directed at the reversal of anaphylactoid features and/or controlling nausea and vomiting. Airway support, reversal of bronchospasm and maintenance of vital functions may also be required. If a patient exhibits a severe anaphylactoid reaction but still needs treatment on the basis of a plasma paracetamol measurement, an antihistamine such as chlorpheniramine or diphenhydramine (Bailey and McGuigan, 1998) (Table 1.2) may be given orally and the infusion recommenced at a lower rate. Alternatively, oral NAC/methionine may be administered provided that there is no contraindication, although this is rarely done in practice. Donovan *et al.* (1986) reported sudden onset of respiratory distress with resultant fatal cardiac arrest in a patient with pre-existing chronic obstructive pulmonary disease who was given probably too much NAC (20-h i.v. regimen) for paracetamol overdose. Other deaths after accidental i.v. NAC overdosage have been reported (Flanagan and Meredith, 1991).

4.16.2 Additional potential uses of sulphydryl donors

The use of NAC in acute poisoning with halogenated hydrocarbons such as chloroform, carbon tetrachloride and 1,2-dichloropropane has been discussed (Flanagan and Meredith, 1991). These compounds are potent hepatorenal toxins – the fatal dose in an adult may be as little as 5–10 mL. There is a clear theoretical rationale for the use of NAC in the treatment of poisoning with either chloroform or 1,2-dichloropropane. Phosgene ($COCl_2$) is an important metabolite of chloroform. Phosgene depletes GSH to form diglutathionyl dithiocarbonate (GS-CO-SG) and also binds to cell macromolecules and causes tissue necrosis. 1,2-Dichloropropane administration is also associated with hepatic GSH depletion in rats (Imberti *et al.*, 1990). NAC could thus be used to replenish intracellular GSH and thereby may mitigate the hepatorenal toxicity of the parent compounds as with paracetamol. Intratracheal NAC protects against the toxicity of inhaled phosgene in rabbits (Sciuto *et al.*, 1995 – see section 7.4).

With carbon tetrachloride, the mechanism of toxicity, and thus the possible role of NAC in treatment, is more complex. The trichloromethyl free radical ($\cdot CCl_3$) formed initially may bind covalently to macromolecules or react further by several routes. Chloroform is a minor metabolite and may be metabolized to phosgene, but the importance of this is unclear – carbon tetrachloride does not deplete hepatic GSH to the same extent as chloroform in animals. A number of antioxidants/free radical scavengers have been advocated for use as cytoprotective agents in carbon tetrachloride poisoning, including vitamin E and sulphydryl compounds. Hyperbaric oxygen has also been used to treat one patient (Flanagan and Meredith, 1991).

Despite much discussion, NAC has not found wide application in reducing the toxicity of chemotherapeutic agents, or in preventing or ameliorating tissue radiation damage. Other sulphydryl donors, such as amifostine (*S*-[2-(3-aminopropylamino)ethyl] dihydrogen phosphorothioate; ethiophos; WR-2721; Ethyol; CAS 53028-04-9) and mesna (sodium 2-mercaptoethanesulphonate; mesnum; CAS 19767-45-4), are under investigation in this role (Lewis, 1994; Alberts and Bleyer, 1996). Clinical studies have reported no protective effect of NAC in doxorubicin poisoning, and the iron chelator dexrazoxane (section 2.3.7.2) is thought to be effective.

Acute poisoning with acrylonitrile, bromobenzene or naphthalene is very rare and, although there are theoretical arguments for the use of NAC, there are no reports demonstrating the efficacy of NAC in treatment (Flanagan and Meredith, 1991). NAC may be of benefit in acute poisoning with 2-chloroethanol (Kvistad *et al.*, 1983). Oral NAC (140 mg/kg initially and then 70 mg/kg 4-hourly for 17 doses) is claimed to have been effective in treating sodium valproate-induced hepatic damage in three children (Farrell *et al.*, 1989).

NAC has been advocated as treatment for acute poisoning with potassium permanganate, and with sodium dichromate and/or chromate, the clinical course of which can resemble severe untreated paracetamol poisoning, with hepatorenal damage developing some hours after ingestion (Vassallo and Howland, 1988; Young *et al.*, 1996). NAC may also have a protective action against dimethylformamide-induced liver damage (Buylaert *et al.*, 1996) and against pulmonary toxicity caused by inhalation of perfluoroisobutene in rats (Lailey, 1997).

Recently, NAC has been suggested for use in *Amanita phalloides* (death cap mushroom) poisoning (Montanini *et al.*, 1999).

4.17 THIOCTIC ACID

Thioctic acid [lipoic acid; 1,2-dithiolane-3-pentanoic acid; CAS (*d*-form) 1200-22-2; Figure 4.23] is a cofactor in the metabolism of pyruvate to acetylcoenzyme A by the hepatic pyruvate dehydrogenase complex. Administration of thioctic acid has been advocated in poisoning from cyclopeptide-containing fungi such as *Amanita phalloides* and *A. virosa* (Plotzker *et al.*, 1982; Hanrahan and Gordon, 1984). A dose of 75–125 mg in 5 % (w/v) D-glucose i.v. every 6–24 h for up to 1 week has been suggested, increasing to 300–500 mg if hepatic damage becomes obvious. This use is questionable, but thioctic acid is relatively non-toxic.

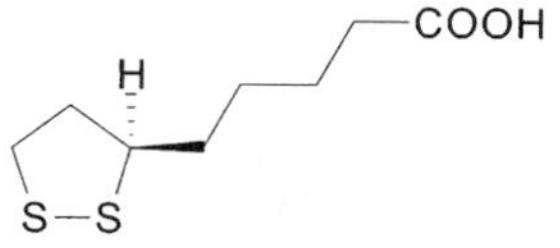

Figure 4.23: Structural formula of thioctic acid (*d*-form)

4.18 ZINC SALTS

Zinc acetate or sulphate (50 mg orally thrice daily) is used in the later stages of treating Wilson's disease as maintenance therapy, and in presymptomatic patients (Brewer, 1995). Zinc acetate is preferred as this is less irritating to the stomach than the sulphate. Zinc induces synthesis of metallothionein in the intestine. Metallothionein has a higher affinity for copper than for zinc, and thus copper absorption is prevented. However, the onset of action of zinc is slow, and therapy with ammonium tetrathiomolybdate (section 2.4.2), D-penicillamine (section 2.2.6) or TETA (section 2.2.6.1) is needed to reduce plasma copper concentrations in symptomatic patients.

REFERENCES

Alberts DS, Bleyer WA. Future development of amifostine in cancer treatment. *Semin Oncol* 1996; 23 (Suppl 8): 90–9.

Anonymous. Acetylcysteine. *Lancet* 1991; 337: 1069–70.

Bailey B, McGuigan MA. Management of anaphylactoid reactions to intravenous N-acetylcysteine. *Ann Emerg Med* 1998; 31: 710–15.

Bailey DJ, Andres JM. Liver injury after oral and rectal administration of N-acetylcysteine for meconium ileus equivalent in a patient with cystic fibrosis. *Pediatrics* 1987; 79: 281–2.

Barceloux DG, Krenzelok EP, Olson K, Watson W. American Academy of Clinical Toxicology practice guidelines on the treatment of ethylene glycol poisoning. *J Toxicol Clin Toxicol* 1999; 37: 537–60.

Bateman DN, Woodhouse KW, Rawlins MD. Adverse reactions to N-acetylcysteine. *Hum Toxicol* 1984; 3: 393–8.

Baud FJ, Bismuth C, Garnier R, Galliot M, Astier A, Maistre G, Soffer M. 4-Methylpyrazole may be an alternative to ethanol therapy for ethylene glycol intoxication in man. *J Toxicol Clin Toxicol* 1986/7; 24: 463–83.

Baud FJ, Galliot M, Astier A, Bien DV, Garnier R, Likforman J, Bismuth C. Treatment of ethylene glycol poisoning with intravenous 4-methylpyrazole. *N Engl J Med* 1988; 319: 97–100.

Baud FJ, Brouard A, Muszynski J, Bismuth C. 4-Methylpyrazole. In: *Les Antidotes*. Baud F, Barriot P, Riou B (eds). Paris: Masson, 1992: 195–205.

Bendich A, Cohen M. Vitamin B_6 safety issues. *Ann NY Acad Sci* 1990; 585: 321–30.

Berning J. Hypokalaemia of barium poisoning [letter]. *Lancet* 1975; i: 110.

Beutler E. Drug-induced hemolytic anaemia. *Pharm Rev* 1969; 21: 73–103.

Bjornsson TD, Blaschke TT. Vitamin K_1 disposition and therapy of warfarin overdose [letter]. *Lancet* 1978; ii: 846–7.

Borgström L, Kågedal B. Dose dependent pharmacokinetics of N-acetylcysteine after oral dosing in man. *Biopharm Drug Dispos* 1990; 11: 131–6.

Borgström L, Kågedal B, Paulsen O. Pharmacokinetics of N-acetylcysteine in man. *Eur J Clin Pharmacol* 1986; 31: 217–22.

Borron SW, Mégarbane B, Baud FJ. Fomepizole in treatment of uncomplicated ethylene glycol poisoning. *Lancet* 1999; 354: 831.

Bray GP, Harrison PM, O'Grady JG, Tredger JM, Williams R. Long-term anticonvulsant therapy worsens outcome in paracetamol-induced fulminant hepatic failure. *Hum Exp Toxicol* 1992; 11: 265–70.

Brent J, McMartin K, Phillips S, Burkhart KK, Donovan JW, Wells M, Kulig K. Fomepizole for the treatment of ethylene glycol poisoning. *N Engl J Med* 1999; 340: 832–8.

Brewer GJ. Interactions of zinc and molybdenum with copper in therapy of Wilson's disease. *Nutrition* 1995; 11 (Suppl 1): 114–16.

British National Formulary, 40th edn. London: British Medical Association and Royal Pharmaceutical Society of Great Britain, September 2000a: 439–40.

British National Formulary, 40th edn. London: British Medical Association and Royal Pharmaceutical Society of Great Britain, September 2000b: 21–3.

Brophy PD, Tenenbein M, Gardner J, Bunchman TE, Smoyer WE. Childhood diethylene glycol poisoning treated with alcohol dehydrogenase inhibitor fomepizole and hemodialysis. *Am J Kidney Dis* 2000; 35: 958–62.

Brown RS, Cohen JH, Braverman LE. Successful treatment of massive acute thyroid hormone poisoning with iopanoic acid. *J Pediatr* 1998; 132: 903–5.

Bruno GR, Howland MA, McKeeking A, Hoffman RS. Long-acting anticoagulant overdose: brodifacoum kinetics and optimal vitamin K dosing. *Ann Emerg Med* 2000; 36: 262–7.

Bruno MK, Cohen SD, Khairallah EA. Antidotal effectiveness of N-acetylcysteine in reversing acetaminophen-induced hepatotoxicity. Enhancement of the proteolysis of arylated proteins. *Biochem Pharmacol* 1988; 37: 4319–25.

Buckley NA, Whyte IM, O'Connell DL, Dawson AH. Oral or intravenous N-acetylcysteine: which is the treatment of choice for acetaminophen (paracetamol) poisoning? *J Toxicol Clin Toxicol* 1999a; 37: 759–67.

Buckley NA, Whyte IM, O'Connell DL, Dawson AH. Activated charcoal reduces the need for N-acetylcysteine treatment after acetaminophen (paracetamol) overdose. *J Toxicol Clin Toxicol* 1999b; 37: 753–7.

Burgunder JM, Varriale A, Lauterberg BH. Effect of N-acetylcysteine on plasma cysteine and glutathione following paracetamol administration. *Eur J Clin Pharmacol* 1989; 36: 127–31.

Buylaert W, Calle P, De Paepe P, Verstrate A, Samyn N, Vogelaers D, Vandenbulcke M, Belpaire F. Hepatotoxicity of N,N-dimethylformamide (DMF) in acute poisoning with the veterinary euthanasia drug T-61. *Hum Exp Toxicol* 1996; 15: 607–11.

Byer AJ, Traylor TR, Semmer JR. Acetaminophen overdose in the third trimester of pregnancy. *J Am Med Assoc* 1982; 247: 3114–15.

Caravati EM. Acute hydrofluoric acid exposure. *Am J Emerg Med* 1988; 6: 143–50.

Charley G, Dean BS, Krenzelok EP. Oral N-acetylcysteine-induced urticaria: a case report [abstract]. *Vet Hum Toxicol* 1987; 29: 477.

Choonara IA, Scott AK, Haynes BP, Cholerton S, Breckenridge AM, Park BK. Vitamin K_1 metabolism in relation to pharmacodynamic response in anticoagulated patients. *Br J Clin Pharmacol* 1985; 20: 643–8.

Chow MT, Di Silvestro VA, Yung CY, Nawab ZM, Leehey DJ, Ing TS. Treatment of acute methanol intoxication with hemodialysis using an ethanol-enriched, bicarbonate base dialysate. *Am J Kidney Dis* 1997; 30: 568–70.

Chugh SN, Kolley T, Kakkar R, Chugh K, Sharma A. A critical evaluation of antiperoxidant effect of intravenous magnesium in acute aluminium phosphide poisoning. *Magnesium Res* 1997; 10: 225–30.

Civil IDS, McDonald MJA. Acute selenium poisoning: case report. *NZ Med J* 1978; 87: 354–6.

Clark RF, Wethern-Kestner S, Vance MV, Gerkin R. Clinical presentation and treatment of black widow spider envenomation: a review of 163 cases. *Ann Emerg Med* 1992; 21: 782–7.

Corke PJ. Superwarfarin (brodifacoum) poisoning. *Anaesth Intens Care* 1997; 25: 707–9.

Crippin JS. Acetaminophen hepatotoxicity: potentiation by isoniazid. *Am J Gastroenterol* 1993; 88: 590–2.

Dargan PI, Wallace CI, Jones AL. Acetaminophen (paracetamol) overdose: an evidence based flowchart to guide management. *Emerg Med J* 2001 (in press).

Dawson AH, Henry DA, McEwen J. Adverse reactions to N-acetylcysteine during treatment for paracetamol poisoning. *Med J Aust* 1989; 150: 329–31.

DiSanto AR, Wagner JG. Pharmacokinetics of highly ionized drugs. II. Methylene blue – absorption, metabolism, and excretion in man and dog after oral administration. *J Pharm Sci* 1972; 61: 1086–90.

Domingo JL, Llobet JM, Tomas JM, Corbella J. Influence of chelating agents on the toxicity, distribution and excretion of vanadium in mice. *J Appl Toxicol* 1986; 6: 337–41.

Donovan JW. Nitrates, nitrites, and other sources of methaemoglobinaemia. In: *Clinical Management of Poisoning and Drug Overdose*, 2nd edn. Haddad LM, Winchester JF (eds). Philadelphia: WB Saunders, 1990: 1419–30.

Donovan JW, Proudfoot AT, Prescott LF. Adverse effects of intravenous N-acetylcysteine [abstract]. *Vet Hum Toxicol* 1986; 28: 487.

Donovan KD, Gerace RV, Dreyer JF. Acebutolol-induced ventricular tachycardia reversed with sodium bicarbonate. *J Toxicol Clin Toxicol* 1999; 37: 481–4.

Ekins BR, Ford DC, Thompson MIB, Bridges RR, Rollins DE, Jenkins RD. The effect of activated charcoal on N-acetylcysteine absorption in normal subjects. *Am J Emerg Med* 1987; 5: 483–7.

Farrell K, Abbott FS, Junker AK, Waddell JS, Pippenger CE. Successful treatment of valproate hepatotoxicity with N-acetylcysteine [abstract]. *Epilepsia* 1989; 30: 700.

Feldwick MG, Noakes PS, Prause U, Mead RJ, Kostyniak PJ. The biochemical toxicology of 1,3-difluoro-2-propanol, the major ingredient of the pesticide gliftor: the potential of 4-methylpyrazole as an antidote. *J Biochem Mol Toxicol* 1998; 12: 41–52.

Fenner PJ, Williamson JA, Burnett JW, Rifkin J. First aid treatment of jellyfish stings in Australia. Response to a newly differentiated species. *Med J Aust* 1993; 158: 498–501.

Ferner RE, Hutchings A, Anton C, Almond S, Jones A, Routledge PA. The origin of errors in dosage: acetylcysteine as a paradigm [abstract]. *Br J Clin Pharmacol* 1999; 47: 581P.

Finch CA. Methemoglobinemia and sulfhemoglobinemia. *N Engl J Med* 1948; 239: 470–8.

Flanagan RJ, Meredith TJ. Use of N-acetylcysteine in clinical toxicology. *Am J Med* 1991; 91 (Suppl 3C); 131S–9S.

Flanagan RJ, Meredith TJ, Ruprah M, Onyon LJ, Liddle A. Alkaline diuresis for acute poisoning with chlorophenoxy herbicides and ioxynil. *Lancet* 1990; 335: 454–8.

Flomenbaum NE. Rodenticides. In: *Goldfrank's Toxicologic Emergencies*, 6th edn. Goldfrank LR, Flomenbaum NE, Lewin NA, Weisman RS, Howland MA, Hoffman RS (eds). Stamford: Appleton and Lange, 1998: 1459–73.

Frommer DA, Kulig KW, Marx JA, Rumack B. Tricyclic antidepressant overdose: a review. *J Am Med Assoc* 1987; 257: 521–6.

Goldfarb DS. Fomepizole for ethylene glycol poisoning [letter]. *Lancet* 1999; 354: 1646.

Graudins A, Burns MJ, Aaron CK. Regional intravenous infusion of calcium gluconate for hydrofluoric acid burns of the upper extremity. *Ann Emerg Med* 1997; 30: 604–7 [see also correspondence 1998; 31: 526–7].

Hanrahan JP, Gordon MA. Mushroom poisoning: case reports and a review of therapy. *J Am Med Assoc* 1984; 251: 1057–61

Harrison PM, Keays R, Bray GP, Alexander GJM, Williams R. Improved outcome of paracetamol-induced fulminant hepatic failure by late administration of acetylcysteine. *Lancet* 1990; 335: 1572–3.

Harrison PM, Wendon JA, Gimson AES, Alexander GJM, Williams R. Improvement by acetylcysteine of hemodynamics and oxygen transport in fulminant hepatic failure. *N Engl J Med* 1991; 324: 1852–7.

Harry P, Turcant A, Bouachour G, Houze P, Alquier P, Allain P. Efficacy of 4-methylpyrazole in ethylene glycol poisoning: clinical and toxicokinetic aspects. *Hum Exp Toxicol* 1994; 13: 61–4.

Harry P, Jobard E, Briand M, Caubet A, Turcant A. Ethylene glycol poisoning in a child treated with 4-methylpyrazole. *Pediatrics* 1998; 102: 31,e31.

Henry JA. Glutathione and HIV infection [letter]. *Lancet* 1990; 335: 235–6.

Hirano M, Matsuki T, Tanishima K, Takeshita M, Shimizu S, Nagamura Y, Yoneyama Y. Congenital methaemoglobinaemia due to NADH methaemoglobin reductase deficiency: successful treatment with oral riboflavin. *Br J Haematol* 1981; 47: 353–9.

Hogaboam CM, Bone-Larson CL, Steinhauser ML, Lukacs NW, Colletti LM, Simpson KJ, Strieter RM, Kunkel SL. Novel CXCR2-dependent liver regenerative qualities of ELR-containing CXC chemokines. *Fed Am Soc Exp Biol J* 1999a; 13: 1565–74.

Hogaboam CM, Simpson KJ, Chensue SW, Steinhauser ML, Lukacs NW, Gauldie J, Strieter RM, Kunkel SL. Macrophage inflammatory protein-2 gene therapy attenuates adenovirus- and acetaminophen-mediated hepatic injury. *Gene Ther* 1999b; 6: 573–84.

Hogaboam CM, Bone-Larson CL, Steinhauser ML, Matsukawa A, Gosling J, Boring L, Charo IF, Simpson KJ, Lukacs NW, Kunkel SL. Exaggerated hepatic injury due to acetaminophen challenge in mice lacking C-C chemokine receptor 2. *Am J Pathol* 2000; 156: 1245–52.

Hogaboam CM, Simpson KJ, Lukacs NW, Kunkel SL, Colletti LM, Streiter RM, Bone-Larson C. *Treatment of Liver Disease and Injury with CXC Chemokines*. World Intellectual Property Organization International Publication No. WO0110899 (published 15 February 2001).

Holdiness MR. Clinical pharmacokinetics of N-acetylcysteine. *Clin Pharmacokinet* 1991; 20: 123–34.

Holford NHG. Clinical pharmacokinetcis of ethanol. *Clin Pharmacokinet* 1987; 13: 273–92.

Hunter D. *The Diseases of Occupations*, 6th edn. London: Hodder and Stoughton, 1978: 469–71.

Imberti R, Mapelli A, Colombo P, Richelmi P, Bertè F, Bellomo G. 1,2-Dichloropropane (DCP) toxicity is correlated with DCP-induced glutathione (GSH) depletion and is modulated by factors affecting intracellular GSH. *Arch Toxicol* 1990; 64: 459–65.

Inoue K, Kera Y, Kiriyama T, Komura S. Suppression of acetaldehyde accumulation by 4-methylpyrazole in alcohol-hypersensitive Japanese. *Japan J Pharmacol* 1985; 38: 43–8.

Ioannides C, Hall DE, Mulder DE, Steele CM, Spickett J, Delaforge M, Parke DV. A comparison of the protective effects of N-acetylcysteine and S-carboxymethylcysteine against paracetamol-induced hepatotoxicity. *Toxicology* 1983; 28: 313–21.

Jacobsen D. New treatment for ethylene glycol poisoning [editorial]. *N Engl J Med* 1999; 340: 879–80.

Jacobsen D, Sebastian CS, Blomstrand R, McMartin KE. 4-Methylpyrazole: a controlled study of safety in healthy human subjects after single, ascending doses. *Alcohol Clin Exp Res* 1988; 12: 516–22.

Jacobsen D, Barron SK, Sebastian CS, Blomstrand R, McMartin KE. Non-linear kinetics of 4-methylpyrazole in healthy human subjects. *Eur J Clin Pharmacol* 1989; 37: 599–604.

Jacobsen D, Sebastian CS, Barron SK, Carriere EW, McMartin KE. Effects of 4-methylpyrazole, methanol/ethylene glycol antidote, in healthy humans. *J Emerg Med* 1990; 8: 455–61.

Jacobsen D, Østensen J, Bredesen L, Ullstein E, McMartin K. 4-Methylpyrazole (4-MP) is effectively removed by haemodialysis in the pig model. *Hum Exp Toxicol* 1996a; 15: 494–6.

Jacobsen D, Sebastian CS, Dies DF, Breau RL, Spann EG, Barron SK, McMartin KE. Kinetic interactions between 4-methylpyrazole and ethanol in healthy humans. *Alcohol Clin Exp Res* 1996b; 20: 804–9.

Jaeger A, Le Tacon S, Bosquet C, Sauder P. Effects of poisons on ion channels [abstract]. *J Toxicol Clin Toxicol* 2000; 38: 160–1.

Jones AL. Mechanism of action and value of N-acetylcysteine in the treatment of early and late acetaminophen poisoning: a critical review. *Clin Toxicol* 1998; 36: 277–85.

Jones AL, Haynes W, MacGilchrist AJ, Webb DJ, Hayes PC. N-Acetylcysteine (NAC) is a potent peripheral vasodilator [abstract]. *Gut* 1994; 35 (Suppl 5): S10.

Jones AL, Hayes PC, Proudfoot AT, Vale JA, Prescott LF. Should methionine be put in every paracetamol tablet? No: the risks are not well enough known. *Br Med J* 1997a; 315: 301–3.

Jones AL, Jarvie DR, Simpson D, Hayes PC, Prescott LF. Pharmacokinetics of N-acetylcysteine are altered in chronic liver disease. *Aliment Pharmacol Ther* 1997b; 11: 787–91.

Kallmann B, Burkart V, Kröncke K-D, Kolb-Bachofen V, Kolb H. Toxicity of chemically generated nitric oxide towards pancreatic islet cells can be prevented by nicotinamide. *Life Sci* 1992; 51: 671–8.

Kaufenberg AJ, Shepherd MF. Role of cimetidine in the treatment of acetaminophen overdose. *Am J Hlth-Syst Pharm* 1998; 55: 1516–19.

Keays R, Harrison PM, Wendon JA, Forbes A, Gove C, Alexander GJM, Williams R. Intravenous acetylcysteine in paracetamol induced fulminant hepatic failure: a prospective controlled trial. *Br Med J* 1991; 303: 1026–9.

Keniston RC, Cabellon S, Yarbrough KS. Pyridoxal 5'-phosphate as an antidote for cyanide, spermine, gentamicin, and dopamine toxicity: an *in vivo* rat study. *Toxicol Appl Pharmacol* 1987; 88: 433–41.

Knudsen K, Abrahamsson J. Epinephrine and sodium bicarbonate independently and additively increase survival in experimental amitriptyline poisoning. *Crit Care Med* 1997; 25: 669–74.

Kowalczyk M, Halvorsen S, Ovrebo S, Bredesen JE, Jacobsen D. Ethanol treatment in ethylene glycol poisoned patients. *Vet Hum Toxicol* 1998; 40: 225–8.

Krenzelok EP. Should methionine be put in every paracetamol tablet? Yes: but perhaps only in developing countries. *Br Med J* 1997; 315: 303–4.

Kretzschmar M, Klinger W. The hepatic glutathione system – influence of xenobiotics. *Exp Pathol* 1990; 38: 145–64.

Kvistad PH, Bolle R, Wickstrøm E. Acute poisoning by ethylene chlorohydrin. Intoxication by ingestion of film cement in two children. *Hum Toxicol* 1983; 2: 311–13.

Lailey AF. Oral N-acetylcysteine protects against perfluoroisobutene toxicity in rats. *Hum Exp Toxicol* 1997; 16: 212–16.

Lauterberg BH, Velez ME. Glutathione deficiency in alcoholics: risk factor for paracetamol hepatotoxicity. *Gut* 1988; 29: 1153–7.

Lewis C. A review of the use of chemoprotectants in cancer chemotherapy. *Drug Safety* 1994; 11: 153–62.

LeWitt PA. The neurotoxicity of the rat poison vacor: a clinical study of 12 cases. *N Engl J Med* 1980; 302: 73–7.

Lheureux P, Even-Adin D, Askenasi R. Current status of antidotal therapies in acute human intoxications. *Acta Clin Belg* 1990; 13 (Suppl): 29–47.

Lin JH, Levy G. Sulfate depletion after acetaminophen administration and replenishment by infusion of sodium sulfate or N-acetylcysteine in rats. *Biochem Pharmacol* 1981; 30: 2723–5.

Lindros KO, Stowell A, Pikkarainen P, Salaspuro M. The disulfiram(Antabuse)–alcohol reaction in male alcoholics: its efficient management by 4-methylpyrazole. *Alcohol Clin Exp Res* 1981; 5: 528–30.

Litovitz T. The alcohols: ethanol, methanol, isopropanol, ethylene glycol. *Pediatr Clin N Am* 1986; 33: 311–23.

Love JN, Howell JM, Newsome JT, Skibbie DF, Dickerson LW, Henderson KJ. The effect of sodium bicarbonate on propranolol-induced cardiovascular toxicity in a canine model. *J Toxicol Clin Toxicol* 2000; 38: 421–8.

McAuley DF, Hanratty CG, McGurk C, Nugent AG, Johnston GD. Effect of methionine supplementation on endothelial function, plasma homocysteine and lipid peroxidation. *Clin Toxicol* 1999; 37: 435–40.

McCabe JL, Cobaugh DJ, Menegazzi JJ, Fata J. Experimental tricyclic antidepressant toxicity: a randomised, controlled comparison of hypertonic saline solution, sodium bicarbonate, and hyperventilation. *Ann Emerg Med* 1998; 32: 329–33.

McClain CJ, Price S, Barve S, Devalarja R, Shedlofsky S. Acetaminophen hepatotoxicity: an update. *Curr Gastroenterol Rep* 1999; 1: 42–9.

Mackway-Jones K, Thomas M. Alkalinisation in the management of tricyclic antidepressant overdose. *J Accid Emerg Med* 1999; 16: 139–40.

McLean AEM, Day PA. The effect of diet on the toxicity of paracetamol and the safety of paracetamol–methionine mixtures. *Biochem Pharmacol* 1975; 24: 37–42.

McMartin KE, Heath A. Treatment of ethylene glycol poisoning with intravenous 4-methypyrazole [letter]. *N Engl J Med* 1989; 320: 125.

McMartin KE, Jacobsen D, Sebastian S, Barron SK, Blomstrand R. Safety and metabolism of 4-methylpyrazole in human subjects [abstract]. *Vet Hum Toxicol* 1987; 29: 471.

Mansouri A. Methemoglobinemia. *Am J Med Sci* 1985; 289: 200–9.

Mant TGK, Tempowski JH, Volans GN, Talbot JCC. Adverse reactions to acetylcysteine and effects of overdose. *Br Med J* 1984; 289: 217–19.

Mardel S, Phair I, O'Dwyer F, Henry JA. Intravenous pyridoxine in acute ethanol intoxication. *Hum Exp Toxicol* 1994; 13: 321–3.

Meredith TJ, Jacobsen D, Haines JA, Berger J-C (ed.). Antidotes for poisoning by paracetamol. IPCS/CEC Evaluation of Antidotes Series, Volume 3. Cambridge: Cambridge University Press, 1995.

Miller LF, Rumack BH. Clinical safety of high oral doses of acetylcysteine. *Semin Oncol* 1983; 10 (Suppl 1): 76–85.

Miners JO, Drew R, Birkett DJ. Mechanism of action of paracetamol protective agents in mice *in vivo*. *Biochem Pharmacol* 1984; 33: 2995–3000.

Mitchell JR. Acetaminophen toxicity [editorial]. *N Engl J Med* 1988; 319: 1601–2.

Montanini S, Sinardi D, Pratico C, Sinardi AU, Trimarchi G. Use of acetylcysteine as the life-saving antidote in *Amanita phalloides* (death cap) poisoning: case report on 11 patients. *Arzneimittelforschung* 1999; 49: 1044–7.

Moore DF, Bentley AM, Dawling S, Hoare AM, Henry JA. Folinic acid and enhanced renal elimination in formic acid intoxication. *Clin Toxicol* 1994; 32: 199–204.

Nadler JE, Green H, Rosenbaum A. Intravenous injection of methylene blue in man with reference to its toxic symptoms and effect on the electrocardiogram. *Am J Med Sci* 1934: 188: 15–21.

Newton EH, Shih RD, Hoffman RS. Cyclic antidepressant overdose: a review of current management strategies. *Am J Emerg Med* 1994; 12: 376–9.

Nzerue CM, Harvey P, Volcy J, Berdzenshvili M. Survival after massive ethylene glycol poisoning: role of an ethanol enriched, bicarbonate-based dialysate. *Int J Artif Organs* 1999; 22: 744–6.

Olsson B, Johansson M, Gabrielsson J, Bolme P. Pharmacokinetics and bioavailability of reduced and oxidized N-acetylcysteine. *Eur J Clin Pharmacol* 1988; 34: 77–82.

Park BK, Scott AK, Wilson AC, Haynes BP, Breckenridge AM. Plasma disposition of vitamin K_1 in relation to anticoagulant poisoning. *Br J Clin Pharmacol* 1984; 18: 655–62.

Parker D, White JP, Paton D, Routledge PA. Safety of late acetylcysteine treatment of paracetamol poisoning. *Hum Exp Toxicol* 1990; 9: 25–7.

Perry HE, Shannon MW. Efficacy of oral versus intravenous N-acetylcysteine in acetaminophen overdose: results of an open-label, clinical trial. *J Pediatr* 1998; 132: 149–52.

Perry PM, Meinhard E. Necrotic subcutaneous abscesses following injections of methylene blue. *Br J Clin Pract* 1974; 28: 289–91.

Pertoldi F, D'Orlando L, Mercante WP. Electromechanical dissociation 48 hours after atenolol overdose: usefulness of calcium chloride. *Ann Emerg Med* 1998; 31: 777–81.

Pirotte JH. Apparent potentiation by phenobarbital of hepatotoxicity from small doses of acetaminophen. *Ann Intern Med* 1984; 101: 403.

Plotzker R, Jensen DM, Payne JA. *Amanita virosa* acute hepatic necrosis: treatment with thioctic acid. *Am J Med Sci* 1982; 283: 79–82.

Prescott LF. Paracetamol overdose: pharmacological considerations and clinical management. *Drugs* 1983; 25: 290–314.

Prescott LF. Paracetamol, alcohol and the liver. *Br J Clin Pharmacol* 2000; 49: 291–301.

Prescott LF, Illingworth RN, Critchley JAJH, Stewart MJ, Adam RD, Proudfoot AT. Intravenous N-acetylcysteine: treatment of choice for paracetamol poisoning. *Br Med J* 1979; 2: 1097–100.

Prescott LF, Donovan JW, Jarvie DR, Proudfoot AT. The disposition and kinetics of intravenous N-acetylcysteine in patients with paracetamol overdosage. *Eur J Clin Pharmacol* 1989; 37: 501–6.

Prosser PR, Karam JH. Diabetes mellitus following rodenticide ingestion in man. *J Am Med Assoc* 1978; 239: 1148–50.

Proudfoot AT. Antidotes: benefits and risks. *Toxicol Lett* 1995; 82/83: 779–83.

Reed DJ. Glutathione: toxicological implications. *Annu Rev Pharmacol Toxicol* 1990; 30: 603–31.

Renzi FP, Donovan JW, Martin TG, Morgan L, Harrison EF. Concomitant use of activated charcoal and N-acetylcysteine. *Ann Emerg Med* 1985; 14: 568–72.

Reynard K, Riley A, Walker BE. Respiratory arrest after N-acetylcysteine for paracetamol overdose [letter]. *Lancet* 1992; 340: 675.

Riggs BS, Bronstein AC, Kulig K, Archer PG, Rumack BH. Acute acetaminophen overdose during pregnancy. *Obstet Gynecol* 1989; 74: 247–53.

Roe DA, McCormick DB, Lin R-T. Effects of riboflavin on boric acid toxicity. *J Pharm Sci* 1972; 61: 1081–5.

Rosevear SK, Hope PL. Favourable neonatal outcome following maternal paracetamol overdose and severe fetal distress. *Br J Obstet Gynaecol* 1989; 96: 491–3.

■ CHAPTER 4 ■

Ryan JM, McCarthy G, Plunkett PK. Regional intravenous calcium – an effective method of treating hydrofluoric acid burns to limb peripheries. *J Accid Emerg Med* 1997; 14: 401–4.

Schaumberg H, Kaplan J, Windebank A, Vick N, Rasmus S, Pleasure D, Brown MJ. Sensory neuropathy from pyridoxine abuse: a new megavitamin syndrome. *N Engl J Med* 1983; 309: 445–8.

Sciuto AM, Strickland PT, Kennedy TP, Gurtner GH. Protective effects of N-acetylcysteine treatment after phosgene exposure in rabbits. *Am J Respir Crit Care Med* 1995; 151: 768–72.

Seeff LB, Cuccherini BA, Zimmerman HJ, Adler E, Benjamin SB. Acetaminophen hepatotoxicity in alcoholics: a therapeutic misadventure. *Ann Intern Med* 1986; 104: 399–404.

Simpson KJ, Lukacs NW, McGregor AH, Harrison DJ, Strieter RM, Kunkel SL. Inhibition of tumour necrosis factor alpha does not prevent experimental paracetamol-induced hepatic necrosis. *J Pathol* 2000; 190: 489–94.

Singalavanija A, Ruangvaravate N, Dulayajinda D. Potassium iodate toxic retinopathy: a report of five cases. *Retina* 2000; 20: 378–83.

Sjödin K, Nilsson E, Hallberg A, Tunek A. Metabolism of N-acetyl-L-cysteine: some structural requirements for the deacetylation and consequences for the oral bioavailability. *Biochem Pharmacol* 1989; 38: 3981–5.

Smilkstein MJ, Knapp GL, Kulig KW, Rumack BH. Efficacy of oral N-acetylcysteine in the treatment of acetaminophen overdose. Analysis of the national multicenter study (1976 to 1985). *N Engl J Med* 1988; 319: 1557–62.

Smilkstein MJ, Bronstein AC, Linden C, Augenstein WL, Kulig KW, Rumack BH. Acetaminophen overdose: a 48-hour intravenous N-acetylcysteine treatment protocol. *Ann Emerg Med* 1991; 20: 1058–63.

Smith RP. The significance of methemoglobinemia in toxicology. In: *Essays in Toxicology*. Blood FR (ed.). New York: Academic Press, 1969: 83–113.

Stambach T, Haire K, Soni N, Booth J. Saturday night blue – a case of near fatal poisoning from the abuse of amyl nitrite. *J Accid Emerg Med* 1997; 14: 339–40.

Steele CW, Spink WW. Methylene blue in the treatment of poisonings associated with methaemoglobinaemia: report of two cases. *N Engl J Med* 1933; 208: 1152–3.

Stenflo J, Suttie JW. Vitamin K-dependent formation of γ-carboxyglutamic acid. *Annu Rev Biochem* 1977; 46: 157–72.

Tanen DA, Ruha A-M, Curry SC, Graeme KA, Reagan CG. Hypertonic sodium bicarbonate is effective in the acute management of verapamil toxicity in a swine model. *Ann Emerg Med* 2000; 36: 547–53.

Underwood EJ (ed.). Molybdenum. In: *Trace Elements in Human and Animal Nutrition*. New York: Academic Press, 1977: 109–31.

Vale JA, Proudfoot AT. Paracetamol (acetaminophen) poisoning. *Lancet* 1995; 346: 547–52.

Vale JA, Meredith TJ, Goulding R. Treatment of acetaminophen poisoning: the use of oral methionine. *Arch Intern Med* 1981; 141: 394–6.

Vance MV, Curry SC, Kunkel DB, Ryan PJ, Ruggeri SB. Digital hydrofluoric acid burns: treatment with intraarterial calcium infusion. *Ann Emerg Med* 1986; 15: 890–6.

Vassallo S, Howland MA. Severe dichromate poisoning: survival after therapy with iv N-acetylcysteine and hemodialysis. *Vet Hum Toxicol* 1988; 30: 347.

Vassiliadis J, Graudins A, Dowsett RP. Triethylene glycol poisoning treated with intravenous ethanol infusion. *J Toxicol Clin Toxicol* 1999; 37: 773–6.

Velvart J. Arterial perfusion for hydrofluoric acid burns. *Hum Toxicol* 1983; 2: 233–8.

Walsh TS, Hopton P, Philips BJ, Mackenzie SJ, Lee A. The effect of N-acetylcystine on oxygen transport and uptake in patients with fulminant hepatic failure. *Hepatology* 1998; 27: 1332–40.

Wason S, Lacouture PG, Lovejoy FH. Single high-dose pyridoxine treatment for isoniazid overdose. *J Am Med Assoc* 1981; 246: 1102–4.

Wax PM, Hoffman RS. Sodium bicarbonate. In: *Contemporary Management in Critical Care*. Vol. 1 (Part 3): *Critical Care Toxicology*. Hoffman RS, Goldfrank LR (eds). New York: Churchill Livingstone, 1991: 81–108.

Wieth JO, Funder J. Treatment of bromide poisoning. Comparison of forced halogen turnover and haemodialysis. *Lancet* 1963; ii: 327–9.

Williams JR, Challis FE. Methylene blue as an antidote for anilin dye poisoning: case report with confirmatory experimental study. *J Lab Clin Med* 1933; 19: 166–71.

Wilson WL, Bottiglieri, NG. Phase I studies with pyrazole. *Cancer Chemother Rep* 1962; 21: 137–41.

Yarborough BE, Wood JP. Isoniazid overdose treated with high-dose pyridoxine. *Ann Emerg Med* 1983; 12: 303–5.

Young RJ, Critchley JAJH, Young KK, Freebairn RC, Reynolds AP, Lolin YI. Fatal acute hepatorenal failure following potassium permanganate ingestion. *Hum Exp Toxicol* 1996; 15: 259–61.

■ CHAPTER 4 ■

Pharmacological Antidotes

Contents

5.1 α-ADRENOCEPTOR ANTAGONISTS

Phenoxybenzamine (CAS 59-96-1) and phentolamine (Rogitine, Alliance; CAS 50-60-2; Figure 5.1) are, respectively, long- and short-acting α-adrenoceptor antagonists and cause peripheral vasodilatation. Phentolamine also has a direct action on vascular smooth muscle. These drugs are used to treat severe hypertension due to amphetamines, cocaine, clonidine, methylphenidate, monoamine oxidase inhibitors (MAOIs), oxedrine and phenylephrine. The use of β-blockers in such instances would lead to unopposed α-stimulation and hence worsened hypertension.

Phenoxybenzamine hydrochloride (1 mg/kg) is given i.v. in 250–500 mL 5 % (w/v) D-glucose over at least 2 h, while 2–5 mg phentolamine mesilate is given slowly by i.v. injection, repeated as necessary. In a child 20–100 μg/kg phentolamine mesilate is given i.v. as a loading dose, then $10–40 \ \mu g \ kg^{-1} \ h^{-1}$ as a maintenance dose if necessary (maximum $1 \ mg \ kg^{-1} \ d^{-1}$).

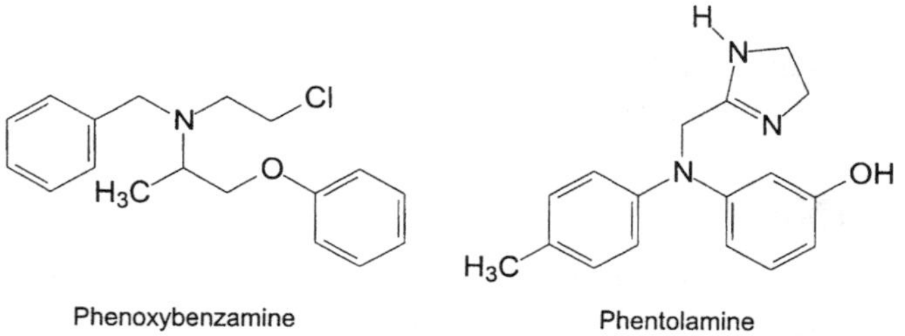

Figure 5.1: Structural formulae of phenoxybenzamine and phentolamine

5.2 β-ADRENOCEPTOR ANTAGONISTS

Propranolol (CAS 525-66-6; Figure 5.2) is a non-selective β-adrenoceptor blocking drug and suppresses sympathetic overactivity, reducing rate-related myocardial ischaemia. Propranolol has been used to control tachycardia, agitation and tremor after thyroxine overdose (Roesch *et al.*, 1985). Propranolol is also said to reverse hypokalaemia due to overdosage with β-adrenoceptor stimulants such as ephedrine, thyroxine and theophylline (Amin and Henry, 1985). In adults, propranolol hydrochloride (1–2 mg i.v. over 1 min initially, repeated every 2 min up to 5–10 mg, or 40 mg orally 6- to 8-hourly) is given, after atropine (0.6–1.2 mg i.v.). Propranolol is contraindicated for use in asthmatic patients or patients with chronic obstructive airways disease. Caution should be exercised in its use in patients with hepatic impairment as it normally undergoes extensive first-pass metabolism in the liver.

Esmolol (CAS 81147-92-4; Figure 5.2) is a short-acting cardioselective β_1-adrenoceptor blocker. It is commonly used to treat supraventricular tachycardia in theophylline or methylenedioxymethamphetamine (MDMA) poisoning (Jones and Dargan, 2001). The adult dose is 40 mg esmolol hydrochloride i.v. over 1 min, repeated as necessary. Esmolol can also be used to control hypertension where use of a longer acting β-blocker might be inappropriate, as in an elderly patient in whom some degree of chronic airway obstruction is a possibility. The infusion dose (esmolol hydrochloride) for an adult is 4 mg/min up to a maximum of 12 mg/min. It is ineffective in the management of ventricular tachycardia. Like propranolol, esmolol is contraindicated if the patient is known to have chronic airway obstruction or asthma.

■ CHAPTER 5 ■

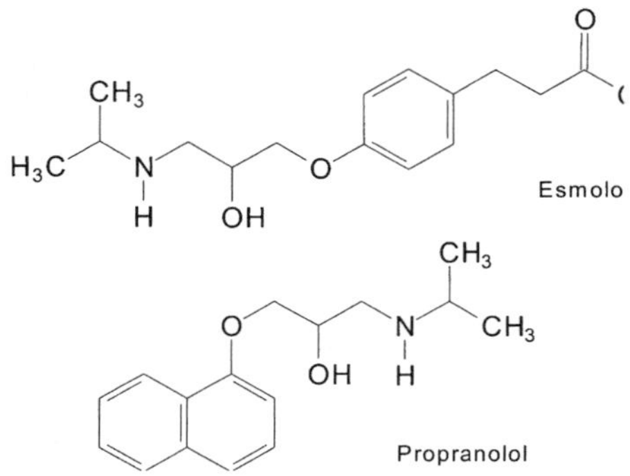

Figure 5.2: Structural formulae of esmolol and propranolol

Sotalol is not a suitable β-blocker for use in poisoned patients as it prolongs the QT interval and may precipitate ventricular arrhythmias.

5.3 ATROPINE

Atropine, an alkaloid extracted from *Atropa belladonna*, is a racemic mixture of hyoscyamine (Figure 5.3), of which *l*-hyoscyamine is almost entirely responsible for its antimuscarinic properties. The related compound hyoscine (scopolamine; Figure 5.3) has muscle relaxant properties. The activity of atropine towards different muscarinic receptor subtypes has been studied (Trovero *et al.*, 1998). Atropine is used to overcome the muscarinic features of anticholinesterase poisoning such as may be seen after exposure to carbamate and organophosphorus (OP) insecticides or OP nerve agents, i.e. nausea, vomiting, abdominal cramps, diarrhoea, bronchorrhoea, bronchospasm, miosis, bradycardia and involuntary micturition. In OP poisoning, atropine is usually used in combination with a cholinesterase reactivator such as pralidoxime (sections 5.9.2 and 7.3.2). Some compounds having greater antimuscarinic action than atropine, such as benactyzine (CAS 302-40-9), show greater protection in experimental OP poisoning when combined with a cholinesterase reactivator, but these compounds have not been used clinically in this role (Das Gupta *et al.*, 1991).

Atropine (sulphate)

CAS registry number (free base)	5908-99-6 (51-55-8)
Relative formula mass (free base)	676.8 (289.4)
pK_a (20 °C)	9.9
Oral absorption (%)	95
Presystemic metabolism	Negligible
Plasma half-life (h) (range)	2–5
Volume of distribution (L/kg)	1–6
Plasma protein binding (%)	50

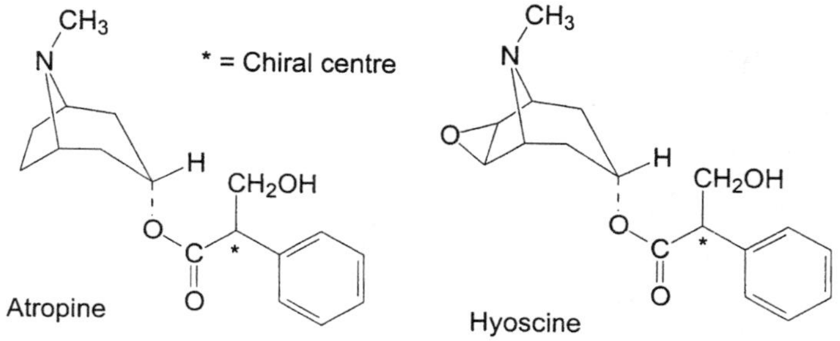

Figure 5.3: Structural formulae of atropine (hyoscyamine) and hyoscine (scopolamine)

In anticholinesterase poisoning the dose of atropine is titrated against clinical improvement, and in particular the heart rate (Heath and Meredith, 1992). At the doses used, atropine has little or no effect at the nicotinic receptors of the autonomic ganglia and neuromuscular junctions, where accumulation of acetylcholine in OP poisoning causes weakness, and eventually paralysis, of skeletal muscles, including those responsible for respiration; mechanical ventilation is then required (section 5.9.1). In severe poisoning, atropine sulphate should be given in an initial dose of 0.015–0.05 mg/kg (2 mg in adults) i.v. (i.m. or s.c. in less severe cases) followed by further doses at 5–10 min intervals until the clinical features of full atropinization become apparent. A dry mouth, a heart rate of 70–80 beats per minute, and reduction of bronchial secretions as judged by auscultation are the most reliable clinical features. Full atropinization should be continued for 2–3 d and large doses of the drug may be required (1–2 g atropine may be needed in a single day).

Features of atropine overdose are those of anticholinergic excess, i.e. dilated pupils (mydriasis), paralysed accommodation (cycloplegia), flushed dry skin, tachycardia, fever, ileus, disorientation, delirium, urinary retention and excessive drying of secretions. Adequate oxygenation is important as atropine can precipitate ventricular fibrillation in the presence of hypoxia. Atropine should be used with caution in the presence of

---

Atropine in clinical toxicology – I

- Atropine can reverse muscarinic features of carbamate and OP poisoning including nausea, vomiting, abdominal cramps, diarrhoea, bronchorrhoea, bronchospasm, miosis, bradycardia, involuntary micturition
- Atropine has little effect at nicotinic receptors, where accumulation of acetylcholine may paralyse skeletal muscles including those involved in respiration
- In severe OP poisoning in an adult, 2 mg atropine sulphate should be given i.v. and repeated as necessary
- Clinical features of atropinization include dry mouth, flushed red skin, dilated pupils and a heart rate of 70–80 beats/minute
- Adequate oxygenation important as atropine can cause ventricular fibrillation if hypoxia is present

---

Atropine in clinical toxicology – II

- Doses of 1–2 g/d atropine sulphate for several days may be needed in severe OP poisoning
- Features of atropine overdose include cycloplegia, tachycardia, fever, ileus, disorientation, delirium, urinary retention
- Physostigmine should not be used to reverse atropinization if an anticholinesterase is present
- Additional uses of atropine may include:
    - physostigmine overdose
    - poisoning with synthetic choline esters such as carbachol
    - after ingestion of *Amanita muscaria* or other fungi if muscarinic features are present

---

glaucoma, hypertension, hyperthermia and hypothyroidism, although in life-threatening OP poisoning such issues are peripheral. Physostigmine (section 5.8) should not be used to reverse atropinization if an anticholinesterase is present because of the risk of precipitating bronchospasm and cardiac arrhythmias.

In addition to its use in anticholinesterase poisoning, atropine may be indicated if physostigmine has been administered to excess, if synthetic choline esters (for example carbachol, urecholine) have been administered and after ingestion of *Amanita muscaria*, *Clitocybe* or *Inocybe* fungi if clear muscarinic features are present. Atropine (0.6 mg i.v. or s.c.) may also be given before intubation is performed after overdosage with β-adrenoceptor blocking drugs such as propranolol with the aim of preventing cardiovascular collapse due to vagal stimulation during the procedure.

5.4 BENZATROPINE AND DIPHENHYDRAMINE (TREATMENT OF DRUG-INDUCED DYSTONIAS)

Benzatropine [benztropine; (1R,3r,5S)-3-benzhydryloxytropane; Cogentin, MSD; Figure 5.4] and also diphenhydramine (Figure 5.4) can reverse dystonias associated with treatment with neuroleptics such as haloperidol, phenothiazines and thioxanthines, and with metoclopramide, by competitive inhibition of muscarinic receptors and blockade of dopamine reuptake. An example is oculogyric crisis, which is common in young women given i.v. metoclopramide. Benzatropine is also effective in drug-induced Parkinsonism as well as in true Parkinson's disease.

Benzatropine mesilate (mesylate, methanesulphonate) (either i.m. or i.v. at doses of 1–2 mg) or diphenhydramine (1–3 mg/kg i.m. or slowly i.v. up to 50 mg) rapidly reverse acute dystonias in adults (Hasan *et al.*, 1999). Patients with dystonias who have been poisoned by long-acting neuroleptics should be given continuation oral therapy for 3 days to prevent relapse (benzatropine 1–2 mg twice daily, diphenhydramine 25 mg thrice daily – one dose only is usually adequate in the case of metoclopramide toxicity). Benzatropine toxicity arises from its anticholinergic activity and diphenhydramine is the preferred agent in patients expected to tolerate anticholinergics poorly, such as

	Benzatropine (mesilate)	Diphenhydramine (hydrochloride)
CAS registry number	132-17-2	147-24-0
Relative formula mass (free base)	403.5 (307.4)	291.8 (255.4)
pK_a	10.0	9.0 (25 °C)
Oral absorption (%)	–	> 90
Presystemic metabolism (%)	–	50
Plasma half-life (h) (mean, range)	–	3.3 (2.4–8)
Volume of distribution (L/kg)	–	c. 3
Plasma protein binding (%)	–	85–98

those with pre-existing cardiovascular disease. Benzatropine is contraindicated in patients with glaucoma or with prostatic hypertrophy.

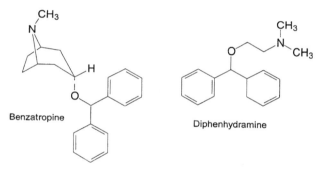

Figure 5.4: Structural formulae of benzatropine and diphenhydramine

5.5 BENZYLPENICILLIN

High-dose benzylpenicillin sodium (penicillin G; CAS 69-57-8; Figure 5.5), 250 mg/kg i.v. daily in divided doses, has been advocated in treating death-cap mushroom (*Amanita phalloides*) poisoning. One suggestion is that benzylpenicillin displaces *Amanita* toxins from binding sites on plasma albumin, thereby facilitating their excretion in urine. Alternatively, benzylpenicillin may inhibit hepatic uptake of the toxins (Hruby *et al.*, 1983). The evidence of efficacy is sparse, although, as the toxicity of benzylpenicillin is so low, it is often given. A history of penicillin allergy is an absolute contraindication to use of benzylpenicillin.

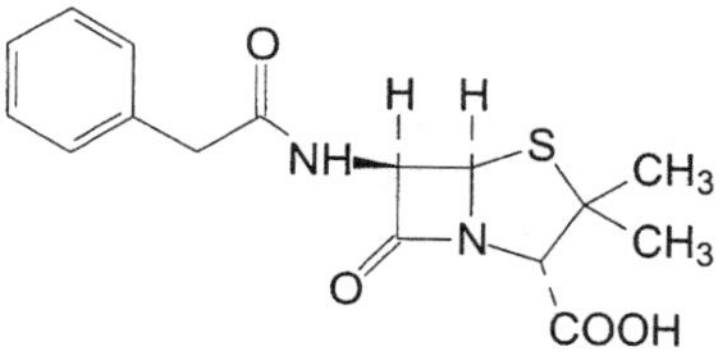

Figure 5.5: Structural formula of benzylpenicillin

5.6 CALCITONIN

Calcitonin (CAS 9007-12-9) is a peptide hormone (formula weight *c.* 4,500). Salmon calcitonin (4 U/kg twice daily i.m., 15 days) was used to treat hypervitaminosis D in an 8-month-old boy who had been given 300,000 IU vitamin D orally four times over 60 days. He had presented with nausea and vomiting and had failed to respond to conventional treatment (Mete *et al.*, 1997). His serum calcium was 3.95 mmol/L (15.8 mg/dL) on admission and 2.45 mmol/L (9.8 mg/L) after calcitonin treatment.

5.7 CALCIUM CHANNEL AGONISTS

The calcium entry promoter 4-aminopyridine (4-AP; CAS 504-24-5; Figure 5.6) has been used in conjunction with haemodialysis in treating severe poisoning with verapamil (ter Wee *et al.*, 1985). The investigational calcium entry promoter BAYK8644 (methyl [1,4-dihydro-2,6-dimethyl-5-nitro-4-(2-(trifluoromethyl)phenyl]pyridine-3-carboxylate; CAS 71145-04-4; Figure 5.6) was found to be effective in treating verapamil poisoning in rabbits (Korstanje *et al.*, 1987) but was less effective than 4-AP in treating verapamil poisoning in rats (Tuncok *et al.*, 1998).

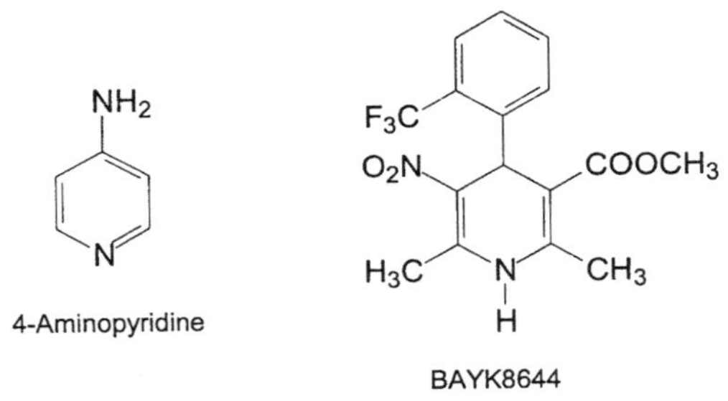

Figure 5.6: Structural formulae of 4-aminopyridine and BAYK8644

5.8 CHOLINESTERASE INHIBITORS

The active site of acetylcholinesterase (AChE) is thought to be based on the hydroxyl moiety of serine. An adjacent anionic site based on the imidazole group of histidine attracts the positively charged quaternary nitrogen atom of acetylcholine and brings the serine hydroxyl into juxtaposition with the electrophilic carbon atom of the carbonyl group of the molecule. Choline is split off, leaving the acetylated enzyme, which then undergoes hydrolysis, and the enzyme is regenerated (Figure 5.7). The time taken for a molecule of acetylcholine to undergo this reaction is about 80 µs.

Edrophonium (Figure 5.8) is a quaternary ammonium compound that is available as either the chloride (CAS 116-38-1) or the bromide. It is a reversible cholinesterase inhibitor and has actions similar to those of neostigmine, except that the effect of edrophonium on skeletal muscle is claimed to be particularly prominent. Edrophonium may be preferred to neostigmine in reversing intense block due to the short-acting competitive agent mivacurium. Edrophonium has also been suggested for reversal of neuromuscular blockade in patients poisoned with anticholinesterase nerve agents who require surgery (Karalliedde *et al.*, 1991). Its action is rapid in onset and of short

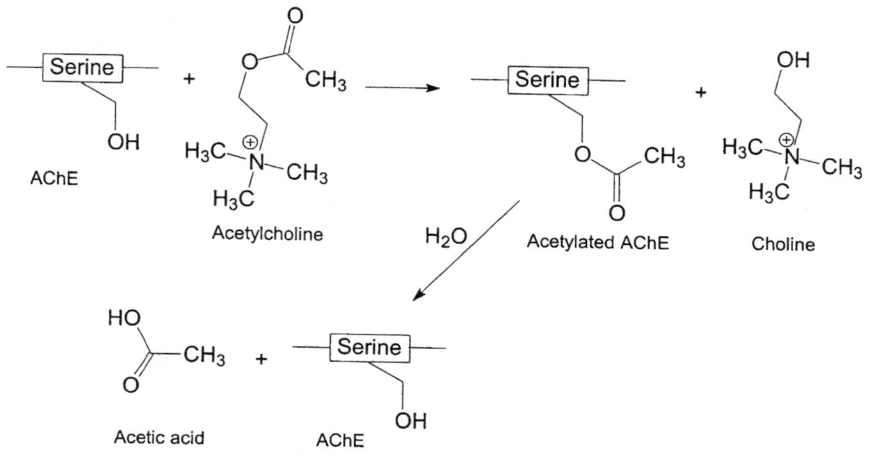

Figure 5.7: Schematic of the hydrolysis of acetylcholine by acetylcholinesterase

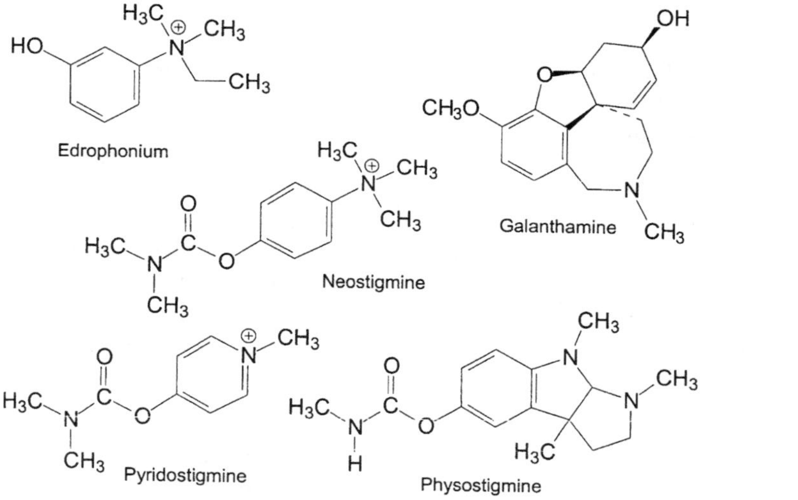

Figure 5.8: Structural formulae of edrophonium, galanthamine, neostigmine, pyridostigmine and physostigmine

duration. Studies in mice have suggested that edrophonium may have a role in preventing reinhibition of AChE after reactivation by certain oximes (obidoxime, trimedoxime – see section 5.9.2) if used in the treatment of OP pesticide poisoning (Luo *et al.*, 1999a,b).

Galanthamine (galantamine; CAS 357-70-0; Figure 5.8) is found in Caucasian snowdrop (Voronov's snowdrop, *Galanthus woronowii*) and other *Galanthus* species. Galanthamine, possibly Homer's 'moly' (section 1.4), is an orally active reversible cholinesterase inhibitor with actions similar to those of neostigmine but with a longer

■ CHAPTER 5 ■

plasma half-life (Bickel *et al.*, 1991). It is under investigation for use in Alzheimer's disease and other conditions where it is thought that prolonged cholinesterase inhibition might be beneficial.

Neostigmine (Figure 5.8) reversibly inactivates cholinesterases via carbamylation of the active site, giving rise to cholinergic reactions that commence after 0.5–1 h and last for about 4 h. Neostigmine is a quaternary ammonium compound and, unlike physostigmine, does not cross the blood–brain barrier. It is given i.m. to terminate the effects of competitive neuromuscular blocking drugs such as tubocurarine. Adverse effects include bradycardia, increased salivation, anorexia, nausea and vomiting, abdominal cramps and diarrhoea.

Pyridostigmine (Figure 5.8) is an anticholinesterase with actions similar to those of neostigmine but slower in onset and of longer duration. Like neostigmine, it is a quaternary ammonium compound and penetration into the CNS is poor. It is thought to be less satisfactory than neostigmine in reversing neuromuscular blockade due to drugs such as tubocurarine, and is used mainly in the treatment of myasthenia gravis. However, pyridostigmine has also been given prophylactically to protect against attack with anticholinesterase chemical warfare agents (section 7.3.5). Pyridostigmine binds reversibly to AChE and provides a protected store from which active AChE is later regenerated. Pyridostigmine prophylaxis greatly enhances the efficacy of atropine (section 5.3) and pralidoxime (section 5.9.2) against soman exposure, but it is not effective alone and may not be uniformly effective against other OP nerve agents. An oral dose of 30 mg pyridostigmine bromide 8-hourly provides optimum protection – although adverse effects are common at this dosage the ability to perform military duties is not impaired (Keeler *et al.*, 1991; section 7.3.5).

Physostigmine (eserine; Figure 5.8) reversibly inactivates cholinesterases via carbamylation of the active site, giving rise to cholinergic reactions that last for several hours. Unlike neostigmine, physostigmine does cross the blood–brain barrier, and thus central effects occur. Physostigmine can be used to treat serious poisoning with atropine, hyoscine, tricyclic and tetracyclic antidepressants and other anticholinergics, as discussed in recent reports (Schmidt and Lang, 1997; Sopchak *et al.*, 1998). However, the risks of administration generally outweigh the possible benefits. Thus,

	Neostigmine (bromide)	Physostigmine (sulphate)	Pyridostigmine (bromide)
CAS registry number	114-80-7	64-47-1	101-26-8
Relative formula mass	303.2	648.8	261.1
pK_a	12.0	1.8, 7.9	–
Oral absorption (%)	< 40	Good	Low
Presystemic metabolism (%)	–	11–37	–
Plasma half-life (range)	1 (0.4–1.3) h	20 (12–40) min	0.4–1.9
Volume of distribution (L/kg)	0.1–1.1	0.2–1.2	0.53–1.8
Plasma protein binding (%)	Negligible	–	Negligible

physostigmine does not affect the mortality rate in poisoning with tricyclic and tetracyclic antidepressants, and may exacerbate the risk of grand mal seizures and arrhythmias (Aquilonius and Hedstrand, 1978; Knudsen and Heath, 1984). Similarly, although i.v. physostigmine has been shown to reverse the central effects of baclofen, including coma, within 2 min of administration (Müller-Schwefe and Penn, 1989), it is not always effective and there may be major side-effects, including bradycardia, urinary retention and increased airway secretions. Further relative contraindications to the use of physostigmine include the presence of cardiovascular disease, gastrointestinal obstruction or asthma.

Anticholinesterases such as neostigmine have been used in treating snake bite and in patients poisoned with tetrodotoxin. Edrophonium given i.v. has produced an increase in motor power in patients with respiratory distress and paresis or reduced muscle power following ingestion of puffer fish (*Sphaeroides maculatus* or *Arothron stellatus*) (Chew *et al.*, 1984). Recovery was thought to be accelerated by subsequent treatment with neostigmine. In mild poisoning, neostigmine i.m. alone has brought about improvement in paraesthesia and numbness. There have been no controlled trials in this area, however.

5.9 CHOLINESTERASE REACTIVATORS

5.9.1 Organophosphorus anticholinesterases

OP insecticides were developed in the 1930s as replacements for nicotine, pyrethrum and rotenone. The OP insecticide tetraethylpyrophosphate (TEPP) was marketed in Germany in 1944. More toxic, more volatile, but less persistent OPs were also developed as chemical warfare agents in Germany at this time (section 7.1). Nowadays, more than 100 OP insecticides are used worldwide (Johnson *et al.*, 2000). Although OP insecticides and chemical warfare agents (nerve agents) have many complex actions, their principal effect is inhibition of cholinesterases, particularly acetylcholinesterase (AChE, EC 3.1.1.7) (Minton and Murray, 1988; Wagner, 1997). This leads to accumulation of acetylcholine at muscarinic receptors (cholinergic effector cells), nicotinic receptors (skeletal neuromuscular junction and autonomic ganglia) and in the CNS. OP insecticides are well absorbed by ingestion, inhalation and through the skin; with chemical warfare agents exposure is normally by inhalation or through the skin. The onset, severity and duration of poisoning are dependent on the route of exposure and the agent involved. The onset of clinical effects is usually within 1–2 h but can be as early as 5 min after exposure or delayed for up to 12 h.

Features of acute OP poisoning include muscarinic effects (vomiting, abdominal pain, diarrhoea, miosis, sweating, hypersalivation and dyspnoea due to broncho-constriction and excessive bronchial secretions), nicotinic effects (muscle fasciculation, tremor and later weakness) and CNS effects (anxiety, headache, loss of memory, drowsiness and coma). Although bradycardia would be predicted from the mechanism of action, tachycardia occurs in some 30 % of cases. Later, flaccid muscle paralysis with paralysis of limb muscles, respiratory muscles and sometimes extraocular muscles occurs. Respiratory muscle paralysis, bronchoconstriction and the presence of copious respiratory secretions contribute to respiratory failure, but depression of respiratory drive is probably the single most important factor. Coma occurs in severely poisoned patients; rarely hyperglycaemia, complete heart block and arrhythmias also occur. However, respiratory complications are the major cause of death in severely poisoned patients. In animals, diaphragm muscle fibre necrosis can be demonstrated 24 h after exposure to a variety of OPs (Cavaliere *et al.*, 1998).

5.9.1.1 Delayed features in OP poisoning

Some 10–40 % of patients poisoned with OP insecticides develop the so-called 'intermediate syndrome' (Johnson *et al.*, 2000). This is characterized by cranial nerve and brain stem lesions and a proximal neuropathy commencing 1–4 days after exposure and lasting for some 3 weeks. Respiratory depression is a complication, and ventilatory support is required as the 'intermediate syndrome' is said to be unresponsive to atropine and oximes. The syndrome has been said to be due to inadequate oxime therapy, but the aetiology is probably more complicated. Treatment with glycopyrrolate in addition to atropine and oximes has been advocated in such cases (Choi *et al.*, 1998).

OP-induced delayed neuropathy is rare and starts 2–5 weeks after massive exposure to only a few OPs and is the result of degeneration of large myelinated motor and sensory fibres (Johnson *et al.*, 2000). An initial flaccidity and muscle weakness in the arms and legs gives rise to a clumsy shuffling gait and is followed later by spasticity, hypertonicity, hyperreflexia and clonus. In many patients, recovery is limited to the arms and hands, and damage to lower extremities such as foot drop is permanent. The OPs that can give rise to delayed neuropathy have been phased out in most developed countries. Early antidotal treatment (see below) is ineffective in preventing the onset of neuropathy in susceptible individuals.

5.9.1.2 Assessment of severity and management

In general, clinical features are more helpful than red cell AChE measurements in assessing the severity of intoxication and the prognosis. There is wide inter-individual variation in cholinesterase activity, although there is a rough correlation between cholinesterase activity and clinical effects ($\sim$ 50 % cholinesterase activity in subclinical poisoning, 20–50 % activity in mild poisoning and < 10 % activity in severe poisoning). An ECG should be carried out in all OP-poisoned patients, and blood glucose, urea and electrolytes should be monitored.

The management of acute poisoning with OPs includes clearing the airway, ensuring adequate ventilation and giving high-flow oxygen. After dermal exposure, soiled clothing should be removed and placed in double-sealed bags and the skin thoroughly washed with soap and water. If the compound has been ingested, gastric lavage may be undertaken if the patient presents within approximately 1 h of ingestion. Activated charcoal (50 g in an adult) should be left in the stomach. If possible, it is wise to confirm the diagnosis by measuring cholinesterase activity, preferably in both red cells and plasma. Patients who are severely poisoned with OPs should be managed in an intensive care unit. Convulsions and twitching should be controlled with intravenous diazepam (10–20 mg for an adult, 0.2 mg/kg for a child), which may also have additional benefits (section 7.3.3).

Sodium bicarbonate (section 4.15) was found to decrease mortality by 85 % in dogs poisoned with an OP (Cordoba *et al.*, 1983) and has been used to treat arrhythmias in patients with OP poisoning. The adult i.v. dose is 50 mL of 8.4 % (w/v) sodium bicarbonate (50 mmol). Subsequent doses may be given to maintain blood pH at 7.4–7.5. There are anecdotal reports of efficacy (Johnson *et al.*, 2000).

Atropine (section 5.3) reduces bronchorrhoea, bronchospasm, salivation and abdominal colic and should be repeated every 10 min until signs of atropinization (flushed red skin, tachycardia, dilated pupils and dry mouth) develop. Up to 30 mg of atropine or more may be required in the first day, and therapy may have to be continued for a prolonged period. Atropine in conjunction with supportive measures has been used successfully to treat severe OP poisoning (de Silva *et al.*, 1992).

Cholinesterase reactivators, such as the oximes pralidoxime and obidoxime, are helpful if given before the OP–cholinesterase enzyme complex 'ages'. In the UK, pralidoxime should be given in addition to atropine to every symptomatic patient by slow i.v. injection. Clinical improvement (cessation of convulsions and fasciculation, improved muscle power and recovery of consciousness) usually occurs within 20–30 min. The need for further therapy is guided by clinical observation together with monitoring of red cell AChE activity. If necessary, further doses of pralidoxime can be given (see below). Side-effects are seen at high rates of administration (more than 500 mg/min). They include tachycardia, muscular rigidity, neuromuscular blockade, hypertension and laryngospasm. Haemoperfusion and haemodialysis are of no benefit in OP poisoning.

5.9.2 Mechanism of action and use of cholinesterase reactivators

The toxicity of OP insecticides and of carbamate insecticides is due to inhibition of cholinesterase with consequent accumulation of acetylcholine at nicotinic and muscarinic receptors in autonomic ganglia, neuromuscular junctions, smooth muscle, glands and the CNS (Ballantyne and Marrs, 1992; Johnson *et al.*, 2000). OP nerve agents, such as tabun, sarin and soman, act similarly (section 7.3). The excess of acetylcholine at synapses leads to stimulation and later inhibition of neurotransmission. As discussed above, atropine (section 5.3) blocks the effects of anticholinesterase agents at muscarinic receptors, whereas asoxime, obidoxime (LüH-6; Toxogonin) and pralidoxime (2-pyridine aldoxime methyl; 2-PAM) and some other oximes (Table 5.1; Figures 5.9 and 5.10) can reactivate phosphorylated cholinesterase and form inert complexes with many OPs (some exceptions are given in Table 5.2).

OPs react with cholinesterase to produce, for example, phosphorylated enzyme. With some OPs, hydrolysis at the phosphorylated site occurs over a period of hours and active enzyme is regenerated. However, with OPs such as di-isopropyl phosphofluoridate (DFP), hydrolysis does not occur to any marked extent and return of enzyme activity is dependent upon synthesis of new enzyme. Oximes used in treatment can react with the phosphorylated enzyme to form an oxime–OP complex, thus regenerating active enzyme (Figure 5.11). The speed of this reaction varies depending on the nature of the phosphoryl group. Pralidoxime, for example, is a more potent reactivator of cholinesterase after some OPs than others (Sterri *et al.*, 1979). Pralidoxime has no effect against AChE inhibited by soman (section 7.3.2).

Ideally, an oxime should be given simultaneously with atropine to treat OP poisoning but, if not readily available, the oxime should be administered as soon as possible after atropine (Bismuth *et al.*, 1992). Phosphorylated or phosphonylated cholinesterase appears to 'age' so that it becomes resistant to reactivation by oximes. This probably results from the loss of an alkyl or alkoxy group to produce the much more stable

TABLE 5.1
Classification of oximes evaluated for use in OP insecticide and nerve agent poisoning

Class	Subclass	Examples	CAS registry number (may sometimes refer to various salts)
Monopyridinium oximes	–	Pralidoxime iodide (2-PAM, 2-PAMI)	94-63-3
		Pralidoxime methanesulphonate/ mesilate (P$_2$S, PAMM)	154-97-2
		Pralidoxime methylsulphate (Contrathion)	1200-55-1
		Pralidoxime chloride (2-PAMCl, Protopam chloride)	51-15-0
		Pyrimidoxime dibromide	69445-02-9
		Obidoxime dichloride (BH-6, LüH-6, Toxogonin)	114-90-9
Bispyridinium dioximes	–	Trimedoxime dibromide (obidoxime + methyl, TMB-4)	56-97-3
		Methoxime dichloride (MMB-4)	61444-84-6
Bispyridinium [Hagedorn (H)] oximes	Carboxamides	Asoxime (HI-6, HJ-6) dichloride	34433-31-3
		BI-6 dibromide	–
		HS-6 dichloride	22625-23-6
		HS-7 dibromide	34211-36-4
	Dioxime	HS-3 dichloride	25487-36-9
	Dioxime carboxamide	HLö-7 diiodide	120103-35-7
	Mono-oxime	HS-14 dichloride	34211-28-4
	Benzoyl	HGG-12 dichloride	83972-73-0
	Cyclohexylcarboxy	HGG-42 dichloride	71752-85-7

TABLE 5.2
OP pesticides against which oximes have limited efficacy

Crotoxyphos (Ciodrin)	Morphothion
Demeton	Schradan
Dimethoate	Prothoate
Dimefox	Triamiphos
Methyl-phenkapton	

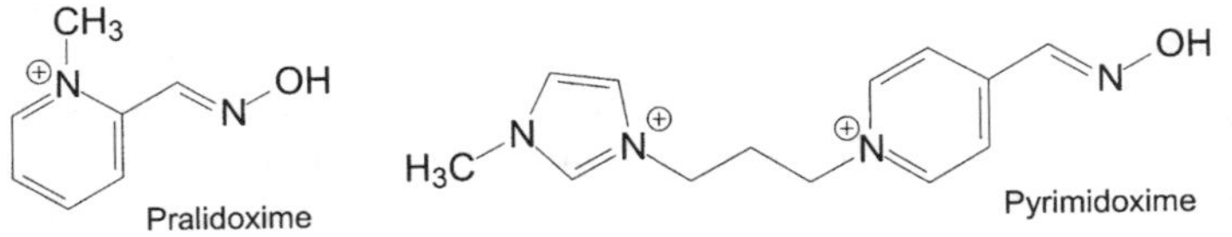

Figure 5.9: Structural formulae of the monopyridinium oximes pralidoxime and pyrimidoxime

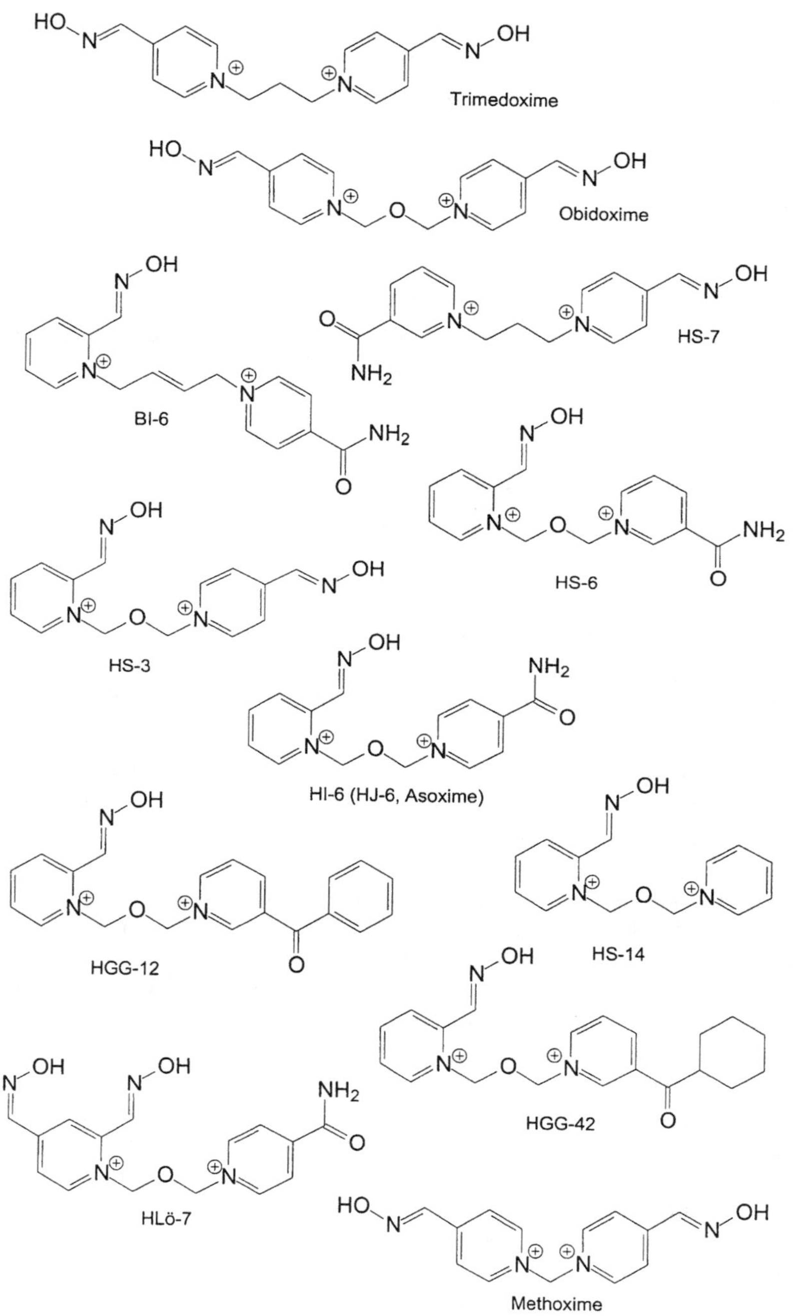

Figure 5.10: Structural formulae of some bipyridinium oximes

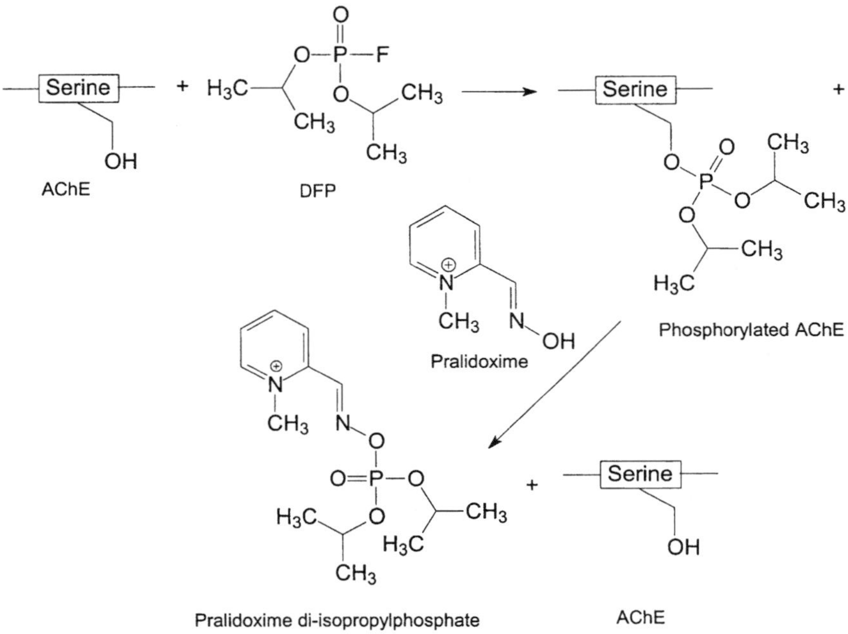

Figure 5.11: Schematic of the reaction of di-isopropyl phosphofluoridate (DFP) with acetylcholinesterase and subsequent reactivation of the enzyme with pralidoxime

monoalkyl- or monoalkoxy-phosphoryl–enzyme complex. The rate of 'ageing' is different with different OPs, and different people have different sensitivities to OPs.

Reactivation by some oximes has been reported to be faster in the presence of quaternary ammonium AChE ligands such as 1,1'-(oxybis(methylene))bis(4-(1,1-dimethylethyl)pyridinium) dichloride (SAD-128; CAS 40225-02-3) and decamethonium bromide (CAS 541-22-0). This phenomenon was first observed in experiments with human erythrocyte AChE using soman and sarin to obtain inhibited enzyme (Harris *et al.*, 1978). It was found that SAD-128 slowed the ageing of soman-inhibited AChE and thereby extended the period during which obidoxime and trimedoxime were able to restore enzyme activity before ageing took place. A similar effect has been observed in the presence of other monoquaternary and bisquaternary ligands, such as tetramethylammonium, suxamethonium, hexamethonium and edrophonium (Luo *et al.*, 1998). For sarin-inhibited AChE, it was suggested that the enhancement of reactivation could not simply be attributed to delayed 'ageing' because of the slow ageing of the AChE–sarin conjugate compared with that of the AChE–soman complex. Explanations such as decreasing the rate of inhibition by parent OP or conformational changes due to tight binding of the quaternary ammonium ligands at the peripheral site of the enzyme were suggested (Harris *et al.*, 1978). However, recent studies in mice have suggested that, with obidoxime or trimedoxime, the cholinesterase inhibitor edrophonium (section 5.8) may act by preventing reinhibition of AChE by phosphorylated oxime formed during the oxime–OP inhibited AChE reactivation sequence (Luo *et al.*, 1999b). Edrophonium may have a practical role in preventing reinhibition of AChE after reactivation by obidoxime and trimedoxime if these compounds are used in the treatment of OP pesticide poisoning (Luo *et al.*, 1999a).

It is thought that oximes such as pralidoxime and obidoxime have no beneficial effect in carbamate poisoning as the oxime–carbamate–enzyme complex formed does not hydrolyse rapidly to leave the regenerated enzyme. Indeed, this process is thought to be slower for the oxime complex than for the carbamaylated enzyme alone (Figure 5.12). Furthermore, work in animals suggests that pralidoxime and obidoxime may exacerbate toxicity in poisoning with some carbamates, especially carbaryl (Natoff and Reiff, 1973; Sterri *et al.*, 1979), although this work has not been validated in humans. Be this as it may, there have been two reports of carbamate (aldicarb and methomyl) poisoning in which administration of pralidoxime was thought to be associated with clinical improvement (Burgess *et al.*, 1994; Ekins and Geller, 1994), and the whole topic has been reviewed (Kurtz, 1990; Mortensen, 1990).

5.9.2.1 Clinical use of cholinesterase reactivators

Oximes in general are most effective when given within 24 h of OP exposure, and should preferably be given within a few hours (Johnson *et al.*, 2000). They are less effective if given more than 36–48 h after exposure. The effects of pralidoxime are most prominent at skeletal neuromuscular junctions, and muscle weakness and fasciculation should improve within 10 min of oxime administration; little effect is seen at autonomic receptor sites and almost none in the CNS. The efficacy of each oxime is also dependent on the compound involved. OPs against which pralidoxime is said to be effective include amiton, demeton-methyl, diazinon, dichlorvos, disulfoton, dyflos, fenthion, malathion, mevinphos, parathion, parathion-methyl, phosphamidon and TEPP. Agents against which pralidoxime appears to be less effective include dimefox, dimethoate, methyl diazinon, mipafos and schradan.

Obidoxime, a dioxime, has been said to be a more effective reactivator than pralidoxime (Erdmann and Engelhard, 1964; Vasić *et al.*, 1977; Schoene *et al.*, 1988). Like pralidoxime, obidoxime may also detoxify some OPs directly (Finkelstein *et al.*, 1988). Also, like pralidoxime, obidoxime is more effective against some OPs (parathion, for example) and less effective against others (malathion, dimethoate, fenthion). In animals, obidoxime is ineffective against triamphos, mevinphos and demeton-*O*-

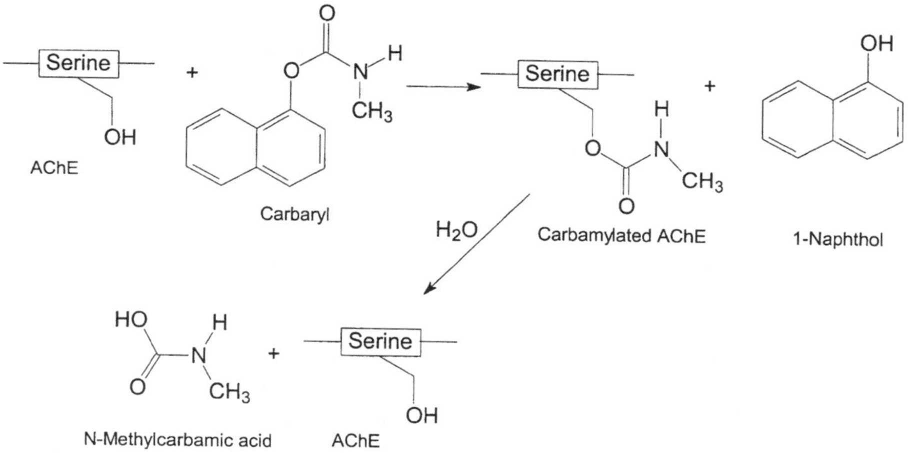

Figure 5.12: Schematic of the reaction of carbaryl with acetylcholinesterase

methylsulphoxide (Hahn and Henschler, 1969). Low-dose obidoxime has an anticholinergic, atropine-like effect, while high-dose obidoxime can inhibit AChE activity and lead to mild cholinergic signs (Schoene *et al.*, 1988). However, concern about the possible hepatic toxicity of obidoxime has limited clinical use of the drug (Finkelstein *et al.*, 1989).

Parenteral administration of pralidoxime to volunteers can cause heaviness of the eyes, blurred vision and difficulty in accommodation. Patients should be warned about its effects before it is given if they are conscious (Holland and Parkes, 1976). Rapid i.v. administration of pralidoxime has been associated with apparently dose-related dizziness, blurred vision, diplopia, headache, drowsiness, nausea, tachycardia, muscle rigidity, neuromuscular blockade, hypertension, hyperventilation and laryngospasm. Pralidoxime must be used cautiously in patients with myasthenia gravis because it may precipitate a myasthenic crisis in patients under treatment with anti-cholinesterases. In such patients mechanical ventilation is preferable.

A further oxime, 2,3-butanedione monoxime (diacetylmonoxime, DAM; CAS 57-71-6), was once used in the treatment of OP pesticide poisoning but is now considered obsolete.

	Obidoxime (dichloride)	Pralidoxime (chloride)
CAS registry number	114-90-9	51-15-0
Relative formula mass (free base)	359.2 (289.2)	172.6 (137.1)
pK_a (25 °C)	7.6, 8.3	8.0
Oral absorption (%)	Poor	< 30
Presystemic metabolism	Negligible	–
Plasma half-life (min)	83	75
Volume of distribution (L/kg)	0.17	0.6
Plasma protein binding (%)	Very low	Very low

5.9.2.2 Pralidoxime formulation and dosage

Pralidoxime was originally formulated as the iodide (2-pyridine aldoxime methiodide, 2-PAM, 2-PAM iodide, 2-PAMI). The chloride (2-PAM chloride, 2-PAMCl), methanesulphonate (P_2S, 2-PAM mesylate, 2-PAMM) and methyl sulphate salts have replaced the iodide in many countries as they are more soluble in water and produce fewer adverse effects. 2-PAMCl and P_2S are equally effective. Early experiments in cats suggested that plasma pralidoxime concentrations of 4 mg/L or more are required to counteract fully neuromuscular block, bradycardia, hypotension and respiratory failure due to cholinesterase inhibition (Vale and Meredith, 1986). The duration of action is 1.5–2 h after parenteral administration. If the poison is still present, prolonged administration may be necessary – atropine and pralidoxime were continued for 30 and 37 days, respectively, in one patient poisoned with fenthion (Merrill and Mihm, 1982). Pralidoxime is primarily excreted by glomerular filtration and active transport in the kidney, hence reduced dosage may be needed if renal failure is present, but only if the glomerular filtration rate (GFR) is less than 30 mL/min (Sidell and Groff, 1971; Vale and Meredith 1986). Heat and exercise decreased the renal excretion of pralidoxime in volunteers (Swartz and Sidell, 1972). Pralidoxime is not significantly bound to plasma protein.

The bioavailability of pralidoxime after oral doses of P_2S or 2-PAMCl is 20–30 % (Thompson et al., 1987). The administration of aqueous 2-PAMI (71–143 mg/kg) to volunteers produced pralidoxime concentrations above 4 mg/L 3 h after dosing, concentrations which were maintained above 4 mg/L for a further 2 h (Kondritzer et al., 1968). The administration of 5 g (71 mg/kg in 10 tablets) 2-PAMCl 4-hourly produced plasma pralidoxime concentrations above 4 mg/L, though most subjects experienced gastrointestinal symptoms such as diarrhoea and vomiting (Sidell et al., 1969). The terminal elimination half-life of pralidoxime in these studies was 1.7–2.7 h (Kondritzer et al., 1968; Sidell et al., 1969). However, the delay in obtaining therapeutically effective plasma concentrations and the oxime-induced side-effects are arguments against the use of oral therapy in OP poisoning. In addition, for military purposes, the need to wear a face mask precludes the use of oral pralidoxime except in prophylaxis.

In volunteers, i.m. injection of more than 7.5 mg/kg 2-PAMCl was required to produce plasma pralidoxime concentrations above 4 mg/L (Sidell and Groff, 1971). This concentration was reached within 5–10 min and sustained for 1 h. The plasma half-life of pralidoxime was 1.3 h. P_2S (20–30 mg/kg) i.m. produced peak pralidoxime concentrations of 8–25 mg/L after 5–20 min, although the rate of absorption and the maximal plasma concentration varied considerably between resting subjects, perhaps because of different depths of injection. Therapeutic pralidoxime concentrations were maintained for 90–170 min. In a further study, therapeutic pralidoxime concentrations in humans were maintained for more than 6 h after i.m. 2-PAMCl (30 mg/kg). There is no significant difference in the rate of uptake of P_2S as judged by plasma concentrations following a single i.m. injection of P_2S (500–750 mg) and atropine (2 mg) or P_2S (500–750 mg) alone (Holland et al., 1975; Vale and Meredith, 1986).

Sidell and Groff (1971) administered 2-PAMCl (2.5–10 mg/kg) i.v. to volunteers and found that doses above 7.5 mg/kg were necessary to produce plasma pralidoxime concentrations of more than 4 mg/L for 1 h. The plasma half-life of pralidoxime was 1.2 h. Injection of 2-PAMCl i.v. (15–30 mg/kg) gave pralidoxime concentrations of more than 4 mg/L for 6 h. In the same study, i.v. P_2S (45 mg/kg) produced 'therapeutic' plasma pralidoxime concentrations for only 4 h (Vale and Meredith, 1986). However, plasma pralidoxime concentrations up to 20 mg/L may be needed to achieve enzyme reactivation in serious OP poisoning.

Administration of 2-PAM to children poisoned with OP pesticides [25 mg/kg loading dose in 0.9 % (w/v) sodium chloride i.v. over 15–30 min, followed by i.v. infusion of 10–20 mg kg^{-1} h^{-1} for 18–60 h] has been advocated on the basis of clinical experience in seven patients (Farrer et al., 1990). A pralidoxime infusion (500 mg/h) was used in the treatment of a 2-year-old boy who had ingested chlorpyriphos (Tush and Anstead, 1997).

In summary, plasma pralidoxime concentrations of 4 mg/L and above may be achieved by giving pralidoxime: (i) orally (71 mg/kg) 4-hourly, although adverse effects, including diarrhoea and vomiting, may be limiting; (ii) i.m. (30 mg/kg) 4- to 6-hourly; and (iii) i.v. (30 mg/kg over 5–10 min) 4-hourly (P_2S) and 6-hourly (2-PAMCl). In severe OP poisoning, we would advocate the i.v. route. The rate of i.v. administration should not exceed 500 mg/min otherwise weakness, blurred vision, diplopia, dizziness, headache, nausea and tachycardia may develop. After two bolus doses of P_2S have been given 4 h apart, the drug may be given as an i.v. infusion (8 mg kg^{-1} h^{-1}) in either 5 % (w/v) D-

CHAPTER 5

glucose or 0.9 % (w/v) sodium chloride. It is possible that higher doses of pralidoxime will be needed to achieve AChE reactivation in severe OP poisoning.

5.9.2.3 Obidoxime dosage

Obidoxime chloride is poorly absorbed after oral administration and is normally given parenterally. When given i.m. in doses of 2.5–10 mg/kg, obidoxime reached dose-related peak plasma concentrations of between 5.3 and 26.5 mg/L after 20 min and had a plasma half-life of approximately 80 min (Sidell and Groff, 1970). Up to 90 % of a parenteral dose is excreted unchanged in urine (Sidell *et al.*, 1972), hence the drug should be used with caution in the presence of renal impairment.

Obidoxime has a much smaller V_D than pralidoxime and a longer plasma half-life, and thus plasma concentrations are five times those of pralidoxime after similar (w/w) i.v. doses (Sidell *et al.*, 1972). An i.v. dose of 250 mg obidoxime (4 mg/kg in a typical adult) has proved to be effective and largely free of adverse effects, except hepatotoxicity, in treating OP poisoning. Plasma obidoxime concentrations of 1 mg/L are thought to be effective, and thus the duration of action of obidoxime in the presence of an OP is about 4 h, by which time plasma concentrations have dropped to 1–2 mg/L (Sidell *et al.*, 1972). Obidoxime has a wide therapeutic range, and even neuromuscular blockade due to AChE inhibition is minimal with i.v. doses of 4 mg/kg repeated 4-hourly (Finkelstein *et al.*, 1988). Obidoxime has been given as an initial i.v. bolus (250 mg) followed by i.v. infusion (750 mg/d) to treat OP poisoning in adults (Thiermann *et al.*, 1997; Zilker *et al.*, 1997).

5.9.2.4 Asoxime and other oximes

Asoxime chloride (1-[[[4-(aminocarbonyl)pyridinio]methoxy]methyl]-2-[(hydroxy-imino)methyl] pyridinium dichloride; HI-6; HJ-6; CAS 34433-31-3; Figure 5.10) is one of a family of bispyridinium oximes (H-series oximes, Hagedorn oximes; Table 5.1) which have been shown to reactivate soman-inhibited AChE *in vitro* as well as possessing activity against AChE inhibited by other OPs (Kassa, 1998). The series is named after Professor Hagedorn, the leader of the group that first synthesized these compounds. H-series oximes are thought to act not only by reactivation of AChE, but also via their ganglion blocking, antimuscarinic and post-junctional non-depolarizing actions as well as effects on cardiovascular and respiratory systems (Rousseaux and Dua, 1989).

Obidoxime was more potent and more efficacious than pralidoxime, asoxime and HLö-7 in reactivating AChE after treatment with various OP insecticides and tabun *in vitro* (Worek *et al.*, 1997). However, asoxime was more effective against the OP nerve agents soman, sarin, cyclosarin and VX (*O*-ethyl-*S*-[2-(diisopropylamino)ethyl]methyl phosphonothioate). Asoxime has been found to be relatively non-toxic in laboratory animals (Clement *et al.*, 1988), and has been used (4 g/d i.v. or 500 mg i.m. 4-hourly) with success together with atropine, diazepam and supportive therapy in treating acute OP insecticide poisoning in man (Jovanović *et al.*, 1990; Kušić *et al.*, 1991). The shelf-life of asoxime solutions may be a problem, however (Briggs and Simons, 1986). A *trans*-2-butene analogue of asoxime, BI-6, was found to have lower efficacy against the nerve agent GF (cyclosarin) than the H-series oximes tested (Kassa and Cabal, 1999). Further discussion of OP nerve agents is to be found in section 7.3.

Anticholinesterases: mechanism of action

- In hydrolysing acetylcholine, a serine residue at the cholinesterase active site is acetylated. Hydrolysis is rapid (total reaction time c. 80 μs) and active enzyme is regenerated
- OPs phosphorylate or phosphonylate and carbamates carbamylate the active site of cholinesterase
- With some OPs, hydrolysis at the phosphorylated or phosphonylated site regenerates active enzyme over a period of hours
- With other OPs, no hydrolysis occurs and regeneration of enzyme activity is dependent on synthesis of new AChE
- Carbamylated AChE is regenerated at different rates depending on the carbamate involved

Antidotes to anticholinesterases

- The toxicity of OP insecticides and nerve agents, and of carbamate insecticides, is due to inhibition of cholinesterase
- Acetylcholine accumulates at nicotinic and muscarinic receptors in autonomic ganglia, the CNS and elsewhere
- Death from respiratory failure or circulatory collapse may ensue in severe cases
- Atropine blocks the effects of acetylcholine at muscarinic receptors
- Pralidoxime, obidoxime and other oximes such as asoxime can reactivate phosphorylated or phosphonylated cholinesterase and form inert complexes with OPs
- Oximes are thought to have little beneficial effect in carbamate poisoning

Oximes in anticholinesterase poisoning – I

- Pralidoxime and obidoxime interact with phosphorylated or phosphonylated enzyme to form an oxime–phosphate complex, thus allowing regeneration of active enzyme
- The speed of the reaction varies depending on the nature of the phosphoryl or phosphonyl moiety
- Oximes should be given as soon as possible after atropine as derivatized enzyme 'ages' and within hours becomes resistant to reactivation
- 'Ageing' is due to loss of an alkyl or alkoxy moiety to give a more stable monoalkyl or monoalkoxyphosphate at the cholinesterase active site
- Oxime–carbamate–enzyme complexes may be more stable than carbamate–enzyme complexes, and thus oximes are contraindicated in poisoning with carbamate insecticides

---

Oximes in anticholinesterase poisoning – II

- Oximes should be given as soon as possible and may be ineffective unless given within 36–48 h of exposure
- Pralidoxime and obidoxime do not penetrate the CNS
- OPs against which pralidoxime is effective include amiton, demeton-demethyl, diazinon, dichlorvos, disulfoton, dyflos, fenthion, malathion, mevinphos, parathion, phosphamidon
- Pralidoxime appears to be less effective against dimefox, dimethoate, methyl diazinon, mipafos, schradan
- Obidoxime is sometimes preferred to pralidoxime and may detoxify certain OPs directly
- Obidoxime is more effective than pralidoxime against parathion and less effective against malathion, dimethoate and fenthion

---

5.10 DANTROLENE

Dantrolene (1-{[5-(4-nitrophenyl)furfurylidene]amino}hydantoin, sodium salt; Dantrium, Procter and Gamble; Figure 5.13) was introduced to clinical practice in 1978. It causes skeletal muscle relaxation by preventing calcium flux across the sarcoplasmic reticulum (Meredith *et al.*, 1993), and is effective in controlling hyperthermia and muscular spasm in malignant hyperthermia and in neuroleptic malignant syndrome. Hyperthermia due to or associated with increased muscular rigidity, such as may occur in poisoning with, for example, strychnine, phencyclidine and *Cicuta* species (water hemlock etc.), may also respond to dantrolene. In addition, amphetamines, including 'ecstasy' (methylenedioxymethylamphetamine, MDMA) and its analogues methylenedioxyamphetamine (MDA, 'Adam') and methylenedioxyethyl-amphetamine (MDEA, 'Eve'), MAOIs, lysergic acid diethylamide (LSD) and cocaine can all cause hyperthermia, which is thought to be due to release of serotonin. When accompanied by confusion, muscular rigidity and autonomic dysfunction this is called the 'serotonin syndrome'. Dantrolene may be of benefit in such cases either in addition to conventional cooling therapy and diazepam or when such therapy has failed (Meredith *et al.*, 1993; Denborough and Hopkinson, 1997). Dantrolene would not be expected to

---

Dantrolene (sodium)

CAS registry number (dantrolene)	7261-97-4
Relative formula mass (dantrolene sodium)	337
pK_a	7.5
Oral bioavailability (%)	80
Presystemic metabolism	Variable
Plasma half-life range (h) (mean, range) (oral)	8.7 (4–24)
Volume of distribution (L/kg)	*c.* 1.2
Plasma protein binding (%)	80–90

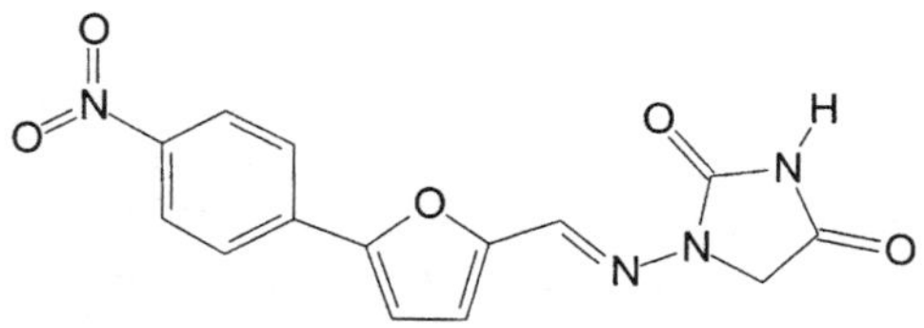

Figure 5.13: Structural formula of dantrolene

be effective in treating hyperthermia due to poisoning with (i) salicylates, dinitrophenol, ioxynil and other compounds that uncouple oxidative phosphorylation and (ii) tricyclic antidepressants and other anticholinergic drugs that reduce sweating and thereby impair heat loss.

5.10.1 Malignant hyperthermia

Malignant hyperthermia results from genetic susceptibility to some anaesthetics (inhalational agents plus suxamethonium) or stress and is usually fatal unless treated appropriately. Usually, while under anaesthesia, the patient develops a rectal temperature in excess of 39 °C. There is a rapid rise in intracellular calcium. The syndrome is characterized by tachycardia, unstable blood pressure, arrhythmias, hyperventilation, hyperthermia, muscular rigidity, cyanosis, hypoxia, respiratory and metabolic acidosis, raised creatinine kinase of muscle origin in plasma, renal failure and hyperkalaemia. The risk of death is predicted from the extent of temperature rise. Once it is recognized, active cooling measures must be employed, together with dantrolene. Untreated, malignant hyperthermia has a mortality in excess of 80 % (Bismuth, 1992).

5.10.2 Neuroleptic malignant syndrome

Neuroleptic malignant syndrome may arise after exposure to an antipsychotic drug after therapeutic dosage or after overdosage. It tends to occur within 24–72 h of starting treatment with the drug. It occurs in 0.2–1 % of patients taking neuroleptics, especially when haloperidol or depot phenothiazines such as fluphenazine are used (Guzé and Baxter, 1985), but has also been described with clozapine and lithium (Pope *et al.*, 1986). It is characterized by confusion, agitation, myoclonus, sweating, renal failure and gross hyperpyrexia. The risk of death is said to be between 20 % and 30 % (Burke *et al.*, 1981). It should be treated by withdrawal of the antipsychotic drug and, in severe cases, by sedation with diazepam and application of cooling measures such as i.v. fluids, and by administration of dantrolene. Diazepam i.v. is very effective at both controlling the patient's agitation and reducing muscular generation of heat. Adequate hydration is also required.

5.10.3 Serotonin syndrome

This may be caused by interaction between MAOIs and many drugs, including selective serotonin reuptake inhibitors (SSRIs), dextromorphan and tricyclic antidepressants

(Gillman, 1998). It can also be seen after overdosage with SSRIs and in amphetamine and MDMA intoxication. It is characterized by confusion, agitation, tremor, myoclonus, sweating, autonomic instability and hyperpyrexia. It should be treated by withdrawal of the serotonergic drug and, in severe cases, sedation with diazepam and application of active cooling measures. Dantrolene can also be used, although recent evidence suggests that it may not be as effective as once thought, possibly because it acts only on peripheral thermogenesis, i.e. muscle spasm. Agents, such as chlorpromazine and ketanserin, which act on central serotonin (5-hydroxtryptamine, 5-HT) receptors may be more effective under such circumstances (Jones and Simpson, 1999).

5.10.4 Dantrolene: clinical use

Peak serum dantrolene concentrations of 4.3–6.5 mg/L were achieved in six patients with malignant hyperthermia treated with 2.5 mg/kg dantrolene sodium i.v. over 10–30 min before surgery (Flewellen and Nelson, 1985). Studies in humans have shown that 2.4–2.5 mg/kg dantrolene sodium i.v. permits muscle relaxation and protects against the risk of hyperthermia (Kolb, 1982; Flewellen et al., 1983). Dantrolene has a large V_D. It is metabolized in the liver by 5-hydroxylation. The resulting metabolite has only half of the activity of the parent compound against muscle contraction. Both dantrolene and 5-hydroxydantrolene are eliminated in urine.

The median plasma half-life of dantrolene is 6 h (range 4–22 h) and that of 5-hydroxydantrolene is 15 h (range 8–29 h) (Lietman et al., 1974; Meyler et al., 1979; Flewellen et al., 1983). When dantrolene sodium was given i.v. at a rate of 0.1 mg/kg (cumulative dose 2.4 mg/kg) every 5 min to 12 volunteers, there was a linear increase in the plasma dantrolene concentration to a peak of approximately 4.2 mg/L at 2.9 h after the first dose. Thereafter, the plasma dantrolene concentration was maintained until 5.5 h after the first dose and then fell to 1.7 mg/L at 20 h and 0.3 mg/L at 48 h. The mean plasma half-life was 12.1 h (Flewellen et al., 1983).

In malignant hyperthermia in adults, dantrolene sodium (total dose 1–10 mg/kg i.v.) together with active cooling measures are effective if treatment is commenced within 6 h of exposure to the precipitating anaesthetic agent. Death may supervene if treatment is delayed for longer (Kolb et al., 1982). A response should be apparent within minutes. In children, the time factor is even more critical as dantrolene administration is often ineffective if delayed for more than 2 h after onset of hyperthermia and children are prone to febrile convulsions. Dosage at a rate of 1 mg kg^{-1} min^{-1} i.v. up to a total of 10 mg/kg or even more is recommended (Meredith et al., 1993). All anaesthetic agents should be discontinued as soon as possible after the presence of malignant hyperthermia is recognized (Kolb et al., 1982). For individuals with proven predisposition to hyperthermia, a prophylactic dantrolene sodium dose of 4–8 mg kg^{-1} d^{-1} can be given starting 1–2 days before surgery, with the last dose given 3–4 h after surgery. Alternatively, 2–5 mg/kg can be given i.v. just before surgery (Bismuth, 1992).

In neuroleptic malignant syndrome, single i.v. doses of dantrolene sodium (less than 3–10 mg/kg) and repeated oral doses (25–600 mg/d) have been used, often in combination with other drugs and supportive therapy such as active cooling, correction of metabolic acidosis and administration of high-flow oxygen (Ward et al., 1986; Harrison, 1988). Dantrolene apparently reduces the pyrexia, usually within 12 h of i.v. therapy and over a somewhat longer period after oral dosage. Most patients also improve clinically, although this tends to lag behind temperature reduction. In some cases, withdrawal of oral dantrolene has been associated with deterioration of the patient's condition and an increase in body temperature. In such circumstances, dantrolene therapy should be reinstituted.

In serotonin syndrome, a minimum dantrolene sodium dose of 1 mg kg^{-1} d^{-1} increasing to a maximum of 10 mg kg^{-1} d^{-1} should be given i.v., titrated to control the degree of hyperpyrexia. If signs of the disorder reappear, further doses can be given. A patient who had taken an overdose of phenelzine was treated successfully with i.v. dantrolene after conventional therapy had failed (Kaplan *et al.*, 1986), as was a patient with carbon monoxide poisoning with hyperthermia and rigidity (ten Holter and Schellens, 1988). In a fatal case of theophylline poisoning with rhabdomyolysis, dantrolene administration was claimed to be useful in controlling the hypermetabolic state, but the evidence in this instance is not convincing (Parr and Willatts, 1991).

It is important that dantrolene administration is accompanied by aggressive supportive therapy, including active cooling techniques, an inspired oxygen concentration of up to 100 % and correction of metabolic acidosis. Serum potassium concentrations should be closely monitored as they increase in hyperthermia as a result of muscle injury. Further supportive therapy may need to be directed towards complications such as respiratory acidosis, cardiac arrhythmias, unstable blood pressure and renal failure induced by rhabdomyolysis (Meredith *et al.*, 1993). Dantrolene is contraindicated if calcium channel blockers are being used.

Dantrolene can cause tissue necrosis due to extravasation during i.v. injection. After high doses, pancreatitis and hepatitis have occurred in 1.8 % of patients. The hepatic reaction is commoner in women over 30 years of age taking oestrogens and in those on prolonged or high-dose therapy with dantrolene, i.e. doses of more than 300 mg/d or treatment for more than 60 days (Utili *et al.*, 1977). Histologically, necrosis of the liver or chronic active hepatitis is seen (Utili *et al.*, 1977). Rarely, cholestasis also occurs (Schneider and Mitchell, 1976). Dantrolene has also been associated with diarrhoea, abdominal cramps, constipation, drowsiness, headache, rash, dysphagia, tachycardia, erratic blood pressure, haematuria, pericarditis and pleural effusion (British National Formulary, 2000a). More rarely its use is associated with hallucinations (Andrews *et al.*, 1975), respiratory depression (Rivera *et al.*, 1975) and leucopenia (Greenspun and Pacho,

CHAPTER 5

Clinical use of dantrolene sodium (*Dantrium*)

- Dantrolene causes skeletal muscle relaxation by preventing Ca^{2+} flux across the sarcoplasmic reticulum
- In adults 1–7 mg/kg i.v. within 6 h is effective in treating malignant hyperthermia (children up to 10 mg/kg i.v. within 2 h)
- Dantrolene sodium (3–10 mg/kg i.v. followed by 25–600 mg/d p.o. as needed) is also effective in neuroleptic malignant syndrome, in which case supportive therapy (central cooling, 100 % oxygen, correction of metabolic acidosis, etc.) is also needed
- Dantrolene may also be useful in poisoning with compounds causing increased muscle rigidity (strychnine) or hyperthermia due to motor overactivity (amphetamines, MAOIs)

1981). In the context of malignant hyperthermia and neuroleptic malignant syndrome the benefits outweigh risks of its use. For treatment of hyperthermia due to serotonin syndrome, such as in subjects with MDMA intoxication, the risk–benefit ratio is much less clear-cut (Jones and Simpson, 1999).

5.11 DAPSONE

Dapsone (Figure 5.14) has been used to inhibit local wound infiltration by polymorphonuclear leucocytes in patients developing a central purplish bleb or vesicle within 6–8 h of being bitten by a brown recluse spider (*Loxosceles reclusa*). In one case an 8 × 8 cm area of erythema resolved when treated with dapsone within 24 h (King and Rees, 1983). One study reported dapsone alone to be as effective as antivenin (section 3.1.4.3) alone or dapsone plus antivenin in bite victims (Rees *et al.*, 1987). A recommended dosing schedule is 50–100 mg dapsone i.v. once or twice daily. Dapsone should only be used in adults with a proven history of brown recluse spider bite; it should not be used in children (Gendron, 1990). There has been one report of methaemoglobinaemia after dapsone used to treat a suspected brown recluse spider bite (Iserson, 1985).

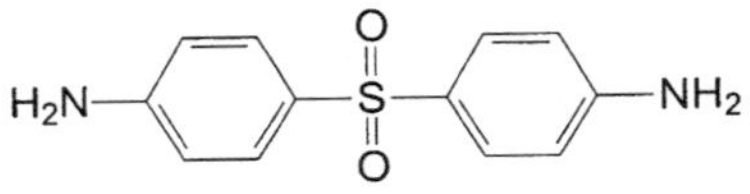

$$H_2N-\!\!\!\bigcirc\!\!\!-\overset{O}{\underset{O}{\overset{\|}{S}}}-\!\!\!\bigcirc\!\!\!-NH_2$$

Figure 5.14: Structural formula of dapsone

Dapsone	
CAS registry number	80-08-0
Relative formula mass (anhydrous)	248.3
pK_a	1.3, 2.5
Oral bioavailability (%)	> 90
Plasma half-life range (h) (mean, range)	27 (12–48)
Plasma protein binding (%)	*c.* 50

5.12 DIAZEPAM

Diazepam (Figure 5.15) (0.1–0.3 mg/kg) given by slow i.v. injection (repeated as necessary) is very effective at controlling convulsions induced by drugs or other poisons (Table 1.2). In addition, diazepam has been said to have a specific protective action in severe chloroquine poisoning. N'Dri *et al.* (1976) reported that some patients who ingested chloroquine and diazepam concomitantly did not have clinical features of chloroquine poisoning. Further studies (Bondurand *et al.*, 1980; Vitris and Aubert, 1983) suggested that diazepam administration reduced cardiovascular mortality in severe poisoning with this agent. Crouzette *et al.* (1983) subsequently reported that diazepam reduces mortality in rats acutely poisoned with chloroquine, while Riou *et al.* (1986)

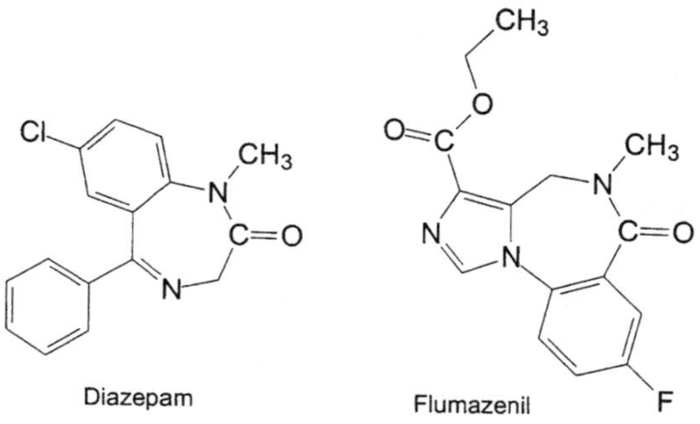

Figure 5.15: Structural formulae of diazepam and flumazenil

demonstrated cardioprotection and increased urinary chloroquine excretion in chloroquine-poisoned pigs after diazepam.

Diazepam (2 mg/kg i.v. over 30 min) together with early mechanical ventilation and i.v. adrenaline (0.25 μg kg^{-1} min^{-1}, and increased until systolic blood pressure > 100 mmHg) for up to 4 days was used to treat 11 patients with severe chloroquine poisoning, all of whom would have been expected to die on the basis of historical control data. Ten patients survived (Riou *et al.*, 1988). Mechanical ventilation was instituted in part because of the respiratory depressant effect of high-dose diazepam. Adrenaline was administered to counteract chloroquine-induced myocardial depression and vasodilatation, effects not counteracted by diazepam. An initial dose of 0.5 μg kg^{-1} min^{-1} is recommended as inotropic support, increased until a systolic blood pressure of 100 mmHg is attained.

The mechanism of the protective effect of diazepam in acute chloroquine poisoning is unknown. Croes *et al.* (1993) reported a patient with severe chloroquine poisoning who had also ingested clorazepate (initial whole-blood chloroquine and plasma nordiazepam concentrations 7.9 and 2.3 mg/L respectively) and in whom mechanical ventilation was instituted. She was treated successfully with diazepam (2 mg/kg over 30 min, followed by 1–2 mg/kg over 24 h) and noradrenaline (0.25 μg kg^{-1} min^{-1} for 18 h). However, despite plasma diazepam + nordiazepam concentrations of 3 mg/L and above, she required additional sedation with piritramide-facilitated mechanical ventilation. Although it is possible that chloroquine antagonized the sedative effects of diazepam, the patient could have acquired tolerance to these effects because of

	Diazepam	*Nordiazepam*
CAS registry number	439-14-5	1088-11-5
Relative formula mass	284.8	270.7
pK_a	3.3	–
Oral absorption (%)	100	50
Presystemic metabolism	Negligible	Negligible
Plasma half-life (h) (mean, range)	30 (20–100)	(30–200)
Volume of distribution (L/kg)	1.1	0.5–2.5
Plasma protein binding (%)	98–99	97

prior use of clorazepate. Recent animal work suggests that barbiturate anaesthesia and isoprenaline infusion may be a more effective combination than diazepam and adrenaline in treating severe chloroquine poisoning (Buckley *et al.*, 1996).

5.13 FLUMAZENIL

5.13.1 Clinical toxicology of benzodiazepines

In general, benzodiazepines are remarkably safe in overdosage, and after deliberate self-poisoning full recovery usually takes place within 24 h. However, performance in skilled tasks such as driving may be impaired for several days as the plasma half-life of some benzodiazepines and their metabolites are long. Poisoning with benzodiazepines may be particularly severe if such drugs are ingested in overdosage (i) together with other CNS depressants such as tricyclic antidepressants, opioids or alcohol or (ii) by susceptible groups of patients such as those with pre-existing respiratory disease or the elderly.

Clinical features of benzodiazepine poisoning include drowsiness and mid-position or dilated pupils, often occurring within 2–3 h of ingestion. Ataxia, dysarthria, nystagmus and confusion can occur. Coma, seldom less than grade 10 on the Glasgow coma scale (GCS) and lasting for < 24 h may follow. Minor hypotension may also occur. Impairment of consciousness should be treated conventionally, with particular attention being paid to maintaining the airway. Observation should be for at least 6 h after ingestion (24 h in more severe cases). Pulse oximetry is useful for monitoring adequacy of ventilation if marked CNS depression is present.

5.13.2 Clinical pharmacology of flumazenil

Flumazenil (RO 15-1788; Anexate, Roche; Figure 5.15), an imidazobenzodiazepine, can reverse the sedative, anticonvulsant, anxiolytic, amnesic, anaesthetic and muscle relaxant effects of therapeutic doses of benzodiazepines by competing at central GABA receptor sites (GABA$_A$) but does not seem to block peripheral (renal, cardiac, etc.) benzodiazepine effects (Hunkeler *et al.*, 1981). Flumazenil also reverses benzodiazepine-induced respiratory depression, increasing the minute volume and the respiratory rate, and has been used to reverse benzodiazepine-induced respiratory depression in neonates (Dixon *et al.*, 1998). It has no inherent convulsive properties and has been used to antagonize benzodiazepine-induced toxicity and to reverse sedation after procedures such as endoscopy (Weinbroum *et al.*, 1991; Höjer, 1994). Even cases of paradoxical reaction to midazolam in elderly patients (confusion and aggression) (Ricou *et al.*, 1986) and first-degree atrioventricular block after alprazolam overdose (Mullins, 1999) have been treated successfully with flumazenil.

Flumazenil also antagonizes the sedative effects of other compounds that act through GABA receptors, such as zopiclone (Hunkeler *et al.*, 1981) and zolpidem, though the clinical course of poisoning with zopiclone would seldom require use of the antidote (Lheureux *et al.*, 1990). Flumazenil has been reported to be effective in countering the central effects of baclofen overdose (Saissy *et al.*, 1992), but this has not been confirmed (Byrnes *et al.*, 1996). The use of flumazenil to reverse the sedative effects of promethazine has been reported (Plant and MacLeod, 1994). Flumazenil (5 mg i.v.) may have a transient effect in ethanol-induced coma (Martens *et al.*, 1990). The use of

Flumazenil

CAS registry number	78755-81-4
Relative formula mass	303.3
pK_a	1.7
Oral absorption (%)	> 95
Presystemic metabolism (%)	70–80
Plasma half-life (h) (mean, range)	0.85 (0.7–1.3)
Volume of distribution (L/kg)	0.95
Plasma protein binding (%)	50

flumazenil in clinical toxicology has been reviewed (Amrein *et al.*, 1987; Brogden and Goa, 1991; Geller *et al.*, 1991; Weinbroum *et al.*, 1991; Hoffman and Warren, 1993; Cone and Stott, 1994).

Flumazenil is active orally, but bioavailability is less than 20 %, and this, together with the delay in attaining a peak serum concentration using the oral route, is why an i.v. preparation is used. Flumazenil is 50 % bound to plasma protein and has a V_D of approximately 1 L/kg. Its plasma half-life is about 1 h (Roncari *et al.*, 1986; Breimer *et al.*, 1991). Less than 1 % of a dose of flumazenil is excreted unchanged in urine. The metabolites do not have pharmacological activity. In the doses used in humans (2–100 mg), flumazenil demonstrates linear kinetics, which are not influenced by the presence of other benzodiazepines in high concentrations. The disposition of flumazenil appears to be similar in healthy young and elderly volunteers (Roncari *et al.*, 1993).

The effect of flumazenil is to shift the dose–response curve for each modality of benzodiazepine agonist effect to the right. Relatively low doses of flumazenil will lighten midazolam-induced hypnosis and muscle relaxation, while progressively higher doses are required to ensure complete reversal of sedation and anxiolysis. When given before or with other benzodiazepines it modifies their effects. For example, 5 mg flumazenil i.v. will block the effect of a subsequent dose of up to 6 mg midazolam, while doses of 6–10 mg midazolam will reverse the antagonist effect of flumazenil (Gath *et al.*, 1984). The duration of action of flumazenil after a single dose of 3.5 mg i.v. was at least 3–5 h (Lheureux and Askenasi, 1988). However, this time is very variable and probably depends on the type of benzodiazepine ingested and the presence of other drugs (Hofer and Scollo-Lavizzari, 1985). Many patients require more than a single dose of the drug.

Use of flumazenil may only be considered in benzodiazepine poisoning after all the contraindications (see below) have been evaluated, and then only in deeply unconscious patients (e.g. GCS < 8). Its routine use in benzodiazepine poisoning cannot be justified. Flumazenil is not licensed for the treatment of benzodiazepine self-poisoning in the UK (Burkhart and Kulig, 1990; Hoffman and Goldfrank, 1995). The vast majority of patients taking benzodiazepines alone are best left to recover without active treatment. Flumazenil is contraindicated if a benzodiazepine has been ingested together with other drugs, particularly tricyclic antidepressants, as it may reduce the seizure threshold and provoke ventricular arrhythmias. Flumazenil may be helpful in the diagnosis of coma of unknown aetiology (Höjer *et al.*, 1990), in the reversal of iatrogenic benzodiazepine poisoning in hospitalized patients or in patients with respiratory depression of such severity that endotracheal intubation and a short period of mechanical ventilation would otherwise be indicated. In elderly benzodiazepine overdose

■ CHAPTER 5 ■

patients or those with pre-existing respiratory disease, it is probably better to accept the need for mechanical ventilation rather than attempt repeated use of flumazenil. However, a single adequate dose of flumazenil may be worth trying. Flumazenil is contraindicated in patients:

- with epilepsy or hypersensitivity to benzodiazepines;
- who have received prolonged treatment with benzodiazepines (because of the risk of precipitating withdrawal reactions);
- in whom reversal of anaesthesia in the presence of neuromuscular blockade is considered (Watanabe et al., 1998);
- with head injury – flumazenil has been reported to cause a marked rise in intracranial pressure in patients with severe head injury (Chiolero et al., 1988);
- who have ingested other drugs, especially tricyclic antidepressants, in overdose.

In one patient who took an overdose of oxazepam and chloral hydrate, the administration of 0.5 mg flumazenil precipitated multifocal ventricular beats with episodes of ventricular tachycardia (Short et al., 1988). In other patients who had co-ingested benzodiazepines and tricyclic antidepressants, flumazenil precipitated convulsions (Passeron et al., 1987; Haverkos et al., 1994). The ability of flumazenil to precipitate seizures in dogs poisoned with amitriptyline has been demonstrated (Lheureux et al., 1992).

If flumazenil is to be given, the recommended method of administration of flumazenil is by titration starting with 0.2 mg i.v. over 30 s followed by incremental doses of 0.3 mg i.v. until the desired end-point is reached. It is usual to give each dose at least 60 s to work before giving a further dose. The normal dose is 0.5 mg i.v. to a maximum of about 5 mg. If there is no response then benzodiazepine poisoning is unlikely to be the cause of the CNS depression. Following benzodiazepine overdose or in critical care situations, doses of 1–3 mg may be required and may need to be repeated (Weinbroum et al., 1996). The maximum recorded dose to date (with good effect) has been 9.4 mg over 10 h in nine separate doses.

The duration of action of flumazenil following a single i.v. dose has varied between 15 and 150 min (Klotz et al., 1984, 1985; Lauven et al., 1985), depending on the relative doses of the agonist and antagonist, their relative receptor binding affinities, half-lives and V_D, and the interval between their administration. Flumazenil may also be given by continuous infusion in 0.9 % (w/v) sodium chloride or 5 % (w/v) D-glucose at a rate of 0.5–1 mg/h for an adult provided there is a response (Bodenham et al., 1988; Chern et al., 1998). It is vital that, once the first dose of flumazenil has been given, the patient is adequately monitored for recurrence of respiratory depression. There are no specific recommendations as to the use of flumazenil except for potentially high-risk groups such as young children. If indicated in children aged 4 years and over, 10 µg/kg may be given i.v. and repeated once.

Adverse reactions to flumazenil may include nausea, vomiting, mild dizziness, facial erythema or flushing, anxiety and headache. Such reactions are most frequent after i.v. doses of more than 5 mg, and usually resolve within a few minutes. Anxiety has also been reported in patients awakening after flumazenil administration, but this is most probably due to the amnesic patient waking up in an unfamiliar clinical environment. Similarly, in elderly patients a tachycardia and brief period of hypertension may be seen on waking (Baud and Brouard, 1992). Convulsions have been reported rarely, and

---

Flumazenil (*Anexate*)

- Flumazenil is an imidazobenzodiazepine that can reverse the sedative, anticonvulsant, anxiolytic, amnesic, anaesthetic and muscle relaxant effects of benzodiazepines
- Flumazenil also reverses respiratory and cardiovascular depression due to benzodiazepines
- It competes at central GABA receptors and hence does not antagonize peripheral benzodiazepine effects (renal, cardiac, etc.)
- it antagonizes the sedative effects of other compounds, such as zopiclone, which act through GABA receptors
- It is a competitive inhibitor – higher doses are needed if large amounts of agonist are present

---

Clinical use of flumazenil

- Flumazenil is occasionally used to antagonize benzodiazepine effects after iatrogenic poisoning in the endoscopy suite or in critical care
- Flumazenil is contraindicated if more than one drug has been taken
- The initial adult dose is 0.2 mg i.v., with further doses of 0.1–0.5 mg being given i.v. if necessary. In overdose patients, 1–2 mg is often needed
- Adverse reactions may include dizziness, facial erythema or flushing, anxiety and headache
- Flumazenil should not be used in patients poisoned with chloral hydrate or tricyclic antidepressants (risk of ventricular dysrhythmias and convulsions respectively)

---

may represent effects of withdrawal in those dependent on benzodiazepines (Prischl *et al.*, 1988). When the effect of flumazenil declines, recurrence of benzodiazepine agonist activity may occur.

5.14 GACYCLIDINE

Gacyclidine (GK 11; *cis*(Pip/Me 1-[1-(2-thienyl)-2-methylcyclohexyl]piperidine; CAS 68134-81-6; Figure 5.16) is an antagonist at brain glutaminergic N-methyl-D-aspartate

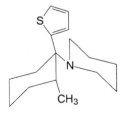

Figure 5.16: Structural formula of gacyclidine

(NMDA) receptors. It has been suggested as an additional neuroprotective agent in OP poisoning (Lallement et al., 1997).

5.15 GLUCAGON

Glucagon (GlucaGen, Novo Nordisk; CAS 9007-92-5; Figure 5.17) is a peptide hormone produced by the pancreas that stimulates gluconeogenesis and glycogenolysis. It is now produced commercially for medicinal use to reverse hypoglycaemia in diabetic patients and for the treatment of poisoning with certain drugs. Glucagon is used in symptomatic β-adrenoceptor blocker poisoning as, although myocardial depression can be antagonized by β-agonists such as isoprenaline, large doses may be required and the safety margin between the desired effect and toxicity is small. Glucagon directly stimulates myocardial adenylate cyclase by a non-β-receptor mechanism, thereby increasing muscle contractility, i.e. it is a positive inotrope (Parmley et al., 1968; Peterson et al., 1984; Critchley and Ungar, 1989; Mansell, 1990; O'Mahony et al., 1990) (Figure 5.18). Glucagon has a small effect on reducing systemic vascular resistance but does not reduce left ventricular end-diastolic pressure.

Despite its efficacy, glucagon is not licensed in the UK for treating β-blocker poisoning, although it is commonly used in such circumstances. Use of dopamine (Toet et al., 1996) or amrinone (Love et al., 1993) together with glucagon to treat β-blocker poisoning may not be advisable. Glucagon may also have a role in treating severe poisoning with calcium channel blockers such as diltiazem (Mahr et al., 1997) and nifedipine (Fant et al., 1997), but there are conflicting reports of efficacy (Pollack, 1993). Glucagon has also been used to treat hypotension encountered in a case of severe poisoning with imipramine (Sener et al., 1995) and dothiepin (Sensky and Olczak, 1999).

Glucagon cannot be given orally as it is broken down by peptidases in the gastrointestinal tract. Glucagon can be administered s.c., i.m. or i.v. Commonly it is given i.v. (initial bolus dose 10 mg in an adult). It should be reconstituted in either 5 % (w/v) D-glucose or 0.9 % (w/v) sodium chloride in treating β-blocker poisoning as the diluent provided (the preparation is intended for giving 1-mg doses to diabetic patients) may contain phenol (2 g/L) as a preservative (Pollack, 1993). Such a glucagon solution has a stability of 14 days if refrigerated (2–8 °C). An i.v. dose of 50–150 μg/kg over 1 min should be followed by 10–50 μg kg^{-1} h^{-1} by i.v. infusion over 5–12 h, titrated to haemodynamic response (Hall-Boyer et al., 1984; Peterson et al., 1984). Glucagon cannot be used to treat β-blocker-induced convulsions. Alternatively, i.v. boluses can be given every 20–30 min (Hall-Boyer et al., 1984). The effects of i.v. glucagon usually begin within 1–3 min and peak at 5–7 min after administration, and last for 15–20 min (Peterson et al., 1984). The plasma half-life is between 3 and 6 min. The drug is largely catabolized by the liver and metabolism is impaired in patients with chronic liver disease, portocaval shunts or obstructive jaundice. Glucagon is excreted by the kidney and undergoes tubular reabsorption, such that in chronic renal failure clearance is reduced (Assan, 1978; Sornay et al., 1988). Higher doses may be needed in some patients; the

1
His-Ser-Gln-Gly-Thr-Phe-Thr-Ser-Asp-Tyr-Ser-Lys-Tyr-Leu-Asp-Ser-Arg

29 |
Thr-Asn-Met-Leu-Trp-Gln-Val-Phe-Asp-Gln-Ala-Arg

Figure 5.17: Schematic representation of glucagon

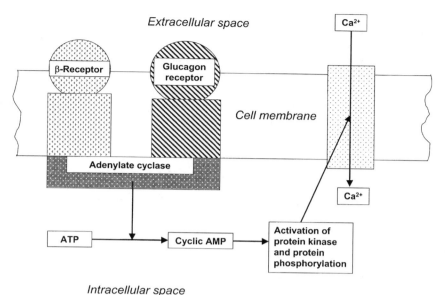

Figure 5.18: Mechanism of action of β-blockers and glucagon

effective dose is often the dose required to make the patient vomit. However, this said, probably no more than 30 mg i.v. should be given to an adult within 10 min.

Children can be given 50–150 µg/kg i.v., or up to 50 µg/kg hourly by i.v. infusion. If glucagon is given s.c. the actions are more prolonged than if given i.v. (Assan, 1978), but nowadays it is preferable to start with a bolus dose and then establish a continuous infusion if required (10–50 µg/kg hourly i.v. over 5–12 h). Isoprenaline (section 5.17) and/or adrenaline may be needed for additional positive inotropic support but are of second-line use in β-blocker poisoning (Weinstein, 1984). Adrenaline is preferred because isoprenaline possesses β_2-agonist activity, and may induce vasodilatation, especially after overdose with cardioselective β-blockers.

Adverse effects of glucagon may include nausea, vomiting, hypokalaemia and hyperglycaemia (which seldom requires treatment) (Pollack, 1993). Rarely, paradoxical hypoglycaemia has been reported, due to stimulation of insulin secretion. Hypersensitivity reactions have also been described previously (Parfitt, 1999). Glucagon is a teratogen in animals, causing cataracts, glaucoma and microphthalmos. Little is know about possible teratogenicity in humans, but it is not listed as a drug to be avoided in pregnancy and its duration of use is short when used to treat β-blocker poisoning. Patients should be placed on a cardiac monitor. Glucagon should not be used in patients with hypoglycaemia due to sulphonylureas, alcohol, phaeochromocytoma or insulinoma. Glucagon potentiates the effect of vitamin K as an anticoagulant (Hall-Boyer *et al.*, 1984).

Other drawbacks to the use of glucagon in the relatively high doses needed to treat β-blocker poisoning are its high cost and limited availability. More recently, a lyophilized preparation (GlucaGen, Novo Nordisk) has become available, which obviates the need for repeated doses from 1-mg syringes (which occasionally led to phenol poisoning in the past). The lyophilized preparation may be stored for up to 3 years if refrigerated. If glucagon fails, adrenaline (section 5.17) is the next step in treating serious β-blocker poisoning.

5.16 HEPARIN

Heparin (CAS 9005-49-6; Figure 5.19) (30,000–50,000 units daily i.v.) is used to reverse hypercoagulation states such as may occur in chronic poisoning with ergotamine or in poisoning with aminocaproic or tranexamic acids. It is not known if low-molecular-weight heparins would be an adequate substitute, but it is likely they would have efficacy in such conditions.

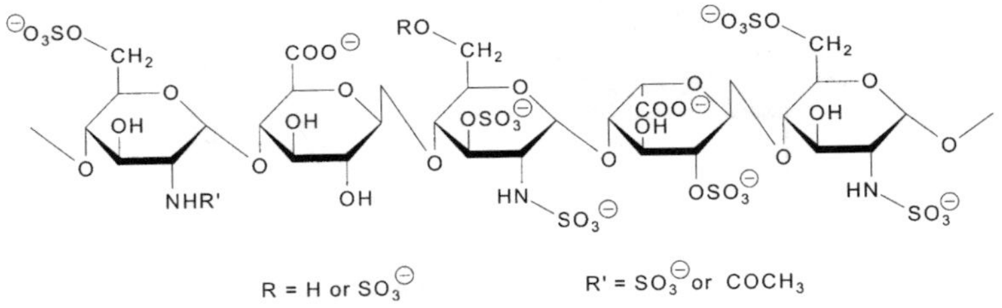

Figure 5.19: Antithrombin binding site of heparin

5.17 INOTROPIC AGENTS

Inotropes are frequently used to treat hypotension and low cardiac output due to acute poisoning with a variety of agents including verapamil (Kalman *et al.*, 1998) once hypovolaemia has been excluded or treated.

Isoprenaline (isoproterenol; Saventrine, Pharmax; Figure 5.20) is a β-adrenoceptor agonist. It is used in addition to glucagon (section 5.15) to treat hypotension or low cardiac output due to β-adrenoceptor blocking drugs, and to treat poisoning by calcium channel-blocking drugs if there is no response to calcium gluconate (section 4.3). The adult dose is 5–10 μg/min by i.v. infusion in either 5 % (w/v) D-glucose or 0.9 % (w/v) sodium chloride, titrated to cardiovascular response (mean arterial blood pressure > 60 mmHg). Much higher doses may be needed in severe cases. In children, 0.02 μg kg^{-1} min^{-1} is given i.v. (maximum of 0.5 μg kg^{-1} min^{-1}). Isoprenaline has the disadvantage that it may reduce the diastolic blood pressure due to vasodilatation, especially following the ingestion of cardioselective β-blockers. It is pro-arrhythmic and therefore should be used with vigilance after overdosage with cardiotoxic agents.

Adrenaline (epinephrine; Figure 5.20) (β$_1$-, β$_2$- and α-receptor agonist) increases heart rate and stroke volume (via peripheral vasoconstriction) and may be used as a positive inotrope. It is very useful when glucagon is ineffective in β-blocker poisoning. Adults and children should be given 1–5 μg kg^{-1} min^{-1}, titrating the dose to cardiovascular response. At low doses, the primary effect is increased cardiac output, while at higher doses there is additional potent vasoconstriction. It is useful in low-output states with low peripheral vasomotor tone and low mean arterial blood pressure. It is the drug of choice in emergency hypotensive states when the overall haemodynamic status is not clear. However, if a drug that sensitizes the myocardium to the action of adrenaline, such as a tricyclic antidepressant or an amphetamine, has been taken, use of adrenaline may precipitate arrhythmias and the dose should therefore be kept as modest as possible.

Noradrenaline (norepinephrine, *N*-demethyladrenaline; Figure 5.20) is often used in combination with adrenaline to treat vasodilatation such as encountered after overdose with calcium channel blockers as it is a potent vasoconstrictor as well as a

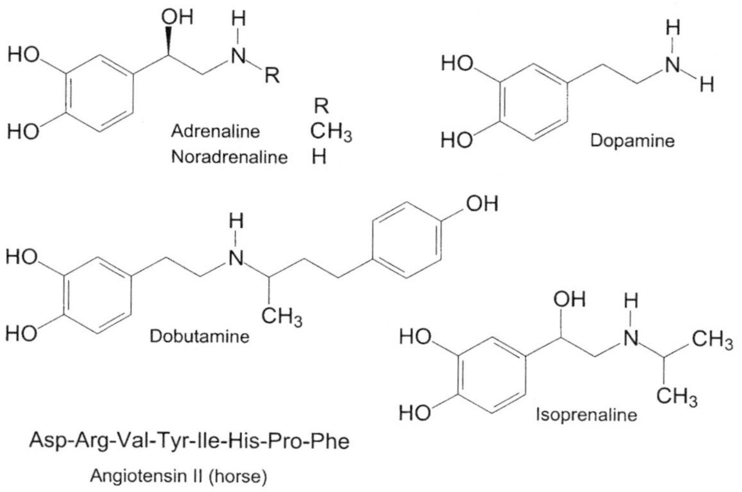

Adrenaline   CH$_3$
Noradrenaline   H

Dopamine

Dobutamine

Isoprenaline

Asp-Arg-Val-Tyr-Ile-His-Pro-Phe

Angiotensin II (horse)

Figure 5.20: Structural formulae of adrenaline and noradrenaline, dopamine, dobutamine, isoprenaline, and schematic representation of angiotensin II

positive inotrope. The dose is 1–5 µg kg^{-1} min^{-1} titrating the dose to cardiovascular response.

Dobutamine (Figure 5.20) (β_1- and less a β_2-agonist) increases heart rate and cardiac output, but causes peripheral and splanchnic vasodilatation. It is used at a dose of 1–20 µg kg^{-1} min^{-1}. It is useful in low cardiac output states when the blood pressure is reasonably maintained. It is not commonly used in managing poisoned patients.

At low doses (up to 5 µg kg^{-1} min^{-1}) the primary action of dopamine is on dopamine receptors, resulting in increased splanchnic and renal perfusion. It may therefore be useful in helping to maintain renal blood flow and promote urine output, though has unproven value in alleviating morbidity or mortality from renal failure. At doses above 5 µg/kg/min, dopamine is a predominant vasoconstrictor and cardiac effects predominate, i.e. it is a positive inotrope.

Angiotensin II (Figure 5.20) has been suggested as an alternative inotrope when conventional drugs prove only partially effective. Its use to treat a severe combined overdose of calcium antagonists and angiotensin-converting enzyme (ACE) inhibitors has been described (Tovar *et al.*, 1997).

5.18 OCTREOTIDE

Octreotide (D-phenylalanyl-L-cysteinyl-L-phenylalanyl-D-tryptophyl-L-lysyl-L-threonyl-*N*-[2-hydroxy-1-(hydroxymethyl)propyl]-L-cysteinamide cyclic (2®7)-disulphide; SMS-201-995; Sandostatin, Novartis; Figure 5.21) is a long-acting octapeptide analogue of somatostatin. It has some opioid antagonist activity (Maurer *et al.*, 1982). Among eight subjects given glipizide (1.45 mg/kg), octreotide (30 ng kg^{-1} min^{-1} i.v.) significantly reduced plasma insulin concentrations, and eliminated the need for exogenous D-glucose in four and reduced the D-glucose requirement in the remainder (Boyle *et al.*, 1993). Diazoxide (300 mg i.v. 4-hourly) was ineffective in reducing plasma insulin and the

CHAPTER 5

	Adrenaline	Dobutamine (hydrochloride)	Dopamine (hydrochloride)	Isoprenaline	Noradrenaline
CAS registry number	51-43-4	49745-95-1	62-31-7	7683-59-2	51-41-2
Relative formula mass (free base)	183.2	337.8 (301.4)	189.6 (153.2)	211.3	169.2
pK_a	8.7, 10.2, 12	9.5	8.8, 10.6	8.6, 10.1, 12	8.6, 9.8, 12
Oral absorption	High	Nil	–	75–95	Good
Presystemic metabolism (%)	Extensive	Extensive	100	Variable	> 95
Plasma half-life (min) (mean, range)	3–10	2	9 (6.7–12)	5	0.6–2.9
Volume of distribution (L/kg)	–	0.1–0.3	0.9	0.5	0.1–0.4
Plasma protein binding (%)	50	–	–	62–74	50

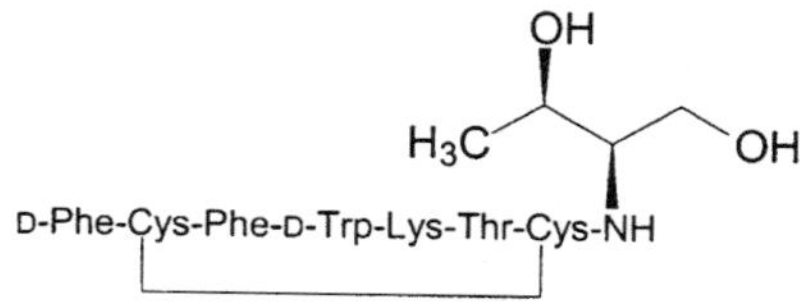

Figure 5.21: Schematic representation of octreotide

Octreotide	
CAS registry number	83150-76-9
Molecular weight	1019.3
pK_a	6.8, 9.7
Oral absorption (%)	Nil
Plasma half-life (i.v., min)	72–98
Volume of distribution (L/kg)	0.3
Plasma protein binding (%)	65

exogenous D-glucose requirement. Subcutaneous octreotide (50 μg 12-hourly) can also suppress stimulated endogenous insulin secretion (Krentz *et al.*, 1993). Octreotide may eliminate the need for prolonged infusion of hypertonic D-glucose and the resultant risks associated with central venous access. It has been used successfully to restore euglycaemia in patients with sulphonylurea poisoning refractory to D-glucose infusion (Spiller, 1999).

The severe hyperinsulinaemia and thus hypoglycaemia that complicates quinine treatment of *Plasmodium falciparum* malaria also responds to octreotide (Phillips *et al.*, 1986). In Thai volunteers, octreotide (100 μg i.m.) suppressed quinine-induced hyperinsulinaemia within 15 min. The effect lasted for 6 h. Octreotide (50 μg i.v. over 15 min followed by 50 μg/h by i.v. infusion, rising to 200 μg/h or reducing to 10 μg/h as appropriate) together with i.v. glucagon and/or D-glucose was effective in treating hyperinsulinaemia and hypoglycaemia in five patients with *P. falciparum* malaria who were treated with quinine (Phillips *et al.*, 1993).

Short-term octreotide (300 μg over 24 h) has been associated with acute pancreatitis in a 55-year-old male patient with acromegaly (Fredenrich *et al.*, 1991) and single doses (100 or 200 μg s.c.) with inducing attacks in two patients with relapsing pancreatitis (Bodemar and Hjortswang, 1996).

5.19 OPIOID ANTAGONISTS

Opioid antagonists are used primarily to reverse the central actions of opioids in overt or suspected poisoning cases that may include perioperative use. Nalorphine (*N*-allylnormorphine; Figure 5.22) was the first opioid antagonist used clinically but has partial agonist activity and is no longer employed (McNicholas and Martin, 1984). Levallorphan is not used nowadays for the same reason. Diprenorphine (Revivon; Figure 5.23) is used as an opioid antagonist in veterinary medicine as it has a longer plasma half-life than naloxone in many species. Naloxone finds greatest use clinically.

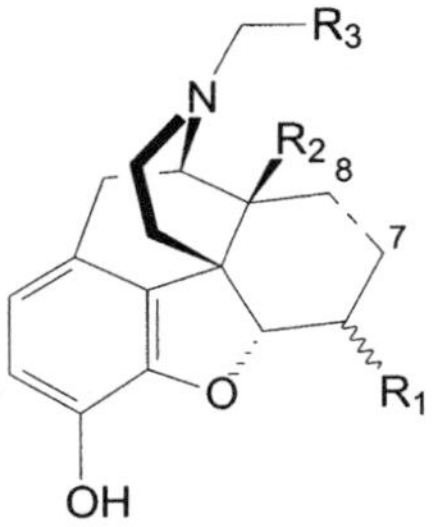

	—R$_1$	R$_2$	R$_3$	Bond$_{7-8}$
Nalbuphine	⋯OH	OH	Cyclobutyl	Single
Nalmefene	=CH$_2$	OH	Cyclopropyl	Single
Nalorphine	⋯OH	H	CH=CH$_2$	Double
Naloxone	=O	OH	CH=CH$_2$	Single
Naltrexone	=O	OH	Cyclopropyl	Single

Figure 5.22: Structural formulae of naloxone and some other opioid partial agonists/antagonists

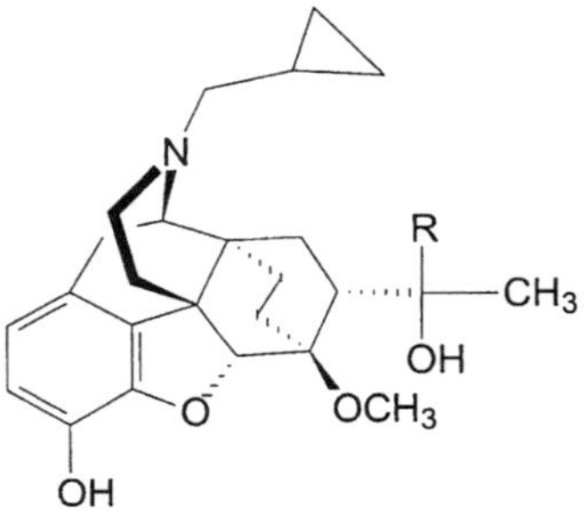

	R
Buprenorphine	C(CH$_3$)$_3$
Diprenorphine	CH$_3$

Figure 5.23: Structural formulae of buprenorphine and diprenorphine

The hallmarks of opioid poisoning are (i) depressed respiration, (ii) pin-point or small pupils, (iii) depressed consciousness and (iv) signs of i.v. drug abuse (e.g. needle track marks). Respiratory arrest, systemic hypotension, pulmonary oedema and hypothermia indicate severe poisoning. Convulsions are common in children. Toxicity can persist for 24–48 h, particularly after ingestion of methadone, a drug that has a particularly long half-life. Steps should be taken to ensure a clear airway and respiratory support if necessary. The need for endotracheal intubation can be avoided by prompt administration of an opioid antagonist.

5.19.1 Nalmefene

Nalmefene (6-desoxy-6-methylenenaltrexone; nalmetrene; CAS 55096-26-9; Revex, Ohmeda; Figure 5.22) is a parenterally active opioid antagonist. At doses in the range 0.1–1 µg/kg it has effectively reversed post-operative opioid-induced respiratory depression without ablating the analgesic response to subsequently administered opioids (Konieczko et al., 1988; Glass et al., 1994). When given at higher doses (0.5–1.6 mg), nalmefene has been shown to be effective in reversing respiratory depression in opioid overdose patients (Kaplan and Marx, 1993). Drowsiness, agitation/irritability and muscle tension were the only adverse effects reported after oral nalmefene (25, 50 or 100 mg) in volunteers (Fudala et al., 1991).

Nalmefene is primarily eliminated (up to 65 %) by conjugation with glucuronic acid with subsequent elimination in urine (Dixon et al., 1986). It is widely distributed with an average steady-state V_D of 1.7 L/kg and has a terminal elimination half-life of approximately 8 h in healthy middle-aged (Gal et al., 1986; Matzke et al., 1996) and elderly (Frye *et al.*, 1996) volunteers. The longer elimination half-life contributes to the observation that nalmefene has a longer duration of action than naloxone (Kaplan *et al.*, 1999) (section 5.19.2), and is more effective in reversing opioid-induced respiratory depression and sedation (Konieczko *et al.*, 1988; Barsan *et al.*, 1989). However, nalmefene is not as yet widely available for clinical use.

5.19.2 Naloxone

Naloxone (17-allylnoroxymorphone; Narcan, Du Pont) (Figure 5.22) is a pure opioid antagonist and is widely used in the treatment of opioid overdosage. It has no agonist activity (Martin, 1976). The precise mechanism of action of naloxone in opiate overdosage is not known, but involves competitive binding at μ (strongest binding), δ and κ CNS opioid receptors (Martin, 1976; Benoist, 1988; Chamberlain and Klein, 1994). Sometimes, at high doses, when CNS effects are seen, naloxone antagonizes GABA receptors and stimulates cholinergic activity (Dingledine *et al.*, 1978). Naloxone has no direct cardiovascular or respiratory actions. It is effective against opiates such as codeine and morphine, and most synthetic opioids such as dextropropoxyphene, diphenoxylate, methadone and pethidine (Buchner *et al.*, 1972). It is also effective against partial agonists such as butorphanol and nalbuphine (Evans *et al.*, 1973; Handal *et al.*, 1983 – see Table 5.3). Oral naloxone at a dose of 10–20 % of that of concurrent opioid analgesia has been suggested for reversal of opioid-induced constipation in cancer patients (Sykes, 1991).

High doses of some synthetic opioids, such as dextropropoxyphene, have been reported to produce toxic effects that are not reversed by naloxone (Barraclough and Lowe, 1982). These effects have been attributed to a direct effect of the drug or its metabolite norpropoxyphene on cardiac cell membranes, but it is possible that not enough naloxone was given to reverse opioid toxicity fully (Barraclough and Lowe, 1982; Hantson *et al.*, 1995). Respiratory depression due to partial agonists (buprenorphine – Figure 5.23, pentazocine) is not, however, readily reversed by naloxone.

Naloxone has been used to treat coma and respiratory depression following clonidine overdose, but in children precipitation of hypertension severe enough to warrant treatment has been reported (Gremse *et al.*, 1986) and its routine use in this situation is not recommended (Chamberlain and Klein, 1994). Inconsistent findings have been obtained when naloxone has been administered after nitrous oxide (Berkowitz *et al.*,

■ CHAPTER 5 ■

	Naloxone (hydrochloride)	Naltrexone (hydrochloride)
CAS registry number	357-08-4	16676-29-2
Molecular weight (free base)	363.8 (327.4)	377.9
pK_a	7.9	8.1
Oral absorption (%)	95	100
Presystemic metabolism (%)	Low	95
Plasma half-life	60–90 min	1.1–10.3 h
Volume of distribution (L/kg)	5	14–16
Plasma protein binding (%)	50	20

TABLE 5.3
Opioid agonists and partial agonists antagonized by naloxone

Alfentanil	Levorphanol
Alletorphine	Lofentanil
Alphaprodine	Loperamide
Anileridine	Meptazinol
Azidomorphine	Methadone
Bezitramide	Metofoline
Buprenorphine	Morphine
Butorphanol	Nalbuphine
Carfentanil	Nicomorphine
Ciramadol	Normethadone
Codeine	Norpipanone
Conorphone	Oxycodone
Dextromoramide	Oxymorphone
Dextropropoxyphene	Pentazocine
Dezocine	Pethidine (Meperidine)
Diamorphine (diacetylmorphine, heroin)	Phenadoxone
Difenoxin	Phenazocine
Dihydrocodeine	Phenoperidine
Diphenoxylate	Picenadol
Dipipanone	Piminodine
Eptazocine	Piritramide
Ethoheptazine	Propiram
Ethylmorphine	Spiradoline
Etorphine	Sufentanil
Fentanyl	Thebacon
Hydrocodone	Tilidine
Hydromorphone	Tonazocine
Ketobemidone	Tramadol
Levomethadone	Trimeperidine
Levomethadyl	

1977; Gillman *et al.*, 1980; Yang *et al.*, 1980). Naloxone has no reliable use in the reversal of ethanol-induced intoxication (Mattila *et al.*, 1981; Guerin and Friedberg, 1982; Nuotto *et al.*, 1983; Chamberlain and Klein, 1994), but may be of value in reversing hypotension due to captopril and other ACE inhibitors (Varon and Duncan, 1991). Reversal of camylofin-induced coma by naloxone in neonates and babies has been reported (Schvartsman *et al.*, 1988), as has reversal of coma induced by sodium valproate in an adult (Montero, 1999).

Oral naloxone has a bioavailability of less than 3 %, and thus the drug has to be given parenterally in order to reverse central opioid effects (Chamberlain and Klein, 1994). Naloxone is available in 1-mL ampoules each containing 0.4 mg naloxone hydrochloride. The contents of the ampoules can be diluted with 0.9 % (w/v) sodium chloride or 5 % (w/v) D-glucose before injection. Naloxone is very lipid soluble (V_D 2.9 L/kg) and rapidly crosses the blood–brain barrier. The plasma half-life of naloxone in adults is 1–2 h (Benoist, 1988). Metabolism is largely via glucuronide formation in the liver and urinary excretion (Benoist, 1988). In neonates, immaturity of glucuronidation is responsible for a more prolonged therapeutic effect than in adults, but this does not occur in children (Benoist, 1988). In adults, the initial dose of naloxone hydrochloride is 0.4 or 0.8 mg *slowly* i.v. or i.m. At least 2.4 mg (bolus dose) is needed to constitute an adequate trial in suspected opioid poisoning; more may be needed to counteract toxicity if a large overdose has been taken (20 mg has been needed in some cases). After i.v. injection, signs of opioid antagonism appear within 1 min if enough drug has been given. In children, the initial dose is 5–10 µg/kg i.v. However, a dose of 0.1 mg/kg has been said to constitute an adequate trial in children (Moore *et al.*, 1980). The drug may be given via an endotracheal tube, or i.m. or s.c. if i.v. access is not available. If these other routes are used then the onset of action may be 5–10 min, or even longer if the patient is hypotensive (Tandberg and Abercrombie, 1982).

Naloxone administration may be repeated if pupillary constriction and respiratory depression (as assessed by respiratory rate and tidal volume) are not reversed within 1–2 min. The dose can be repeated every few minutes as necessary until the level of consciousness and respiratory rate improve. As the half-life of naloxone is much shorter than the half-life of most opioids, naloxone administration may have to be repeated at intervals which may be as short as 20–30 min (Berkowitz, 1976; Hoffman and Goldfrank, 1995), or the drug given by infusion. Infusion of two-thirds of the bolus dose initially required to wake the patient should be given hourly – this can be given diluted in 0.9 % (w/v) sodium chloride and should be titrated to individual patient response (Goldfrank *et al.*, 1986). Treatment may need to be continued for 2–3 days (either by intermittent dosage or by infusion) after overdosage with long-acting opioids such as methadone and normethadone (Gourlay and Coulthard, 1983). Patients must be carefully observed for recurrence of coma and respiratory depression, usually for at least 18–24 h, though the main features of poisoning tend to occur within 1–2 h after the overdose.

When up to 24 mg was given s.c. to adult volunteers naloxone only produced slight drowsiness. At higher doses (up to 4 mg/kg), behavioural disturbances including reluctance to move, sweating, yawning, anxiety, anger, depression, confusion and decreased cognitive function may occur (Martin, 1976; Cohen *et al.*, 1981). Benign transient increases in blood pressure are common after naloxone. However, hypertension, pulmonary oedema and atrial and ventricular dysrhythmias have been associated with post-operative use of naloxone, mostly in patients with known cardiac or pulmonary disease (Chamberlain and Klein, 1994). Two deaths have occurred in previously healthy young adults after naloxone was given i.v. (Andree, 1980). Naloxone use may precipitate fits, especially when large doses are used (Dingledine *et al.*, 1978). There are also a number of isolated reports of anaphylactic reactions to naloxone, but such reactions are seemingly very rare (Goldfrank, 1984).

In opioid-dependent subjects, use of naloxone may precipitate a moderate to severe withdrawal reaction similar to that seen after abrupt withdrawal of opioids such as heroin. The reaction typically appears within minutes of naloxone administration but usually subsides within 2 h or so. It is characterized by abdominal cramps, diarrhoea, piloerection and vasoconstriction causing hypertension (Sun, 1998). Arrhythmias attributed to a rise in catecholamine secretion occur rarely, and are often accompanied by hypoxia or hypercapnia (Michaelis *et al.*, 1974). It is therefore important to ensure adequate oxygenation before naloxone is given (Mills *et al.*, 1988).

■ CHAPTER 5 ■

Naloxone (17-allylnoroxymorphone, Narcan)

- Naloxone is a pure opioid antagonist at the doses used clinically in humans
- Its precise mechanism of action is not known but presumably involves competitive binding at CNS opioid receptors
- It is effective against codeine, heroin, morphine and most synthetic opioids (dextropropoxyphene, diphenoxylate, methadone, pethidine, etc.)
- It is also effective against partial agonists (butorphanol, nalbuphine)
- Diprenorphine (Revivon) is used as an opioid antagonist in veterinary practice as it has a longer plasma half-life in many species

Clinical use of naloxone

- Naloxone is used to reverse the action of opioids – this may include perioperative use
- The normal dose (adults) is 0.4 or 0.8 mg slowly i.v. (or i.m.), titrated according to pupil dilation and response (Glasgow coma scale and respiratory rate)
- It is rapidly metabolized – repeat doses may be needed after 30–60 min, and may need to be continued for 2–3 days (e.g. with methadone)
- It may cause a moderate to severe withdrawal reaction in opioid-dependent subjects
- Naloxone may not reverse respiratory depression due to buprenorphine or pentazocine
- It is relatively safe, although two deaths have been reported in previously healthy young adults after i.v. naloxone

Diagnostic use of naloxone

- Naloxone is given as a diagnostic test in patients with coma/respiratory depression which may be due to opioids
- Lack of response does not always mean that no opioids are present as:
  - brain damage secondary to hypoxia/anoxia may have occurred
  - other drugs may be present
  - insufficient naloxone may have been given (2.4 mg absolute minimum needed for adequate trial in adults)
- Naloxone may have an effect in poisoning with clonidine, but the response is very variable

5.19.3 Naltrexone

Naltrexone (17-cyclopropylmethylnoroxymorphone; Nalorex, Du Pont; Figure 5.22), an analogue of naloxone, is a long-acting opioid antagonist, modifying responses at μ (where it has four times more activity than naloxone), δ and κ receptors (Benoist, 1988). It has twice the opioid antagonist activity of naloxone (Martin *et al.*, 1973) and also weak opioid agonist actions that are clinically insignificant (Gritz *et al.*, 1976). The duration of action of naltrexone is dose related and much longer than that of naloxone. A single dose of naltrexone can be effective for up to 3 days, due in part to the activity and long half-life of its metabolite, β-naltrexone (Verebey *et al.*, 1976). Like naloxone, naltrexone will precipitate an acute withdrawal reaction in patients dependent on opioids. However, naltrexone does not antagonize the effects of phencyclidine, a delta agonist (Moerschbaecher *et al.*, 1988). Despite its low bioavailability (5 % or so) after oral dosage (Meyer *et al.*, 1984), naltrexone is only available commercially in tablet form and is prescribed (one 50-mg tablet daily) to help detoxified opioid addicts to remain abstinent (Miotto *et al.*, 1997). It is not widely available in Europe and tends to be mostly used in the USA.

Recently, naltrexone has been suggested as a possible adjunct to psychosocial treatment of ethanol dependence (Volpicelli, 1995). This additional use of naltrexone was suggested by animal data that demonstrated that ethanol self-administration could be reduced by naltrexone. The underlying mechanism may involve antagonism of the effects of endogenous opioids (McNicholas and Martin, 1984). In alcoholics naltrexone may reduce the pleasure associated with drinking and perhaps the subsequent craving for ethanol (Volpicelli *et al.*, 1995).

5.20 ORG-2766

Org-2766 (CAS 50913-82-1; Figure 5.24) is a 4–9 analogue of corticotrophin (adrenocorticotrophic hormone, ACTH) that protects against the neurotoxicity of cisplatin and of paclitaxel in rats and which is under investigation in man (Lewis, 1994).

H-Met(O₂)-Glu-His-Phe-D-Lys-Phe-OH

Figure 5.24: Schematic representation of Org-2766

5.21 PROCYCLIDINE

Procyclidine (Figure 5.25) is a competitive inhibitor of acetylcholine at muscarinic receptors and is used to treat dystonic reactions caused by antipsychotic drugs and metoclopramide. The i.m. dose is 5–10 mg of procyclidine hydrochloride repeated if necessary after 20 min (maximum 20 mg/d). When given i.v., procyclidine (5 mg) is usually effective within 5 min, but 30 min may be needed before an effect becomes apparent. In some patients, 10 mg or more may be required. In children, 0.5–2 mg (<2

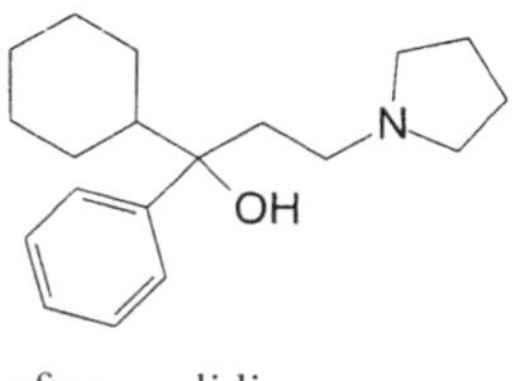

Figure 5.25: Structural formula of procyclidine

Procyclidine (hydrochloride)

CAS registry number	1508-76-5
Molecular weight (free base)	323.9 (287.4)
pK_a	10.7
Oral absorption (%)	100
Presystemic metabolism (%)	25
Plasma half-life (h) mean	12.6
Volume of distribution (L/kg)	1

---

years) or 2–5 mg (2–10 years) procyclidine hydrochloride should be given i.v. (over at least 2 min) or i.m. The dose may be repeated if necessary after 20 min.

5.22 PROTAMINE SULPHATE

Protamine, a basic protein derived from fish sperm, has weak anticoagulant activity. Protamine forms a stable complex with heparin that has no anticoagulant activity and is thus used to stop bleeding after heparin overdose. Protamine has no effect on bleeding caused by coumarin or indandione anticoagulants, hence the use of phytomenadione in these cases (section 4.10). One milligram of protamine i.v. neutralizes 90–115 units of heparin (maximum protamine dose 5 mL of a 10 mg/mL solution over 5 min) if given within 15 min of heparin. If given after this time, less protamine is required as heparin is rapidly excreted. Anaphylactoid reactions (hypotension, dyspnoea, flushing, bradycardia) may occur. The prothrombin time should be monitored after 15 min to assess efficacy. If used in excess, protamine has an anticoagulant effect.

5.23 SILIBININ

The flavonolignan silibinin (3,5,7-trihydroxy-2-[3-(4-hydroxy-3-methoxyphenyl)-2-(hydroxymethyl)-1,4-benzodioxan-6-yl]-4-chromanone; silybin; CAS 22888-70-6; Figure 5.26) is the major component of silymarin, the active principle from the fruit of *Silybum marianum*. It has been suggested that disodium silibinin hemisuccinate at a dose of 5–12.5 mg/kg i.v. in 500 mL 5 % (w/v) D-glucose four times daily can prevent liver damage when given up to 48 h after ingestion of *Amanita phalloides* (Hruby *et al.*, 1983). It is thought that silibinin may act by inhibiting hepatic uptake of α-amanitin. Its efficacy is unproven.

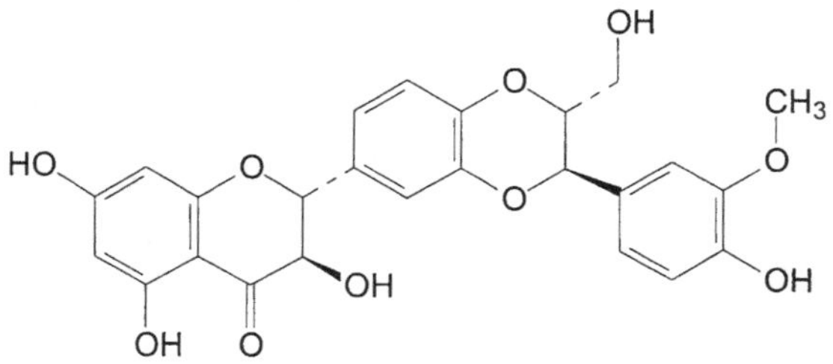

Figure 5.26: Structural formula of silibinin

5.24 SODIUM NITROPRUSSIDE

Sodium nitroprusside (disodium nitrosylpentacyanoferrate; CAS 14402-89-2; Figure 5.27) is a potent, short-acting peripheral vasodilator and as such reverses vasoconstriction and severe hypertension due to amphetamines, ergotamine, MAOIs and methysergide. It is given by i.v. infusion at an initial dose of 0.5–1.5 µg kg^{-1} min^{-1} in either 5 % (w/v) D-glucose or 0.9 % (w/v) sodium chloride. The dose should be increased depending on response by increments of 0.5 µg kg^{-1} min^{-1} every 5 min within a range of 0.5–8 µg/kg/min (British National Formulary, 2000b). The infusion should be protected from light (Palmer and Lasseter, 1975). Adverse effects associated with over-rapid infusion include headache, dizziness, nausea, abdominal pain, palpitations and chest pain. All settle with reduction of the infusion rate. Rarely, reduced platelet count and phlebitis are seen as complications of therapy.

Ideally, an infusion should not be continued for more than 24 h, but in the case of ergotamine especially a longer duration of infusion may be needed. Sodium nitroprusside is metabolized to cyanide and then to thiocyanate, which is excreted via the kidneys and has a long plasma half-life (8 days or so). The treatment of toxicity arising from sodium nitroprusside administration is discussed in section 6.2.4.2. Monitor the blood pressure continuously, and the blood thiocyanate concentration if the duration of treatment exceeds 3 days. Avoid sudden withdrawal; terminate the infusion over 15–30 min. Contraindications to its use include severe hepatic impairment, severe vitamin B$_{12}$ deficiency, Leber's optic atrophy and compensatory hypertension.

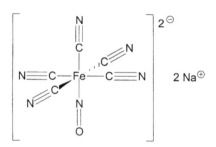

Figure 5.27: Molecular formula of sodium nitroprusside

5.25 TRIMETAZIDINE

It has been suggested that the anti-ischaemic drug trimetazidine (CAS 5011-34-7; Figure 5.28) can protect against the cardiac toxicity of phosphine. Phosphine is a very toxic gas and is widely used as a grain fumigant (Wilson *et al.*, 1980). It is easily produced by hydrolysis of aluminium phosphide. In patients poisoned with aluminium phosphide, elevated malondialdehyde concentrations and lowered reduced glutathione concentrations have been found, indicating the occurrence of oxidative stress in the cardiovascular system (Chugh *et al.*, 1997). Most aluminium phosphide deaths result from cardiovascular collapse. Trimetazidine reduces tissue accumulation of malondialdehyde. One case report suggested that an adult patient's ventricular premature complexes were abolished by oral trimetazidine therapy (20 mg twice daily)

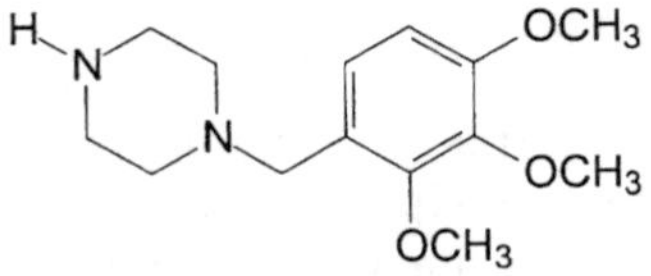

Figure 5.28: Structural formula of trimetazidine

(Dueñas *et al.*, 1999). One case cannot be justification for widespread use and further evaluation is required.

REFERENCES

Amin DN, Henry JA. Propranolol administration in theophylline overdose [letter]. *Lancet* 1985; i: 520–1.

Amrein R, Leishman B, Bentzinger C, Roncarni G. Flumazenil in benzodiazepine antagonism. Actions and clinical use in intoxications and anaesthesiology. *Med Toxicol Adverse Drug Exp* 1987; 2: 411–29.

Andree RA. Sudden death following naloxone administration. *Anesth Analg* 1980; 59: 782–4.

Andrews LG, Muzumdar AS, Pinkerton AC. Hallucinations associated with dantrolene sodium therapy [letter]. *Can Med Assoc J* 1975; 112; 148.

Aquilonius S-M, Hedstrand U. The use of physostigmine as an antidote in tricyclic antidepressant intoxication. *Acta Anaesth Scand* 1978; 22: 40–5.

Assan R. Médicaments hyperglycémiants. In: *Pharmacie Clinique, Bases de la Therapeutique*. Giroud JP, Mathe G, Meyniel G (eds). Paris: Expansion Scientifique Française, 1978: 893–901.

Ballantyne B, Marrs TC (eds). *Clinical and Experimental Toxicology of Organophosphates and Carbamates*. Oxford: Butterworth-Heinemann, 1992.

Barraclough CJ, Lowe RA. Failure of naloxone to reverse the cardiotoxicity of Distalgesic overdose. *Postgrad Med J* 1982; 58: 667–8.

Barsan WG, Seger D, Danzl DF, Ling LJ, Bartlett R, Buncher R, Bryan C. Duration of antagonistic effects of nalmefene and naloxone in opiate-induced sedation for emergency department procedures. *Am J Emerg Med* 1989; 7: 155–61.

Baud FJ, Brouard A. Le flumazénil. In: *Les Antidotes*. Baud F, Barriot P, Riou B (eds). Paris: Masson, 1992; 119–26.

Benoist JM. Analgésiques morphiniques. In *Pharmacologie Clinique. Bases de la Thérapeutique*, 2nd edn. Giroud JP, Mathe G, Meyniel G (eds). Paris: Expansion Scientifique Française, 1988: 813–63.

Berkowitz BA. The relationship of pharmacokinetics to pharmacological activity: morphine, methadone and naloxone. *Clin Pharmacokin* 1976; 1: 219–30.

Berkowitz BA, Finck AD, Ngai SH. Nitrous oxide analgesia: reversal by naloxone and development of tolerance. *J Pharmacol Exp Ther* 1977; 203: 539–47.

Bickel U, Thomsen T, Weber W, Fischer JP, Bachus R, Nitz M, Kewitz H. Pharmacokinetics of galanthamine in humans and corresponding cholinesterase inhibition. *Clin Pharmacol Ther* 1991; 50: 420–8.

Bismuth C. Dantrolène. In: *Les Antidotes*. Baud F, Barriot P, Riou B (eds). Paris: Masson, 1992; 63–86.

Bismuth C, Inns RH, Marrs TC. Efficacy, toxicity and clinical use of oximes in anticholinesterase poisoning. In: *Clinical and Experimental Toxicology of Organophosphates and Carbamates*. Ballantyne B, Marrs TC (eds). Oxford: Butterworth-Heinemann, 1992: 555–77.

Bodemar G, Hjortswang H. Octreotide-induced pancreatitis: an effect of increased contractility of Oddi sphincter. *Lancet* 1996; 348: 1668–9.

Bodenham A, Brownlie G, Dixon JS, Park GR. Reversal of sedation by prolonged infusion of flumazenil (Anexate, Ro 15–1788). *Anaesthesia* 1988; 43: 376–8.

Bondurand A, N'Dri K, Coffi S, Saracino E. L'intoxication à la chloroquine au C.H.U. Abidjan. *Afr Med* 1980; 19: 239–42.

Boyle PJ, Justice K, Krentz AJ, Nagy RJ, Schade DS. Octreotide reverses hyperinsulinemia and prevents hypoglycemia induced by sulphonylurea overdoses. *J Clin Endocrinol Metab* 1993; 76: 752–6.

Breimer LTM, Hennis PJ, Burm AGL, Danhof M, Bovill JG, Spierdijk J, Vletter AA. Pharmacokinetics and EEG effects of flumazenil in volunteers. *Clin Pharmacokinet* 1991; 20: 491–6.

Briggs CJ, Simons KJ. Treatment of organophosphorus poisoning: pharmaceutical aspects of antidotes. In: *Proceedings of the 23rd International Meeting of The International Association of Forensic Toxicologists*. Heyndrickx B (ed.). Ghent: The International Association of Forensic Toxicologists, 1986: 514–23.

British National Formulary. 40th edn. London: British Medical Association and Royal Pharmaceutical Society of Great Britain, 2000a: 473.

British National Formulary. 40th edn. London: British Medical Association and Royal Pharmaceutical Society of Great Britain, 2000b: 85.

Brogden RN, Goa KL. Flumazenil: a reappraisal of its pharmacological properties and therapeutic efficacy as a benzodiazepine antagonist. *Drugs* 1991; 42: 1061–89.

Buchner LH, Cimino JA, Raybin HW, Stewart B. Naloxone reversal of methadone poisoning. *NY State J Med* 1972; 72: 2305–9.

Buckley NA, Smith AJ, Dosen P, O'Connell DL. Effects of catecholamines and diazepam in chloroquine poisoning in barbiturate anaesthetised rats. *Hum Exp Toxicol* 1996; 15: 909–14.

Burgess JL, Bernstein JN, Hurlbut K. Aldicarb poisoning: a case report with prolonged cholinesterase inhibition and improvement after pralidoxime therapy. *Arch Intern Med* 1994; 154: 221–4.

Burke RE, Fahn S, Mayeux R, Weinberg H, Louis K, Willner JH. Neuroleptic malignant syndrome caused by dopamine-depleting drugs in a patient with Huntington disease. *Neurology* 1981; 31: 1022–5.

Burkhart KK, Kulig KW. The diagnostic utility of flumazenil (a benzodiazepine antagonist) in coma of unknown etiology. *Ann Emerg Med* 1990; 19: 319–21.

Byrnes SMA, Watson GW, Hardy PAJ. Flumazenil: an unreliable antagonist in baclofen overdose. *Anaesthesia* 1996; 51: 481–2.

Cavaliere MJ, Puga FR, Calore EE, Calore NMP, Pelegrino J di R, da Rosa AR, Weg R. Protective effect of pralidoxime on muscle fiber necrosis induced by organophosphate compounds. *Clin Toxicol* 1998; 36: 295–300.

Chamberlain JM, Klein BL. A comprehensive review of naloxone for the emergency physician. *Am J Emerg Med* 1994; 12: 650–60.

Chern C-H, Chern T-L, Wang L-M, Hu S-C, Deng J-F, Lee C-H. Continuous flumazenil infusion in preventing complications arising from severe benzodiazepine intoxication. *Am J Emerg Med* 1998; 16: 238–41.

Chew SK, Chew LS, Wang KW, Mah PK, Tan BY. Anticholinesterase drugs in the treatment of tetrodotoxin poisoning. *Lancet* 1984; ii: 108.

Chiolero R-L, Ravussin P, Anderes J-P, Ledermann P, de Tribolet N. The effects of midazolam reversal by RO 15-1788 on cerebral perfusion pressure in patients with severe head injury. *Intensive Care Med* 1988; 14: 196–200.

Choi PT-L, Quinonez LG, Cook DJ, Baxter F, Whitehead L. The use of glycopyrrolate in a case of intermediate syndrome following acute organophosphate poisoning. *Can J Anaesth* 1998; 45: 337–40.

Chugh SN, Kolley T, Kakkar R, Chugh K, Sharma A. A critical evaluation of antiperoxidant effect of intravenous magnesium in acute aluminium phosphide poisoning. *Magnesium Res* 1997; 10: 225–30.

■ CHAPTER 5 ■

Clement JG, Lockwood PA, Thompson HG. The acetylcholinesterase reactivator HI-6 (1-[[[4-(aminocarbonyl)pyridinio]methoxy]methyl]-2-[(hydroxyimino)methyl]pyridinium dichloride): a comparative study of HI-6 samples from various sources. *Arch Toxicol* 1988; 62: 220–3.

Cohen MR, Cohen RM, Pickar D, Weingartner H, Murphy DL, Bunney WE. Behavioural effects after high dose naloxone administration to normal volunteers [letter]. *Lancet* 1981; ii: 1110.

Cone AM, Stott SA. Flumazenil. *Br J Hosp Med* 1994; 51: 346–8.

Cordoba D, Cadavid S, Angulo D, Ramos I. Organophosphate poisoning: modifications in acid base equilibrium and use of sodium bicarbonate as an aid to the treatment of toxicity in dogs. *Vet Hum Toxicol* 1983; 25: 1–3.

Critchley JAJH, Ungar A. The management of acute poisoning due to β-adrenoceptor antagonists. *Med Toxicol Adverse Drug Exp* 1989; 4: 32–45.

Croes K, Augustijns P, Sabbe M, Desmet K, Verbeke N. Diminished sedation during diazepam treatment for chloroquine intoxication. *Pharma World Sci* 1993; 15: 83–5.

Crouzette J, Vicaut E, Palombo S, Girre C, Fournier PE. Experimental assessment of the protective activity of diazepam on the acute toxicity of chloroquine. *J Toxicol Clin Toxicol* 1983; 20: 271–9.

Das Gupta S, Ghosh AK, Chowdhri BL, Asthana SN, Batra BS. Actions and interactions of cholinolytics and cholinesterase reactivators in the treatment of acute organophosphorus toxicity. *Drug Chem Toxicol* 1991; 14: 283–91.

Denborough MA, Hopkinson KC. Dantrolene and 'ecstasy'. *Med J Aust* 1997; 166: 165–6.

Dingledine R, Iversen LL, Breuker E. Naloxone as a GABA antagonist: evidence for iontophoretic, receptor binding and convulsant studies. *Eur J Pharmacol* 1978; 47: 19–27.

Dixon JC, Speidel BD, Dixon JJ. Neonatal flumazenil therapy reverses maternal diazepam. *Acta Paediatr* 1998; 87: 225–6.

Dixon R, Howes J, Gentile J, Hsu H-B, Hsiao J, Garg D, Weidler D, Meyer M, Tuttle R. Nalmefene: intravenous safety and kinetics of a new opioid antagonist. *Clin Pharmacol Ther* 1986; 39: 49–53.

Dueñas A, Pérez-Castrillon JL, Cobos MA, Herreros V. Treatment of the cardiovascular manifestations of phosphine poisoning with trimetazidine, a new antiischemic drug [letter]. *Am J Emerg Med* 1999; 17: 219–20.

Ekins BR, Geller RJ. Methomyl-induced carbamate poisoning treated with pralidoxime chloride. *West Med J* 1994; 161: 68–70.

Erdmann WD, Engelhard H. Pharmacologic/toxicologic investigations of a new esterase reactivator – the dichloride of bis-[4-hydroxyiminomethyl-pyridinium-(1)-methyl]-ether. *Arzneim Forsch* 1964; 14: 5–11.

Evans LEJ, Roscoe P, Swainson CP, Prescott LF. Treatment of drug overdose with naloxone, a specific narcotic antagonist. *Lancet* 1973; i: 452–5.

Fant JS, James LP, Fiser RT, Kearns GL. The use of glucagon in nifedipine poisoning complicated by clonidine ingestion. *Pediatr Emerg Care* 1997; 13: 417–19.

Farrer HC, Wells TG, Kearns GL. Use of continuous infusion of pralidoxime for treatment of organophosphate poisoning in children. *J Pediatr* 1990; 116: 658–61.

Finkelstein Y, Taitelman U, Biegon A. CNS involvement in acute organophosphate poisoning: specific patterns of toxicity, clinical correlates and antidotal treatment. *It J Neuro Sci* 1988; 9: 437–46.

Finkelstein Y, Kushnir A, Raikhlin-Eisenkraft B, Taitelman U. Antidotal therapy of severe acute organophosphate poisoning: a multihospital study. *Neurotoxicol Teratol* 1989; 11: 593–6.

Flewellen EH, Nelson TE. Intravenous dantrolene pharmacokinetics in malignant hyperthermia suspect patients [abstract]. *Anesthesiology* 1985; 63: A300.

Flewellen EH, Nelson TE, Jones WP, Arens JF, Wagner DL. Dantrolene dose response in awake man: implications for management of malignant hyperthermia. *Anesthesiology* 1983; 59: 275–80.

Fredenrich A, Sosset C, Bernard JL, Sadoul JL, Freychet P. Acute pancreatitis after short-term octreotide [letter]. *Lancet* 1991; 338: 52–3.

Frye RF, Matzke GR, Jallad NS, Wilhelm JA, Bikhazi GB. The effect of age on the pharmacokinetics of the opioid antagonist nalmefene. *Br J Clin Pharmacol* 1996; 42: 301–6.

Fudala PJ, Heishman SJ, Henningfield JE, Johnson RE. Human pharmacology and abuse potential of nalmefene. *Clin Pharmacol Ther* 1991; 49: 300–6.

Gal TJ, DiFazio CA, Dixon R. Prolonged blockade of opioid effect with oral nalmefene. *Clin Pharmacol Ther* 1986; 40: 537–42.

Gath I, Weidenfeld J, Collins GI, Hadad H. Electrophysiological aspects of benzodiazepine antagonists, Ro 15-1788 and Ro 15-3505. *Br J Clin Pharmacol* 1984; 18: 541–7.

Gendron BP. *Loxosceles reclusa* envenomation. *Am J Emerg Med* 1990; 8: 51–4.

Geller E, Crome P, Schaller MD, Marchant B, Ectors M, Scollo-Lavizzari G. Risks and benefits of therapy with flumazenil (Anexate®) in mixed drug intoxications. *Eur Neurol* 1991; 31: 241–50.

Gillman MA, Kok L, Lichtigfeld FJ. Paradoxical effect of naloxone on nitrous oxide analgesia in man. *Eur J Pharmacol* 1980; 61: 175–7.

Gillman PK. Serotonin syndrome: history and risk. *Fundam Clin Pharmacol* 1998: 12: 482–91.

Glass PS, Jhaveri RM, Smith LR. Comparison of potency and duration of action of nalmefene and naloxone. *Anaesth Anal* 1994; 78: 536–41.

Goldfrank LR. The several uses of naloxone. *Emerg Med* 1984; 16: 105–16.

Goldfrank L, Weisman RS, Errick JK, Lo M-W. A dosing nomogram for continuous infusion of intravenous naloxone. *Ann Emerg Med* 1986; 15: 566–70.

Gourlay GK, Coulthard K. The role of naloxone infusions in the treatment of overdoses of long half-life narcotic agonists: application to normethadone. *Br J Clin Pharmacol* 1983; 15: 269–72.

Greenspun B, Pacho A. Leukopenia with dantrolene sodium [abstract]. *Arch Phys Med Rehabil* 1981; 62: 521.

Gremse DA, Artman M, Boerth RC. Hypertension associated with naloxone treatment for clonidine poisoning. *J Pediatr* 1986; 108: 776–8.

Gritz ER, Shiffman SM, Jarvik ME, Schlesinger J, Charuvastra VC. Naltrexone: physiological and psychological effects of single doses. *Clin Pharmacol Ther* 1976; 19: 773–6.

Guerin JM, Friedberg G. Naloxone and ethanol intoxication [letter]. *Ann Intern Med* 1982; 97: 932.

Guzé BH, Baxter LR. Neuroleptic malignant syndrome. *N Engl J Med* 1985; 313: 163–6.

Hahn HL, Henschler D. Reactivation of phosphorylated cholinesterases by obidoxime (Toxogonin) in vivo [in German]. *Arch Toxicol* 1969; 24: 147–63.

Hall-Boyer K, Zaloga GP, Chernow B. Glucagon: hormone or therapeutic agent? *Crit Care Med* 1984; 12: 584–9.

Handal KA, Schauben JL, Salamone FR. Naloxone. *Ann Emerg Med* 1983; 12: 438–45.

Hantson P, Evenepool M, Ziade D, Hassoun A, Mahieu P. Adverse cardiac manifestations following dextropropoxyphene overdose: can naloxone be helpful? *Ann Emerg Med* 1995; 25: 263–6.

Harris LW, Heyl WC, Stitcher DL, Broomfield CA. Effects of 1,1′-oxydimethylene bis-(4-tert-butylpyridinium chloride) (SAD-128) and decamethonium on reactivation of soman- and sarin-inhibited cholinesterase by oximes. *Biochem Pharmacol* 1978; 27: 757–61.

Harrison GG. Dantrolene – dynamics and kinetics. *Br J Anaesth* 1988; 60: 279–86.

Hasan MY, Schauben JL, Holmes CH. Management of neuroleptic malignant syndrome with anticholinergic medication. *Vet Hum Toxicol* 1999; 41: 79–81.

Haverkos GP, DiSalvo RP, Imhoff TE. Fatal seizures after flumazenil administration in a patient with mixed overdose. *Ann Pharmacother* 1994; 28: 1347–9.

Heath AJW, Meredith T. Atropine in the management of anticholinesterase poisoning. In: *Clinical and Experimental Toxicology of Organophosphates and Carbamates*. Ballantyne B, Marrs TC (eds). Oxford: Butterworth Heinemann, 1992: 543–54.

■ CHAPTER 5 ■

Hofer P, Scollo-Lavizzari G. Benzodiazepine antagonist Ro 15-1788 in self-poisoning: diagnostic and therapeutic use. *Arch Intern Med* 1985; 145: 663–4.

Hoffman RS, Goldfrank LR. The poisoned patient with altered consciousness: controversies in the use of a 'coma cocktail'. *J Am Med Assoc* 1995; 274: 562–9.

Hoffman EJ, Warren EW. Flumazenil: a benzodiazepine antagonist. *Clin Pharm* 1993; 12: 641–56.

Höjer J. Management of benzodiazepine overdose. *CNS Drugs* 1994; 2: 7–17.

Höjer J, Baehrendtz S, Matell G, Gustafsson LL. Diagnostic utility of flumazenil in coma with suspected poisoning: a double blind, randomised controlled study. *Br Med J* 1990; 301: 1308–11.

Holland P, Parkes DC. Plasma concentrations of the oxime pralidoxime mesylate (P2S) after repeated oral and intramuscular administration. *Br J Ind Med* 1976; 33: 43–6.

Holland P, Parkes DC, White RG. Pralidoxime mesylate absorption and heart rate response to atropine sulphate following intramuscular administration of solution mixtures. *Br J Clin Pharmacol* 1975; 2: 333–8.

ten Holter JBM, Schellens RLLAM. Dantrolene sodium for treatment of carbon monoxide poisoning. *Br Med J* 1988; 296: 1772–3.

Hruby K, Csomos G, Fuhrmann M, Thaler H. Chemotherapy of *Amanita phalloides* poisoning with intravenous silibinin. *Human Toxicol* 1983; 2: 183–95.

Hunkeler W, Möhler H, Pieri L, Polc P, Bonetti EP, Cumin R, Schaffner R, Haefely W. Selective antagonists of benzodiazepines. *Nature* 1981; 290: 514–16.

Iserson KV. Methemoglobinemia from dapsone therapy for a suspected brown recluse spider bite. *J Emerg Med* 1985; 3: 285–8.

Johnson MK, Jacobsen D, Meredith TJ, Eyer P, Heath AJ, Ligtenstein DA, Marrs TC, Szincz L, Vale JA, Haines JA. Evaluation of antidotes for poisoning by organophosphorus pesticides. *Emerg Med* 2000; 12: 22–37.

Jones AL, Dargan PI. *Textbook of Toxicology*. Edinburgh: Churchill Livingstone, 2001: 51, 89.

Jones AL, Simpson KJ. Mechanisms and management of hepatotoxicity in ecstasy (MDMA) and amphetamine intoxications. *Aliment Pharmacol Ther* 1999; 13: 129–33.

Jovanović D, Randjelović S, Joksović D. A case of unusual suicidal poisoning by the organophosphorus insecticide dimethoate. *Hum Exp Toxicol* 1990; 9: 49–51.

Kalman S, Berg S, Lisander B. Combined overdose with verapamil and atenolol: treatment with high doses of adrenergic agonists. *Acta Anaesthesiol Scand* 1998; 42: 379–82.

Kaplan JL, Marx JA. Effectiveness and safety of intravenous nalmefene for emergency department patients with suspected narcotic overdose: a pilot study. *Ann Emerg Med* 1993; 22: 187–90.

Kaplan RF, Feinglass NG, Webster W, Mudra S. Phenelzine overdose treated with dantrolene sodium. *J Am Med Assoc* 1986; 255: 642–4.

Kaplan JL, Marx JA, Calabro JJ, Gin-Shaw SL, Spiller JD, Spivey WL, Gaddis GM, Zhao N, Harchelroad FP. Double-blind, randomised study of nalmefene and naloxone in emergency department patients with suspected narcotic overdose. *Ann Emerg Med* 1999; 34: 42–50.

Karalliedde L, Gauci CA, Carter M. Chemical weapons [letter]. *Br Med J* 1991; 302: 474.

Kassa J. A comparison of the therapeutic efficacy of conventional and modern oximes against supralethal doses of highly toxic organophosphates in mice. *Acta Med (Hradec Králové)* 1998; 41: 19–21.

Kassa J, Cabal J. A comparison of the efficacy of actylcholinesterase reactivators against cyclohexyl methylphosphonofluoridate (GF agent) by *in vitro* and *in vivo* methods. *Pharmacol Toxicol* 1999; 84: 41–5.

Keeler JR, Hurst CG, Dunn MA. Pyridostigmine used as a nerve agent pretreatment under wartime conditions. *J Am Med Assoc* 1991; 266: 693–5.

King LE, Rees RS. Dapsone treatment of a brown recluse bite. *J Am Med Assoc* 1983; 250: 648.

Klotz U, Ziegler G, Reimann IW. Pharmacokinetics of the selective benzodiazepine antagonist Ro15–1788 in man. *Eur J Clin Pharmacol* 1984; 27: 115–17.

Klotz U, Ziegler G, Ludwig L, Reimann IW. Pharmacodynamic interaction between midazolam and a specific benzodiazepine antagonist in humans. *J Clin Pharmacol* 1985; 25: 400–6.

Knudsen K, Heath A. Effects of self-poisoning with maprotilene. *Br Med J* 1984; 288: 601–3.

Kolb ME, Horne ML, Martz R. Dantrolene in human malignant hyperthermia. A multicenter study. *Anesthesiology* 1982; 56: 254–62.

Kondritzer AA, Zvirblis P, Goodman A, Paplanus SH. Blood plasma levels and elimination of salts of 2-PAM in man after oral administration. *J Pharm Sci* 1968; 57: 1142–6.

Konieczko KM, Jones JG, Barrowcliffe MP, Jordan C, Altman DG. Antagonism of morphine-induced respiratory depression with nalmefene. *Br J Anaesth* 1988; 61: 318–23.

Korstanje C, Jonkman FAM, van Kemenade JE, van Zweiten PA. Bay K 8644, a calcium entry promoter, as an antidote in verapamil intoxication in rabbits. *Arch Int Pharmacodyn Ther* 1987; 287: 109–19.

Krentz AJ, Boyle PJ, Justice KM, Wright AD, Schade DS. Successful treatment of severe refractory sulfonylurea-induced hypoglycemia with octreotide. *Diabet Care* 1993; 16: 184–6.

Kurtz PH. Pralidoxime in the treatment of carbamate intoxication. *Am J Emerg Med* 1990; 8: 68–70.

Kušić R, Jovanović D, Randjelović S, Joksović D, Todorović V, Bošković B, Jokanović M, Vojvodić V. HI-6 in man: efficacy of the oxime in poisoning by organophosphorus insecticides. *Hum Exp Toxicol* 1991; 10: 113–18.

Lallement G, Mestries JC, Privat A, Brochier G, Baubichon D, Carpentier P, Kamenka JM, Sentenac-Roumanou H, Burckhart M-F, Peoc'h M. GK 11: promising additional neuroprotective therapy for organophosphate poisoning. *NeuroToxicology* 1997; 18: 851–6.

Lauven PM, Schwilden H, Stoeckel H, Greenblatt DJ. The effect of a benzodiazepine antagonist Ro 15-1788 in the presence of stable concentrations of midazolam. *Anesthesiology* 1985; 63: 61–4.

Lewis C. A review of the use of chemoprotectants in cancer chemotherapy. *Drug Safety* 1994; 11: 153–62.

Lietman PS, Haslam RHA, Walcher JR. Pharmacology of dantrolene sodium in children. *Arch Phys Med Rehabil* 1974; 55: 388–92.

Lheureux P, Askenasi R. Les récepteurs des benzodiazépines et leurs antagonistes: intérêt et applications en clinique. *Réan Soins Intens Méd Urg* 1988; 4: 17–27.

Lheureux P, Debailleul G, De Witte O, Askenasi R. Zolpidem intoxication mimicking narcotic overdose: response to flumazenil. *Hum Exp Toxicol* 1990; 9: 105–7.

Lheureux P, Vranckx M, Leduc D, Askenasi R. Flumazenil in mixed benzodiazepine/tricyclic antidepressant overdose: a placebo-controlled study in the dog. *Am J Emerg Med* 1992; 10: 184–8.

Love JN, Leasure JA, Mundt DJ. A comparison of combined amrinone and glucagon therapy to glucagon alone for cardiovascular depression associated with propranolol toxicity in a canine model. *Am J Emerg Med* 1993; 11: 360–3.

Luo C, Ashani Y, Doctor BP. Acceleration of oxime-induced reactivation of organophosphate-inhibited fetal bovine serum acetylcholinesterase by monoquaternary and bisquaternary ligands. *Mol Pharmacol* 1998; 53: 718–26.

Luo C, Saxena A, Ashani Y, Leader H, Radić Z, Taylor P, Doctor BP. Role of edrophonium in prevention of the re-inhibition of acetylcholinesterase by phosphorylated oxime. *Chem Biol Interact* 1999a; 119–120: 129–35.

Luo C, Saxena A, Smith M, Garcia G, Radić Z, Taylor P, Doctor BP. Phosphoryl oxime inhibition of acetylcholinesterase during oxime reactivation is prevented by edrophonium. *Biochemistry* 1999b; 38: 9937–47.

McNicholas LF, Martin WR. New and experimental therapeutic roles for naloxone and related opioid antagonists. *Drugs* 1984; 27: 81–93.

Mahr NC, Valdes A, Lamas G. Use of glucagon for acute intravenous diltiazem toxicity. *Am J Cardiol* 1997; 79: 1570–1.

Mansell PI. Glucagon in the management of deliberate self-poisoning with propranolol [letter]. *Arch Emerg Med* 1990; 7: 238–40

Martens F, Köppel C, Ibe K, Wagemann A, Tenczer J. Clinical experience with the benzodiazepine antagonist flumazenil in suspected benzodiazepine or ethanol poisoning. *Clin Toxicol* 1990; 28: 341–56.

Martin WR. Naloxone. *Ann Intern Med* 1976; 85: 765–8.

Martin WR, Jasinski DR, Mansky PA. Naltrexone, an antagonist for the treatment of heroin dependence. *Arch Gen Psychiatr* 1973; 28: 784–91.

Mattila MJ, Nuotto E, Seppälä T. Naloxone is not an effective antagonist of ethanol [letter]. *Lancet* 1981; i: 775–6.

Matzke GR, Frye RF, Alexander ACM, Reynolds R, Dixon R, Johnston J, Rault RM. The effect of renal insufficiency and hemodialysis on the pharmacokinetics of nalmefene. *J Clin Pharmacol* 1996; 36: 144–51.

Maurer R, Gaehwiler BH, Buescher HH, Hill RC, Roemer D. Opiate antagonistic properties of an octapeptide somatostatin analog. *Proc Natl Acad Sci USA* 1982; 79: 4815–17.

Meredith TJ, Jacobsen D, Haines JA, Berger J-C. (eds) *Naloxone, Flumazenil and Dantrolene as Antidotes. IPCS/CEC Evaluation of Antidotes Series*, Volume 1. Cambridge: Cambridge University Press, 1993.

Merrill DG, Mihm FG. Prolonged toxicity of organophosphate poisoning. *Crit Care Med* 1982; 10: 550–1.

Mete E, Dilmen U, Energin M, Özkan B, Güler I. Calcitonin therapy in vitamin D intoxication. *J Tropic Paediatr* 1997; 43: 241–2.

Meyer MC, Straughn AB, Low M-W, Schary WL, Whitney CC. Bioequivalence, dose-proportionality, and pharmacokinetics of naltrexone after oral administration. *J Clin Psychiatr* 1984; 45: 15–19.

Meyler WJ, Mols-Thürkow HW, Wesseling H. Relationship between plasma concentration and effect of dantrolene sodium in man. *Eur J Clin Pharmacol* 1979; 16: 203–9.

Michaelis LL, Hickey PR, Clark TA, Dixon WM. Ventricular irritability associated with the use of naloxone hydrochloride: two case reports and laboratory assessment of the effect of the drug on cardiac excitability. *Ann Thorac Surg* 1974; 18: 608–14.

Mills CA, Flacke JW, Miller JD, Davis LJ, Bloor BC, Flacke WE. Cardiovascular effects of fentanyl reversal by naloxone at varying arterial carbon dioxide tensions in dogs. *Anesth Analg* 1988; 67: 730–6.

Minton NA, Murray VSG. A review of organophosphate poisoning. *Med Toxicol Adverse Drug Exp* 1988; 3: 350–75.

Miotto K, McCann MJ, Rawson RA, Frosch D, Ling W. Overdose, suicide attempts and death among a cohort of naltrexone-treated opioid addicts. *Drug Alc Depend* 1997; 45: 131–4.

Moerschbaecher JM, Devia C, Brocklehurst C. Differential antagonism by naltrexone of the effects of opioids on a fixed-ratio discrimination in rats. *J Pharmacol Exp Ther* 1988; 244: 237–46.

Montero FJ. Naloxone in the reversal of coma induced by sodium valproate. *Ann Emerg Med* 1999; 33: 357–8.

Moore RA, Rumack BH, Conner CS, Peterson RG. Naloxone: underdosage after narcotic poisoning. *Am J Dis Child* 1980; 134: 156–8.

Mortensen ME. Pharmacological and toxicological considerations in the treatment of carbamate intoxications. *Am J Emerg Med* 1990; 8: 83–4.

Müller-Schwefe G, Penn RD. Physostigmine in the treatment of intrathecal baclofen overdose. Report of three cases. *J Neurosurg* 1989; 71: 273–5.

Mullins ME. First-degree atrioventricular block in alprazolam overdose reversed by flumazenil. *J Pharm Pharmacol* 1999; 51: 367–70.

Natoff IL, Reiff B. Effect of oximes on the acute toxicity of anticholinesterase carbamates. *Toxicol Appl Pharmacol* 1973; 25: 569–75.

N'Dri KD, Palis R, Saracino E, NyoUma A, Bondurand A. A propos de 286 intoxications a la chloroquine. *Afr Med* 1976; 15: 103–5.

Nuotto E, Palva ES, Lahdenranta U. Naloxone fails to counteract heavy ethanol intoxication [letter]. *Lancet* 1983; ii: 167.

O'Mahony D, O'Leary P, Molloy MG. Severe oxprenolol poisoning: the importance of glucagon infusion. *Hum Exp Toxicol* 1990; 9: 101–3.

Palmer RF, Lasseter KD. Sodium nitroprusside. *N Engl J Med* 1975; 292: 294–7.

Parfitt K (ed.). *Martindale: The Complete Drug Reference*, 32nd edn. London: Pharmaceutical Press, 1999: 982–3.

Parmley WW, Glick G, Sonnenblick EH. Cardiovascular effects of glucagon in man. *N Engl J Med* 1968; 279: 12–17.

Parr MJA, Willatts SM. Fatal theophylline poisoning with rhabdomyolysis. A potential role for dantrolene treatment. *Anaesthesia* 1991; 46: 557–9.

Passeron D, Peschaud JL, Kienlen J, du Cailar J. A preliminary report on the use of the benzodiazepine antagonist (flumazenil) in overdose [abstract; in French]. *Ann Fr Anesth Réanimat* 1987; 5: 26A.

Peterson CD, Leeder JS, Sterner S. Glucagon therapy for β-blocker overdose. *Drug Intell Clin Pharm* 1984; 18: 394–8.

Phillips RE, Warrell DA, Looareesuwan S, Turner RC, Bloom SR, Quantrill D, Moore RA. Effectiveness of SMS 201–995, a synthetic, long-acting somatostatin analogue, in treatment of quinine-induced hyperinsulinaemia. *Lancet* 1986; i: 713–16.

Phillips RE, Looareesuwan S, Molyneux ME, Hatz C, Warrell DA. Hypoglycaemia and counterregulatory hormone responses in severe falciparum malaria: treatment with Sandostatin. *Q J Med* 1993; 86: 233–40.

Plant JR, MacLeod BD. Response of a promethazine-induced coma to flumazenil. *Ann Emerg Med* 1994; 24: 979–82.

Pollack CV. Utility of glucagon in the emergency department. *J Emerg Med* 1993; 11: 195–205.

Pope HG, Cole JO, Choras PT, Fulwiler CE. Apparent neuroleptic malignant syndrome with clozapine and lithium. *J Nerv Ment Dis* 1986; 174: 493–5.

Prischl F, Donner A, Grimm G, Smetana R, Hruby K. Value of flumazenil in benzodiazepine self-poisoning. *Med Toxicol Adverse Drug Exp* 1988; 3: 334–9.

Rees R, Campbell D, Rieger E, King LE. The diagnosis and treatment of brown recluse spider bites. *Ann Emerg Med* 1987; 16: 945–9.

Ricou B, Forster A, Brückner A, Chastonay P, Gemperle M. Clinical evaluation of a specific benzodiazepine antagonist (RO 15-1788). Studies in elderly patients after regional anaesthesia under benzodiazepine sedation. *Br J Anaesth* 1986; 58: 1005–11.

Riou B, Rimailho A, Gaillot M, Bourdon R, Huet Y. Treatment of chloroquine poisoning with diazepam: preliminary results of an experimental study. *Intensive Care Med* 1986; 12: S175.

Riou B, Barriot P, Rimailho A, Baud FJ. Treatment of severe chloroquine poisoning. *N Engl J Med* 1988; 318: 1–6.

Rivera VM, Breitbach WB, Swanke L. Dantrolene in amyotrophic lateral sclerosis [letter]. *J Am Med Assoc* 1975; 233: 863–4.

Roesch C, Becker PG, Sklar S. Management of a child with acute thyroxine ingestion. *Ann Emerg Med* 1985; 14: 1114–15.

Roncari G, Ziegler WH, Guentert TW. Pharmacokinetics of the new benzodiazepine antagonist Ro 15-1788 in man following intravenous and oral administration. *Br J Clin Pharmacol* 1986; 22: 421–8.

Roncari G, Timm U, Zell M, Zumbrunnen R, Weber W. Flumazenil kinetics in the elderly. *Eur J Clin Pharmacol* 1993; 45: 585–7.

Rousseaux CG, Dua AK. Pharmacology of HI-6, an H series oxime. *Can J Physiol Pharmacol* 1989; 67: 1183–9.

Saissy JM, Vitris M, Demazière J, Seck M, Marcoux L, Gaye M. Flumazenil counteracts intrathecal baclofen-induced central nervous system depression in tetanus. *Anesthesiology* 1992; 76: 1051–3.

CHAPTER 5

Schmidt W, Lang K. Life-threatening dysrhythmias in severe thioridazine poisoning treated with physostigmine and transient atrial pacing. *Crit Care Med* 1997; 25: 1925–30.

Schneider R, Mitchell D. Dantrolene hepatitis. *J Am Med Assoc* 1976; 235: 1590–1.

Schoene K, König A, Oldiges H, Krügel M. Pharmacokinetics and efficacies of obidoxime and atropine in paraoxon poisoning. *Arch Toxicol* 1988; 61: 387–91.

Schvartsman S, Schvartsman C, Barsanti C. Camylofin intoxication reversed by naloxone [letter]. *Lancet* 1988; ii: 1246.

Sener EK, Gabe S, Henry JA. Response to glucagon in imipramine overdose. *Clin Toxicol* 1995; 33: 51–3.

Sensky PR, Olczak SA. High-dose intravenous glucagon in severe tricyclic poisoning. *Postgrad Med J* 1999; 75: 611–12.

Short TG, Maling T, Galletly DC. Ventricular arrhythmia precipitated by flumazenil. *Br Med J* 1988; 296: 1070–1.

Sidell FR, Groff WA. Toxogonin: blood levels and side effects after intramuscular administration in man. *J Pharm Sci* 1970; 59: 793–7.

Sidell FR, Groff WA. Intramuscular and intravenous administration of small doses of 2-pyridinium aldoxime methochloride to man. *J Pharm Sci* 1971; 60: 1224–8.

Sidell FR, Groff WA, Ellin RI. Blood levels of oxime and symptoms in humans after single and multiple oral doses of 2-pyridine aldoxime methochloride. *J Pharm Sci* 1969; 58: 1093–8.

Sidell FR, Groff WA, Kaminskis A. Toxogonin and pralidoxime: kinetic comparison after intravenous administration to man. *J Pharm Sci* 1972; 61: 1765–9.

de Silva HJ, Wijewickrema R, Senanayake N. Does pralidoxime affect outcome of management in acute organophosphorus poisoning? *Lancet* 1992; 339: 1136–8.

Sopchak CA, Stork CM, Cantor RM, Ohara PE. Central anticholinergic syndrome due to Jimson weed physostigmine: therapy revisited? [letter]. *J Toxicol Clin Toxicol* 1998; 36: 43–5.

Sornay E, Broussolle C, Terreaux F, Martin C, Orgiazzi J, Noel G. Le glucagon est-il un hyperglycémiant sans risque? [letter]. *Presse Med* 1988; 17: 165.

Spiller HA. Management of sulfonylurea ingestions. *Pediatr Emerg Care* 1999; 15: 227–30.

Sterri SH, Rognerud B, Fiskum SE, Lyngaas S. Effect of toxogonin and P2S on the toxicity of carbamates and organophosphorus compounds. *Acta Pharmacol Toxicol* 1979; 45: 9–15.

Sun HL. Naloxone-precipitated acute opioid withdrawal syndrome after epidural morphine. *Anesth Analg* 1998; 86: 544–5.

Swartz RD, Sidell FR. Effects of heat and exercise on the elimination of pralidoxime in man. *Clin Pharmacol Ther* 1973; 14: 83–9.

Sykes NP. Oral naloxone in opioid-associated constipation [letter]. *Lancet* 1991; 337: 1475.

Tandberg D, Abercrombie D. Treatment of heroin overdose with endotracheal naloxone. *Ann Emerg Med* 1982; 11: 443–5.

Thiermann H, Mast U, Klimmek R, Eyer P, Hibler A, Pfab R, Felgenhauer N, Zilker T. Cholinesterase status, pharmacokinetics and laboratory findings during obidoxime therapy in organophosphate poisoned patients. *Hum Exp Toxicol* 1997; 16: 473–80.

Thompson DF, Thompson GD, Greenwood RB, Trammel HL. Therapeutic dosing of pralidoxime chloride. *Drug Intell Clin Pharm* 1987; 21: 590–3.

Toet AE, Wemer J, Vleeming W, te Biesebeek JD, Meulenbelt J, de Wildt DJ. Experimental study of the detrimental effect of dopamine/glucagon combination in D,L-propranolol intoxication. *Hum Exp Toxicol* 1996; 15: 411–21.

Tovar JL, Bujons I, Ruiz JC, Ibañez L, Salgado A. Treatment of severe combined overdose of calcium antagonists and converting enzyme inhibitors with angiotensin II [letter]. *Nephron* 1997; 77: 239.

Trovero F, Brochet D, Breton P, Tambuté A, Bégos A, Bizot J-C. Pharmacological profile of CEB-1957 and atropine toward brain muscarinic receptors and comparative study of their efficacy against sarin poisoning. *Toxicol Appl Pharmacol* 1998; 150: 321–7.

Tuncok Y, Apaydin S, Gelal A, Ates M, Guven H. The effects of 4-aminopyridine and Bay K 8644 on verapamil-induced cardiovascular toxicity in anesthetized rats. *Clin Toxicol* 1998; 36: 301–7.

Tush GM, Anstead MI. Pralidoxime continuous infusion in the treatment of organophosphate poisoning. *Ann Pharmacother* 1997; 31: 441–4.

Utili R, Biotnott JK, Zimmerman HJ. Dantrolene associated hepatic injury: Incidence and character. *Gastroenterology* 1977; 72: 610–16.

Vale JA, Meredith TJ. Antidotal therapy: pharmacokinetic aspects. In: *New Concepts and Developments in Toxicology.* Chambers PL, Gehring P, Sakai F (eds). Amsterdam: Elsevier, 1986: 329–38.

Varon J, Duncan SR. Naloxone reversal of hypotension due to captopril overdose. *Ann Emerg Med* 1991; 20: 1125–7.

Vasić BV, Milošević MP, Terzić MR. Acetylcholine content and cholinesterase activity in the ponto-medullary region of brain in rats treated with armin and obidoxime. *Biochem Pharmacol* 1977; 26: 601–2.

Verebey K, Volavka J, Mulé SJ, Resnick RB. Naltrexone: disposition, metabolism and effects after acute and chronic dosing. *Clin Pharmacol Ther* 1976; 20: 315–28.

Vitris M, Aubert M. Intoxications à la chloroquine: Notre expérience à propos de 80 cas. *Dakar Med* 1983; 28: 593–602.

Volpicelli JR. Naltrexone in alcohol dependence. *Lancet* 1995; 346: 456.

Volpicelli JR, Watson NT, King AC, Sherman CE, O'Brien CP. Effect of naltrexone on alcohol 'high' in alcoholics. *Am J Psychiatr* 1995; 152: 613–15.

Wagner SL. Diagnosis and treatment of organophosphate and carbamate intoxication. *Occup Med* 1997; 12: 239–49.

Ward A, Chaffman MO, Sorkin EM. Dantrolene. A review of its pharmacodynamic and pharmacokinetic properties and therapeutic use in malignant hyperthermia, the neuroleptic malignant syndrome and an update of its use in muscle spasticity. *Drugs* 1986; 32: 130–68.

Watanabe S, Satumae T, Takeshima R, Taguchi N. Opisthotonus after flumazenil administered to antagonize midazolam previously administered to treat developing local anesthetic toxicity [letter]. *Anesth Analg* 1998; 86: 675–81.

ter Wee PM, Kremer Hovinga TK, Uges DRA, van der Geest S. 4-Aminopyridine and haemodialysis in the treatment of verapamil intoxication. *Hum Toxicol* 1985; 4: 327–9.

Weinbroum A, Halpern P, Geller E. The use of flumazenil in the management of acute drug poisoning – a review. *Intensive Care Med* 1991; 17: S32–8.

Weinbroum A, Rudick V, Sorkine P, Nevo Y, Halpern P, Geller E, Niv D. Use of flumazenil in the treatment of drug overdose: a double-blind and open clinical study in 110 patients. *Crit Care Med* 1996; 24: 199–206.

Weinstein RS. Recognition and management of poisoning with beta-adrenergic blocking agents. *Ann Emerg Med* 1984; 13: 1123–31.

Wilson R, Lovejoy FH, Jaeger RJ, Landrigan PL. Acute phosphine poisoning aboard a grain freighter: epidemiologic, clinical, and pathological findings. *J Am Med Assoc* 1980; 244: 148–50.

Worek F, Bäcker M, Thiermann H, Szinicz, Mast U, Klimmek R, Eyer P. Reappraisal of indications and limitations of oxime therapy in organophosphate poisoning. *Hum Exp Toxicol* 1997; 16: 466–72.

Yang JC, Clark WC, Ngai SH. Antagonism of nitrous oxide analgesia by naloxone in man. *Anesthesiology* 1980; 52: 414–17.

Zilker T, Felgenhauer N, Hibler A, Pfab R, Thiermann H, Worek F, Eyer P. Factors influencing the efficacy of obidoxime in organophosphate pesticides poisoning [editorial]. *Przeglad Lekarski* 1997; 54: 662–4.

Antidotes to Carbon Monoxide, Cyanide and Hydrogen Sulphide

Contents

6.1 CARBON MONOXIDE POISONING

6.1.1 Introduction

The commonest source of inhaled carbon monoxide is incomplete combustion of fossil fuels. In smoke inhalation, however, poisoning may be due to hydrogen sulphide and cyanide as well as carbon monoxide. In smoke inhalation it is important also to look for inhalational injury of the upper airways (Lee-Chiong, 1999).

Carbon monoxide combines with haemoglobin (Hb) to form carboxyhaemoglobin (COHb), the affinity of haemoglobin for carbon monoxide being 200–300 times greater than that for oxygen. Thus the oxygen-carrying capacity of the blood is reduced and its ability to deliver oxygen to tissues is also decreased as the oxyhaemoglobin dissociation curve is moved to the left. In addition, carbon monoxide inhibits cytochrome aa_3 and, thereby, cellular respiration. These effects are compounded by the haemodynamic actions of carbon monoxide, which lead to reduced cardiac output and tissue perfusion.

COHb readily dissociates when the partial pressure of carbon monoxide in the alveolar air falls below that in venous blood. This situation may be induced by reducing the partial pressure of inspired carbon monoxide to zero and increasing the inspired oxygen tension (Gréhant, 1901a,b; Figure 6.1). The blood half-life of carbon monoxide is 250 min when breathing air at normal atmospheric pressure (760 mmHg), but this can be reduced to 50 min if 100 % oxygen is given (Pace *et al.*, 1950). However, the blood carbon monoxide half-life can range up to 164 min in poisoned patients given 100 % oxygen at atmospheric pressure (normobaric oxygen, NBO) (Levasseur *et al.*, 1996). Administration of hyperbaric oxygen (HBO) (2.5 atm) reduces the half-life to 22 min and also increases the amount of oxygen dissolved in blood from 0.25 to 3.8 vol % – this is sufficient to allow tissue respiration to proceed in the absence of oxygenated Hb. Hyperbaric oxygen also dissociates CO from cytochrome aa_3 and other tissue cytochromes.

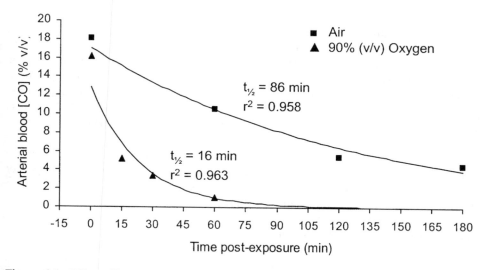

Figure 6.1: Effect of breathing 90 % (v/v) oxygen (atmospheric pressure) on the elimination of carbon monoxide in dogs exposed to 1 % (v/v) carbon monoxide, approximately 15 min (Gréhant, 1901a)

Chronic (subacute) carbon monoxide poisoning may occur as a result of a blocked flue or incomplete combustion of domestic gas in a poorly ventilated room (Crawford *et al.*, 1990). Clinical features of poisoning are vague and mimic those of influenza, and patients and clinicians alike often miss the diagnosis (Maynard and Waller, 1999). Patients usually recover quickly once the source of exposure is removed.

6.1.2 Antidotal treatment of acute carbon monoxide poisoning

Oxygen (100 %, delivered at atmospheric pressure) is an effective treatment for acute carbon monoxide poisoning, and few acutely poisoned patients who survive to reach hospital, except the elderly or those with pre-existing cardiovascular disease, die.

There have been only five controlled trials of hyperbaric oxygen for the treatment of acute carbon monoxide poisoning (Raphael *et al.*, 1989; Ducassé *et al.*, 1995; Thom *et al.*, 1995; Mathieu *et al.*, 1996; Scheinkestel *et al.*, 1999). The results reported range from apparent benefit to possible harm. The studies are difficult to compare because the hyperbaric treatments were different, some studies included patients poisoned in fires and who therefore may have been exposed to additional toxins, and objective end-points were sometimes lacking. In the one study that suggested a poorer outcome in those treated with HBO compared with normobaric oxygen, 46 % of patients did not return for follow-up at 1 month (Scheinkestel *et al.*, 1999). HBO is currently reserved for those who have been unconscious at any stage since exposure, those with blood COHb concentrations exceeding 40 % at any time and those with neurological or psychiatric features suggesting poisoning or patients who are pregnant. However, the logistical problems posed by transporting such patients to hyperbaric facilities remain. There is no evidence that treatment with hyperbaric oxygen would be of any value after chronic carbon monoxide poisoning.

Neuropsychiatric disturbances (intellectual deterioration, memory impairment, cerebral, cerebellar and mid-brain damage such as Parkinsonism and akinetic mutism, and personality changes such as irritability, violence, verbal aggressiveness, impulsiveness, and moodiness) may develop some weeks after apparent full recovery (Howard *et al.*, 1987; Meert *et al.*, 1998). At present, there are no reliable prognostic indicators of who will develop sequelae, though those who have been unconscious for a prolonged period of time may be at greater risk (Mathieu *et al.*, 1985). Hyperbaric oxygen may reduce the incidence of neuropsychiatric sequelae from *c.* 40 % to less than 5 % (Mathieu *et al.*, 1985; Myers *et al.*, 1985; Norkool and Kirkpatrick, 1985), although this remains controversial (Weaver, 1999).

Neuropsychiatric sequelae after acute carbon monoxide poisoning may be due to oxidative damage as oxygen tension rises in a reducing environment (hypoxic/reperfusion injury) (Werner *et al.*, 1985). Such sequelae develop in about 12 % of victims, especially those over 50 years of age. Of these, 80 % will have made a full recovery within a year. Howard *et al.* (1987) reported a 26-year-old man who had been comatose for 35 h after carbon monoxide poisoning (COHb 25 % at 40 h); his cardiorespiratory status was satisfactory and he was not given supplemental oxygen. The patient remained unrousable for 4 days, but on day 5 he was given i.v. NAC (300 mg/kg over 20 h) together with the xanthine oxidase inhibitor allopurinol (100 mg/d, 14 days) via a nasogastric tube. Signs of recovery were apparent 8 h post infusion; a full recovery was made over 3 weeks. There was no evidence of neurological or mental impairment on examination

6 weeks later. Meert *et al.* (1998) reported that delayed neurological toxicity was uncommon in children treated with normobaric oxygen. If neuropsychiatric sequelae from acute carbon monoxide poisoning are due to hypoxic/reperfusion injury, then cytoprotective therapy before, or very soon after, oxygen is administered is worthy of consideration. However, the role of NAC and allopurinol, and of other antioxidants such as vitamin E (tocopherol) is unproven.

6.2 CYANIDE POISONING

6.2.1 Introduction

In acute cyanide poisoning, the time of onset of toxicity is determined by the nature of the cyanide involved (hydrogen cyanide acts most rapidly, followed by inorganic cyanides, aliphatic organocyanides such as acetonitrile and acrylonitrile, and finally cyanogenic glycosides). Exposure may occur by inhalation, skin absorption or ingestion. Hydrogen cyanide has been employed as a chemical warfare agent (section 7.2). Ingestion of cyanide salts may lead to inhalation of hydrogen cyanide as the gas may be released on contact with acidic stomach contents.

Cyanide toxicity is attributed to cellular hypoxia resulting from inhibition of cytochrome oxidase, the terminal member of the mitochondrial electron transport chain, as cyanide ion binds strongly to the haem moiety of the enzyme. In the presence of cyanide, electron transfer is blocked, the tricarboxylic acid cycle is paralysed and cellular respiration ceases. There are endogenous cyanide detoxification mechanisms, the most important of which involve sulphur transferases, namely rhodanese and mercaptopyruvate:cyanide sulphur transferase (Marrs, 1988). Although these systems have low capacity and are thus easily overwhelmed, contrary to popular belief most patients do not die within minutes of ingestion of inorganic salts such as sodium cyanide and therefore antidote administration, in addition to general supportive measures, is a rational option (Hall *et al.*, 1987). Antidotes to cyanide ion or hydrogen cyanide ('cyanide') are often given in combination (Ballantyne and Marrs, 1987; Meredith *et al.*, 1993).

After exposure to hydrogen cyanide, the most important measure is removal from continued exposure, although care must be taken to minimize the risk of poisoning in those attending the victim. After ingestion of cyanide salts, limiting further absorption from the stomach by giving activated charcoal is a rational option. There is no evidence that gastric lavage alters outcome after ingestion of cyanide salts. Similarly, there is no evidence that the traditional oral cyanide antidote prepared by freshly mixing solutions A (ferrous sulphate and citric acid) and B (sodium carbonate) to give a 'ferrous hydroxide' suspension has any clinical value. This mixture was administered with the aim of forming non-toxic iron/cyanide complexes with cyanide in the stomach but also acted sometimes as an emetic.

As suggested above, cyanide forms stable complexes of low toxicity with certain metal ions, notably iron(III) and cobalt(III), but also silver(II), palladium(II), chromium(III) and rhodium(III) (Hambright, 1986). Two metal ions have been exploited as cyanide antidotes: iron (in methaemoglobin) and cobalt. Although stroma-free methaemoglobin has been used to treat cyanide poisoning in animal studies, in humans methaemoglobin is invariably generated *in vivo* by giving nitrites (amyl nitrite and/or sodium nitrite) or 4-dimethylaminophenol (DMAP) (Marrs, 1988). Aminophenones, particularly 4-aminopropiophenone (*para*-aminopropiophenone, PAPP), can form methaemoglobin *in vivo* and have also been studied in cyanide poisoning. However, because they require metabolic activation before beginning to produce methaemoglobin it is thought that aminophenones make better prophylactic than post-poisoning treatments for cyanide poisoning. These and some similar compounds are considered further in section 7.2.

In summary, rational antidotal therapy of cyanide poisoning aims to (i) by-pass the toxic effects of cyanide by giving oxygen; (ii) form methaemoglobin to chelate cyanide by giving nitrites or DMAP; (iii) give dicobalt edetate or hydroxocobalamin to chelate cyanide; and (iv) maintain or enhance metabolic detoxification of cyanide by giving sodium thiosulphate, a source of sulphane sulphur needed as a substrate by rhodanese. Many of these compounds have drawbacks; thiosulphate is thought to work slowly, nitrites reduce the oxygen-carrying capacity of the blood and dicobalt edetate has unwanted cardiovascular effects. Recent research suggests that with nitrites vasodilatation is a more important mechanism of action than methaemoglobin formation. Because some antidotes (hydroxocobalamin, oxygen, and sodium thiosulphate excepted) are potentially dangerous in the absence of cyanide ion, the diagnosis of serious cyanide poisoning must be beyond doubt before antidotal treatment is commenced. As a minimum requirement, the consciousness of the patient should be impaired before antidotal treatment is considered.

Many other compounds have been studied as potential cyanide antidotes (Marrs, 1988). These include D-glucose, sodium pyruvate (Schwartz *et al.*, 1979), α-ketoglutaric acid, glyceraldehyde and pyridoxal 5'-phosphate (Keniston *et al.*, 1987) as well as a number of drugs such as etomidate, naloxone (Leung *et al.*, 1984) and meclofenoxate (centrophenoxine) (Rump and Edelwejn, 1968). However, not one of these compounds has been used clinically to treat cyanide poisoning.

Antidotal treatment of cyanide poisoning

- Cyanide toxicity is attributed to cellular hypoxia due to inhibition of cytochrome oxidase
- Electron transfer is blocked, the tricarboxylic acid cycle paralysed and cellular respiration ceases
- Antidotal therapy aims to:
  - by-pass toxic effects: give oxygen
  - form methaemoglobin: give nitrites (may act via vasodilatation) or DMAP
  - form cobalt complex: give dicobalt edetate or hydroxocobalamin (vitamin B_{12a})
  - enhance metabolism: give sodium thiosulphate

6.2.2 Oxygen

It appears possible to by-pass the toxicity of cyanide by giving 100 % oxygen (atmospheric pressure), the action of which is probably synergistic with that of other cyanide antidotes. Although in serious cyanide poisoning cytochrome oxidase is inhibited and tissue utilization of oxygen prevented, animal experiments suggest that inhibition of cytochrome oxidase is prevented, and recovery accelerated, in the presence of oxygen

(Wirth, 1937; Gordh and Norberg, 1947; Way *et al.*, 1966; Takano *et al.*, 1980). Administration of high-flow oxygen [at least 60 % (v/v) inspired oxygen through a high-flow mask] may also be valuable when methaemoglobin-forming cyanide antidotes (nitrites or DMAP) have been given, or if co-exposure to carbon monoxide has occurred. Administration of sodium nitrite and sodium thiosulphate in combination has been reported in five smoke inhalation victims with combined carbon monoxide and cyanide intoxication (mean blood cyanide concentration 1.62 mg/L). These patients also received hyperbaric oxygen – one patient died (Hart *et al.*, 1985).

6.2.3 Methaemoglobin formation

Methaemoglobin (oxidized haemoglobin) contains iron in the ferric [iron(III), Fe^{3+}] rather than the ferrous [iron(II), Fe^{2+}] state. Cyanide has a low affinity for haemoglobin, but combines with methaemoglobin to form cyanmethaemoglobin. Almost 40 % of the haemoglobin in the body may be converted to methaemoglobin without clinically significant effects. This represents about 300 g haemoglobin or 1 g iron, which theoretically could chelate 500 mg cyanide ion. Two main groups of methaemoglobin-forming substances have been studied as cyanide antidotes: nitrites and aminophenols. Normally methaemoglobin is reduced to haemoglobin by methaemoglobin reductase, which reduces methaemoglobin concentrations by about 8 % per hour in adults, so that chemically induced methaemoglobinaemia is a temporary phenomenon. This means that the presence of methaemoglobin, and hence the binding of cyanide, is of limited duration. Although there is an endogenous system for the detoxication of cyanide, this does not have sufficient capacity to produce adequate detoxication of cyanide before methaemoglobinaemia is reversed. Thus, a second antidote such as a cobalt-containing compound or sodium thiosulphate is thought to be necessary.

Patients suffering from smoke inhalation and combined carbon monoxide and cyanide intoxication should not be given sodium nitrite unless they are to be treated with high-flow or hyperbaric oxygen. For this reason, alternative antidotal therapy (sodium thiosulphate and/or a cobalt-containing compound) may be preferred. Patients with G-6-PDH deficiency are at particular risk from sodium nitrite because of the risk of severe haemolysis. Patients with hereditary methaemoglobinaemia will attain proportionately higher concentrations of methaemoglobin than other patients given similar doses of nitrites, and methaemoglobinaemia greater than 40 % should not be allowed to develop. Note that commonly used methods for measuring methaemoglobin measure cyanmethaemoglobin as haemoglobin. This will give a falsely optimistic impression of the fraction of haemoglobin that is available to carry oxygen.

Treatment of excess methaemoglobinaemia during the management of cyanide intoxication is controversial. Administration of either methylthioninium chloride or tolonium chloride (section 4.13.2) is sometimes recommended, but this will merely convert cyanmethaemoglobin to haemoglobin with concomitant release of cyanide.

Methylthioninium chloride has itself been investigated as a potential cyanide antidote as it was thought that i.v. injection of the drug quickly generated methaemoglobin *in vivo*. However, Nadler *et al.* (1934) found that 50 mL of a 1 % (w/v) solution i.v. produced less than 10 % methaemoglobinaemia in volunteers. Nevertheless, methylthioninium chloride does appear to have exerted slight but significant effects in antagonizing cyanide toxicity in a number of animal studies (Smith, 1969a). There have also been a

CHAPTER 6

few reports of dramatic clinical improvement in serious cyanide poisoning. In two patients who had ingested at least 1 g potassium cyanide, methylthioninium chloride apparently produced prompt clinical improvement and complete recovery, even though both patients were unconscious and one was apnoeic. In a further patient who was thought to have ingested 6.5 g potassium cyanide, the drug was again successful (Geiger, 1932, 1933). Even Chen and Rose (1956) reported a patient who did not respond to nitrite-thiosulphate but responded dramatically to methylthioninium chloride. Nevertheless, methylthioninium chloride is not now considered a viable cyanide antidote.

6.2.3.1 Nitrites

Organic nitrites such as 'amyl nitrite', principally isoamyl nitrite (isopentyl nitrite, 2-methylbutyl nitrite), and inorganic nitrites, sodium nitrite ($NaNO_2$) for example, produce methaemoglobin *in vivo* and have been used as antidotes in cyanide poisoning for many years. Amyl nitrite was the first nitrite used to antagonize cyanide intoxication (Pedigo, 1888), the drug being given by inhalation. Sodium nitrite (CAS 7632-00-0) was introduced in the early 1930s (Chen *et al.*, 1933a–c), the rationale being that amyl nitrite could be inhaled while sodium nitrite was being prepared for i.v. administration. There is some disagreement about how much methemoglobin amyl nitrite is capable of producing in humans (Paulet, 1954). However, it seems clear that only c. 5 % methaemoglobinaemia can be achieved before profound hypotension and bradycardia occur.

There are three reasons to doubt the traditional rationale, i.e. methaemoglobin formation, for the use of nitrites in cyanide poisoning. Firstly, the antidotal effect of nitrite is very rapid, whereas nitrite-generated methaemoglobin formation is relatively slow (Way, 1984). Secondly, when comparable degrees of methaemoglobinaemia were induced in mice by DMAP, hydroxylamine, or sodium nitrite, cyanide toxicity was better antagonized following sodium nitrite administration (Kruszyna *et al.*, 1982). Thirdly, following pretreatment with methylthioninium chloride (to prevent significant methaemoglobinaemia) the efficacy of sodium nitrite in mice was unchanged (Holmes and Way, 1982). These studies strongly suggest that methaemoglobin formation by nitrites plays a minimal role, if any, in the treatment of cyanide poisoning.

Sodium nitrite causes relaxation of vascular smooth muscle *in vitro* (Kruszyna *et al.*, 1985), and both amyl nitrite and sodium nitrite are potent vasodilators in man (Baskin *et al.*, 1996). It has been suggested, therefore, that vasodilatation with improved myocardial capillary blood flow may underlie the antidotal efficacy of these agents (Way *et al.*, 1987). In this regard, it is noteworthy that chlorpromazine and phenoxybenzamine, both of which have α-adrenoceptor blocking activity, potentiate the antidotal effects of sodium thiosulphate in the treatment of cyanide toxicity (Burrows and Way, 1976; Way and Burrows, 1976; Vick and Froehlich, 1985).

The efficacy of sodium nitrite as a cyanide antidote is not known with certainty, although a protective effect in rats fed potassium cyanide has been described (Odunuga and Adenuga, 1997). Only one case of acute cyanide poisoning treated with sodium nitrite alone has been reported (Meredith *et al.*, 1993). Many other patients have received sodium nitrite and sodium thiosulphate, or amyl nitrite and sodium nitrite plus sodium thiosulphate. In other cases, sodium nitrite has been administered in combination with sodium thiosulphate, methylthioninium chloride, dicobalt edetate and hydroxocobalamin. Animal studies show clear evidence of synergism between sodium nitrite and sodium thiosulphate (Meredith *et al.*, 1993) as well as with oxygen (Way *et al.*, 1972).

Sodium nitrite is rapidly absorbed following oral administration. Some 60 % of absorbed nitrite ion is metabolized while the rest is excreted unchanged in urine. Although nitrite ion disappears from blood quickly, little is known about its fate. Injection of 400 and 600 mg sodium nitrite i.v. in humans produced peak methaemoglobinaemia of 10.1 % and 17.5 % respectively (Meredith *et al.*, 1993).

Sodium nitrite is administered i.v. in an initial adult dose of 300 mg [10 mL of a 3 % (w/v) solution over 3–5 min], usually followed by sodium thiosulphate. Hypotension may occur and is best prevented by diluting the solution with 0.9 % (w/v) sodium chloride and infusing the drug over 20 min. The rate of infusion may be increased if hypotension does not develop. The average paediatric dose is 0.33 mL/kg of a 3 % (w/v) solution (about 10 mg/kg); if anaemia is suspected, a reduced dose should be calculated (Meredith *et al.*, 1993). In both adults and children, the dose (one-half the initial amount) may be repeated after 30 min if clinical improvement is judged inadequate. Excessive methaemoglobinaemia may occur (van Heijst *et al.*, 1987), especially when larger than recommended doses are administered to children. Blood methaemoglobin should be monitored whenever possible to avoid this occurrence, particularly if repeat doses are contemplated.

6.2.3.2 *Dimethylaminophenol*

It has been known since 1913 that aminophenols generate methaemoglobin *in vivo* (Heubner, 1913), this property generally being considered disadvantageous. Kiese and Weger (1969) showed that dimethylaminophenol [4-(*N*,*N*-dimethylamino)phenol; dimetamfenol; DMAP; CAS 619-60-3; Figure 6.2] generated methaemoglobin more rapidly than the other compounds studied. Indeed, DMAP generates methaemoglobin more quickly and in larger amounts than either amyl nitrite or sodium nitrite (Klimmek *et al.*, 1979; Bhattacharya, 1995). In Germany, DMAP has been adopted as the treatment of choice for cyanide poisoning in combination with sodium thiosulphate (Jacobs, 1984).

The mechanism by which DMAP catalyses methaemoglobin formation is complex (Meredith *et al.*, 1993). DMAP auto-oxidizes readily at pH values above 7, and this process is accelerated in the presence of oxyhaemoglobin. The product of auto-oxidation is the 4-(*N*,*N*-dimethylamino)phenoxyl radical (Figure 6.2), which in turn rapidly decays to form DMAP and *N*,*N*-dimethylquinoneimine (Eyer *et al.*, 1975). In the absence of oxyhaemoglobin, this product may hydrolyse to 1,4-benzoquinone and dimethylamine, or to formaldehyde and *N*-methyl-4-aminophenol, and in turn the 1,4-benzoquinone may react with dimethylamine or with *N*-methyl-4-aminophenol to form 2-N-substituted quinone derivatives (Eyer *et al.*, 1974).

The autocatalytic formation of the phenoxyl radical, which is responsible for the oxidation of ferrohaemoglobin to methaemoglobin (ferrihaemoglobin), is terminated by binding of *N*,*N*-dimethylquinoneimine to thiol groups of haemoglobin and to GSH in erythrocytes (Eyer and Kampffmeyer, 1978; Eyer and Lengfelder, 1984). Subsequent metabolism of the DMAP–glutathione conjugate within the erythrocyte in man and in dog yields *S*,*S*-(2-dimethylamino-5-hydroxy-1,3-phenylene)bis-glutathione and *S*,*S*,*S*-(2-dimethylamino-5-hydroxy-1,3,4-phenylene)tris-glutathione (Eyer and Kiese, 1976; Jansco *et al.*, 1981). This is excreted into plasma (Eckert and Eyer, 1986), and subsequent

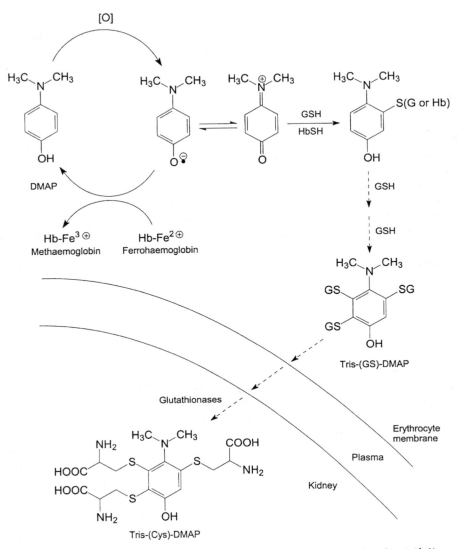

Figure 6.2: Schematic of the catalytic production of methaemoglobin by 4,4′-dimethyl-aminophenol (DMAP) via formation of the corresponding phenoxyl radical/quinoneimine, and the subsequent detoxification of the quinoneimine. Tris-(GS)-DMAP = S,S,S-(2-dimethylamino-5-hydroxy-1,3,4-phenylene)tris-glutathione; tris-(Cys)-DMAP = S,S,S-(2-dimethylamino-5-hydroxy-1,3,4-phenylene)tris-cysteine.

renal metabolism yields S,S,S-(2-dimethylamino-5-hydroxy-1,3,4-phenylene)tris-cysteine, which is excreted in urine. Most of a dose of DMAP is, however, excreted in urine as conjugates with D-glucuronate and with sulphate (Eyer and Gaber, 1978; Jansco et al., 1981; Klimmek et al., 1983).

The dose of DMAP recommended in cyanide poisoning in man is 3–5 mg/kg, which oxidizes 30–50 % of the body's haemoglobin to methaemoglobin (Meredith et al., 1993). Some 50 % of the methaemoglobin to be formed is present within 1–2 min, and the process is complete within 5–10 min. However, most clinicians remain cautious about using DMAP. There is poor dose–response curve reproducibility, attributed to genetic haemoglobin anomalies, which may lead to very high circulating amounts of methaemoglobin after even a single dose of DMAP (Meredith *et al.*, 1993). The need to monitor blood methaemoglobin after the administration of DMAP is often stressed (van Dijk *et al.*, 1987; van Heijst *et al.*, 1987). Children are at particular risk of excessive methaemoglobin formation because of a comparative lack of methaemoglobin reductase activity.

Another complication observed after DMAP administration is haemolysis (van Heijst *et al.*, 1987), and in animals a Heinz-body anaemia has been noted (Marrs *et al.*, 1984). Nephrotoxicity has also been observed in animals (Szinicz, 1984). DMAP is mutagenic in V79 (Chinese hamster) cells *in vitro* (Meredith *et al.*, 1993). The preferred route of administration of DMAP is i.v. because when given i.m. (for example by an auto-injector) it may cause local pain and swelling with fever (Klimmek *et al.*, 1983).

6.2.4 Cobalt-containing compounds

It has long been known that cyanide ion forms stable complexes with cobalt ions (Antal, 1894; Spenzer, 1895). Cobalticyanides and cobaltocyanides are relatively non-toxic, with LD_{50} values in the region of 1 g/kg. Cobalt salts were considered too toxic to use clinically, but Mushett *et al.* (1952) showed that hydroxocobalamin (vitamin B_{12a}) could be used to treat cyanide poisoning in experimental animals. Paulet (1960) studied the antidotal efficacy and toxicity of various other cobalt salts and complexes in cyanide poisoning. He concluded that dicobalt edetate was the most satisfactory cyanide antidote. The combination of sodium nitrite and sodium thiosulphate was superseded by dicobalt edetate in the UK and France on the basis of animal studies that showed the cobalt compound to be more effective and to have a better therapeutic index (Paulet, 1961; Terzic and Milosevic, 1963). Other cobalt salts (chloride, acetate, glutamate, gluconate) and complexes (cobalt histidine, cobamide) have also been studied as potential cyanide antidotes (Marrs, 1987), but not used clinically. Use of sodium cobaltinitrite is a further potential option – this compound can form methaemoglobin as well as providing a source of cobalt ion (Smith, 1969b, 1970).

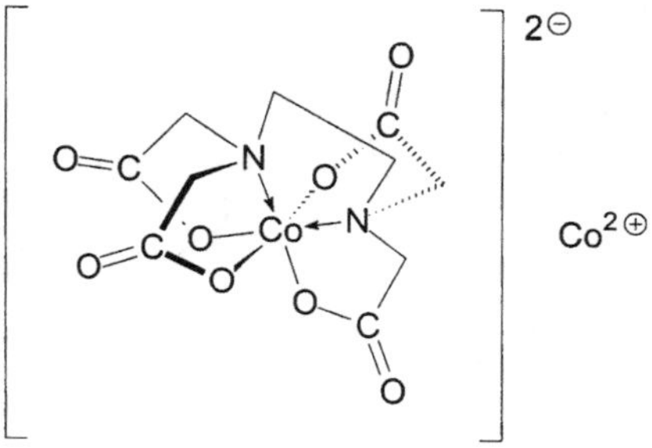

CHAPTER 6

Figure 6.3: Molecular formula of dicobalt edetate (dicobalt ethylenediaminetetra-acetate, dicobalt EDTA)

6.2.4.1 Dicobalt edetate

Dicobalt edetate (dicobalt ethylenediamine-*N*,*N*,*N*′,*N*′-tetra-acetate; dicobalt EDTA; CAS 36499-65-7; Figure 6.3) is now the treatment of choice in the UK for serious cyanide poisoning from all routes of exposure. Dicobalt edetate reacts with cyanide ion to form cobalticyanide $[Co(CN)_6]$ and monocobalt EDTA, both of which are excreted in urine within 24 h (Hillman *et al.*, 1974). Dicobalt edetate has a higher affinity for cyanide ion than cytochrome oxidase and thus will reverse cyanide-induced inhibition of respiration (Nagler *et al.*, 1978). Dicobalt edetate is excreted unchanged in urine in the absence of cyanide ion.

If the patient is thought to be at risk from cyanide toxicity, 600 mg dicobalt edetate should be given i.v. over 1–5 min depending on the patient's condition. A further 300 mg i.v. may be given if the initial response is minimal. The response to dicobalt edetate is rapid, comatose patients generally recovering consciousness within minutes. Electroencephalogram (EEG) abnormalities and oxygen consumption are also normalized. Concomitant administration of glucose (50 mL, 500 g/L D-glucose) has been recommended to mitigate dicobalt edetate toxicity (Meredith *et al.*, 1993).

Dicobalt edetate must not be given to patients who are not suffering from potentially serious cyanide poisoning. Immediate adverse reactions to dicobalt edetate may include vomiting, tachycardia, severe hypotension, vasodilation, chest pain, restlessness, sweating and flushing and facial oedema, especially in periorbital areas, tongue, lips and neck. These effects mostly last for 0.1–3 h; oedema normally resolves within 24 h. Severe facial and pulmonary oedema after dicobalt edetate which resolved slowly over 36 h has been reported in one patient (Dodds and McKnight, 1985). Collapse and convulsions occur rarely. Delayed responses (up to 2 days post treatment) may include facial flushing, nervousness, coarse tremor of the fingers and headache, all of which

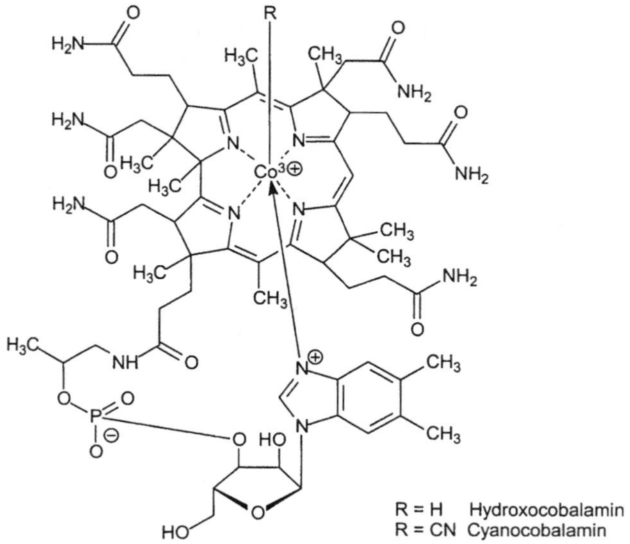

Figure 6.4: Structural formulae of hydroxocobalamin (vitamin B_{12a}) and cyanocobalamin (vitamin B_{12})

resolve in a few days (Nagler *et al.*, 1978). In the absence of cyanide adverse effects are more severe hence the need to confirm severe cyanide poisoning before giving the drug (Bryson, 1978, 1987; McKiernan, 1980).

6.2.4.2 Hydroxocobalamin

Hydroxocobalamin [α-(5,6-dimethylbenzimidazolyl)hydroxocobamide; vitamin B_{12a} (Co^{3+}); CAS 13422-51-0; Figure 6.4] is normally present in minute quantities in humans and plays an essential role as coenzyme B_{12} (cobamamide) once it is activated in the liver. Normally a minor route of cyanide metabolism is reaction with hydroxocobalamin to form cyanocobalamin (vitamin B_{12}). Hydroxocobalamin detoxifies cyanides in foodstuffs, etc., but endogenous supplies quickly become exhausted in cyanide poisoning.

Hydroxocobalamin is an effective antidote to cyanide *in vitro* (Riou *et al.*, 1990). When used as an exogenous antidote in cyanide poisoning, hydroxocobalamin has little in the way of secondary effects, a rapid onset of action and does not reduce blood oxygen transport. Comparative efficacy with other cyanide antidotes has not been evaluated fully, but during an infusion of potassium cyanide (0.1 mg kg^{-1} min^{-1}), a 50 mg/kg bolus of hydroxocobalamin, followed by infusion of 100 mg kg^{-1} h^{-1}, was less effective than thiosulphate in reversing toxicity in dogs (Ivankovitch *et al.*, 1980). The optimum use of hydroxocobalamin is in acute cyanide intoxication, when rapidity of action and absence of side-effects are of value. No toxicity has been observed even when massive doses have been given to guinea pigs (Posner *et al.*, 1976). At therapeutic doses in dogs, no haemodynamic effects were observed, but above 140 mg/kg there was a moderate negative inotropic effect (Riou *et al.*, 1991). The injection of hydroxocobalamin is often associated with a rose coloration of skin and urine. Anaphylaxis has been reported after 1-mg doses of hydroxocobalamin i.m. (James and Warin, 1971), but impurities in the preparations used may have been responsible.

One mole of hydroxocobalamin can theoretically inactivate one mole of cyanide ion (relative formula mass 26.0) via an essentially irreversible reaction (Mushett *et al.*, 1952), but the hydroxocobalamin molecule is much bigger (relative formula mass 1346.4), and thus relatively high doses (w/w) of hydroxocobalamin are needed to treat serious cyanide poisoning (Brouard *et al.*, 1987). Up to 60–70 % of a dose of hydroxocobalamin may be used in chelating cyanide ion (Friedberg *et al.*, 1965). The reaction of hydroxocobalamin with cyanide is more rapid if the blood pH is acidic, and this is often the case in cyanide poisoning (Reenstra and Jenks, 1979; Marques *et al.*, 1988). Hydroxocobalamin infusion is incompatible with reducing agents such as saccharose, sorbitol and ascorbate (Frost *et al.*, 1952). Hydroxocobalamin reacts with thiosulphate, and thus the two compounds should be administered at the very least 1 min apart (Evans, 1964). Hydroxocobalamin forms complexes with nitroprusside that prolong activity at vascular muscle (Hewick *et al.*, 1987).

Use of the 1 g/L solution commonly used to treat pernicious anaemia is impractical in cyanide poisoning – several litres would have to be infused into each patient (Brouard *et al.*, 1987). Nevertheless, cyanide poisoning has been treated successfully with hydroxocobalamin in France in combination with sodium nitrite, sodium thiosulphate, methylthioninium chloride and dicobalt edetate. In the USA, hydroxocobalamin has been used to treat cyanide toxicity arising from infusion of sodium nitroprusside (Cottrell *et al.*, 1978). Hydroxocobalamin (5 g i.v.) may be capable of binding all available cyanide up to a blood cyanide concentration of approximately 1 mg/L (40 μmol/L)

CHAPTER 6

(Demedts *et al.*, 1995; Houeto *et al.*, 1995) and may be able to inactivate intracellular cyanide (Astier and Baud, 1996). Concentrated hydroxocobalamin solutions (5 % w/v, i.e. 5 g in 100 mL) are now becoming more readily available in Europe and the USA. The dose for an adult is 5 g i.v. over 10 min. In some countries, France for example, hydroxocobalamin is combined with thiosulphate in a cyanide antidote kit. Hydroxocobalamin crosses the blood–brain barrier rapidly (Worm-Petersen and Poulsen, 1961). Hydroxocobalamin is rapidly filtered from the plasma by the kidney and tubular reabsorption is negligible, i.e. it behaves just like inulin (Weeke, 1968). The pharmacokinetics of hydroxocobalamin in smoke inhalation victims have been described previously (Houeto *et al.*, 1996).

6.2.5 Sulphane sulphur donors

The major route of detoxification of cyanide *in vivo* is conversion to thiocyanate (Figure 6.5). This reaction requires a source of sulphane sulphur (a divalent sulphur atom bonded to another sulphur atom) and it is catalysed by the sulphane transferases rhodanese (thiosulphate:cyanide sulphur transferase, EC 2.8.1.1) and mercaptopyruvate:cyanide sulphur transferase (EC 2.8.1.2) (Isom and Johnson, 1987). Rhodanese was isolated and named by K. Lang (1933a,b) – Rhodanid is German for thiocyanate. Rhodanese is distributed widely in the body, notably in hepatic mitochondria. Mercaptopyruvate:cyanide sulphur transferase is also widely distributed and is found throughout cells, notably in erythrocytes, liver and kidney.

It seems likely that there is a physiological pool of sulphane sulphur that can act as a source of sulphur for cyanide detoxification (Westley *et al.*, 1983; Way, 1984; Westley, 1988). Thiosulphate can act as a source of sulphane sulphur, but is probably not important normally – sulphane sulphur may also be derived from L-cysteine via mercaptopyruvate, which can then react with its sulphur transferase. The various forms of sulphane sulphur are interconverted by rhodanese and are thought to circulate bound to albumin. NAC may act as an antidote in acute acrylonitrile poisoning by acting as a source of L-cysteine thence sulphane sulphur (Benz *et al.*, 1990; section 4.16.2).

Sodium thiosulphate (sodium hyposulphite; $Na_2S_2O_3$) is used as an antidote in poisoning due to sulphur mustard and nitrogen mustards (section 7.5.2), bromate, chlorate, bromine, iodine, cisplatin and certain drugs [dactinomycin, mechlorethamine (nitrogen mustard), mitomycin] when extravasated (Dorr, 1990; Meredith *et al.*, 1993). However, its principal use is in cyanide poisoning. Use of sodium thiosulphate in cyanide poisoning was first suggested by S. Lang (1895). Combination therapy with sodium

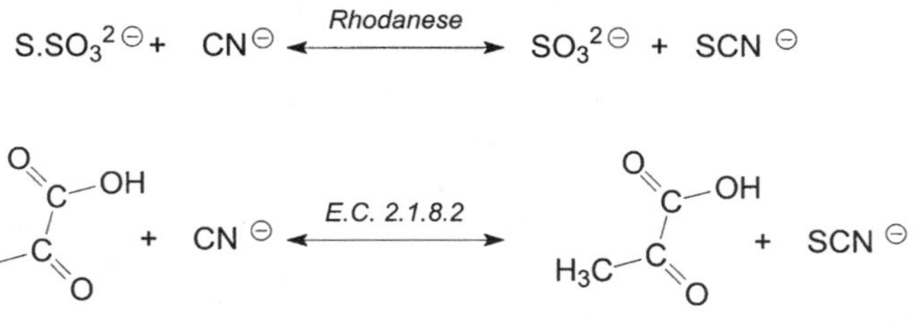

Figure 6.5: Metabolic detoxification of cyanide (EC 2.1.8.2 = 3-mercaptopyruvate:cyanide sulphurtransferase)

TABLE 6.1

Effect of different treatments on outcome in dogs poisoned with sodium cyanide (Chen *et al.*, 1934). MLD = minimum lethal dose

Medication	Number of MLDs of sodium cyanide required to kill
None	●
Nitrogylcerine	●
Methylthioninium chloride	●●●
Sodium thiosulphate	●●●●
Sodium tetrathionate	●●●●
Amyl nitrite	●●●●●
Sodium nitrite	●●●●●
Methylthioninium chloride and sodium tetrathionate	●●●●●●●
Amyl nitrite and sodium thiosulphate	●●●●●●●●●●●●
Sodium nitrite and sodium tetrathionate	●●●●●●●●●●●●●●●●●
Sodium nitrite and sodium thiosulphate	●●●●●●●●●●●●●●●●●●●●●

nitrite and sodium thiosulphate was introduced in the 1930s as a result of the work of Chen *et al.* (1933a–c, 1934) and of Hug (1933, 1934). This combination is sometimes referred to as the 'classical therapy' for cyanide poisoning. A notable feature, in experimental studies, is the marked synergy between sodium nitrite and sodium thiosulphate (Table 6.1).

In the presence of high concentrations of cyanide ion the availability of thiosulphate appears to be a rate-limiting factor in the conversion of cyanide to thiocyanate by rhodanese. Pharmacokinetic studies in volunteers suggest that the total extracellular thiosulphate content of a 70-kg man is about 125 mg (Ivankovich *et al.*, 1983). Rhodanese is present in tissues in large amounts, has a high turnover rate, and catalyses a reaction that, in the case of cyanide, is essentially irreversible. Unfortunately, rhodanese is localized in mitochondria and thiosulphate is thought to penetrate cell membranes slowly, even though a mechanism that transports thiosulphate in rat liver mitochondria has been described (Crompton *et al.*, 1974). Thiosulphate has therefore been assumed to be slow-acting in cyanide poisoning, and has thus always been used in conjunction with other agents that were thought to act more rapidly.

On the other hand, several studies (Ivankovich *et al.*, 1980; Krapez *et al.*, 1981) have indicated that thiosulphate can act very rapidly in cyanide poisoning. Sylvester *et al.* (1983) undertook a pharmacokinetic analysis of cyanide distribution and metabolism, with and without sodium thiosulphate, in mongrel dogs. The mechanism of thiosulphate protection appeared to be due to extremely rapid formation of thiocyanate in the central compartment, thereby limiting the amount of cyanide distributed to tissues. Thiosulphate increased the rate of conversion of cyanide to thiocyanate over 30-fold. These observations are in accord with the sulphane sulphur hypothesis regarding the mechanism of action of thiosulphate (Westley *et al.*, 1983).

Thiosulphate is absorbed poorly after oral administration and is thus normally given i.v. Ivankovich *et al.* (1983) studied the available thiosulphate pool and the pharmacokinetics of administered thiosulphate in volunteers. The mean plasma thiosulphate concentration in 26 healthy volunteers was 11.3 ± 1.1 mg/L and the mean

CHAPTER 6

urine concentration was 2.8 ± 0.2 mg/L ($n = 24$). After i.v. injection of 150 mg/kg thiosulphate to five normal male volunteers, the peak plasma thiosulphate concentration was $1,012 \pm 89$ mg/L at 5 min. The half-life of the distribution phase was 23 min, and that of the elimination phase 182 min. The V_D was 0.15 L/kg. Urine concentration, clearance and the rate of thiosulphate excretion increased markedly after injection. At 3 h, the total amount excreted was $42.6 \% \pm 3.5 \%$ of the injected dose; at 18 h it was $47.4 \% \pm 2.4 \%$. Similar findings were reported in eight cancer patients given thiosulphate by i.v. infusion over 6 h (Shea *et al.*, 1984). 'Therapeutic' doses of thiosulphate therefore elevate the thiosulphate plasma concentration about 100 times, and this may facilitate penetration into cells to allow detoxification of cyanide by rhodanese. Renal excretion is largely by glomerular filtration, although tubular transport may also take place (Sörbo, 1972).

Sodium thiosulphate

CAS registry number	7772-98-7
Relative formula mass (anhydrous)	158.1
pK_a	1.6
Oral absorption	Poor
Plasma half-life (h)	*c.* 3
Volume of distribution (L/kg)	0.15

Sodium thiosulphate has the advantage over other cyanide antidotes (oxygen and hydroxocobalamin excepted) in that it is essentially non-toxic. While it has most often been used in conjunction with sodium nitrite, it is likely in the future to be used with dicobalt edetate or hydroxocobalamin for the treatment of serious cyanide toxicity. Sodium thiosulphate has been most often used as a single cyanide antidote in the context of sodium nitroprusside infusions for hypertension. In these circumstances, concomitant infusion of thiosulphate prevents cyanide accumulation (Schultz *et al.*, 1979; Schulz *et* 1982), although (less desirably) it may also be given as a bolus once cyanide has accumulated (Perschau *et al.*, 1977).

Together with oxygen and necessary supportive therapy, sodium thiosulphate alone is probably adequate treatment for mild to moderate cyanide poisoning. The adult dose is 12.5 g [25 mL of a 50 % (w/v) solution] or 150–200 mg/kg i.v. over 10–15 min. Additional doses may be required depending on the clinical course. Children appear to require a larger initial dose (300–500 mg/kg). To prevent cyanide intoxication during sodium nitroprusside therapy, sodium thiosulphate should be given by simultaneous i.v. infusion in a dose 5–6 times (w/w) that of sodium nitroprusside (Schulz *et al.*, 1979, Schulz *et al.*, 1982; Johanning *et al.*, 1995). In these circumstances it is possible to calculate the appropriate dose of sodium thiosulphate based on the rate of formation of cyanide during sodium nitroprusside therapy.

The adverse effects of sodium thiosulphate are mild. Rapid injection of a hyperosmolar sodium thiosulphate solution has caused nausea and vomiting (Ivankovich *et al.*, 1983). Hypotension has also been reported, perhaps due to the formation of thiocyanate or due to the hyperosmolar nature of the solution (Meredith *et al.*, 1993). Other side-effects attributed to excessive thiocyanate production are nausea, headache and disorientation.

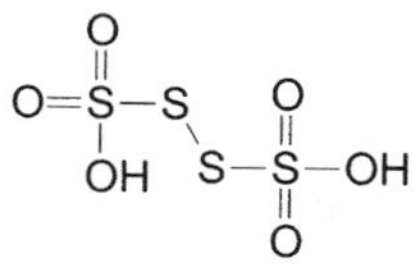

Figure 6.6: Structural formula of disulphanedisulphonic acid

Attempts have been made to improve upon the perceived slow onset of action of sodium thiosulphate by using other sulphane sulphur donors such as sodium ethanethiosulphonate and sodium propanethiosulphonate. By comparison with sodium thiosulphate any superiority observed has been small, but combined with i.v. administration of exogenous sulphur transferases (rhodanese from bovine heart or bacteria, or β-mercaptopyruvate:cyanide sulphur transferase) greater advantage was seen (Frankenberg, 1980). Despite their superiority in animal studies, none of these alternative sulphane sulphur donors have been used clinically. Disulphanedisulphonic acid (tetrathionic acid; thioperoxydisulphuric acid; CAS 13760-29-7; Figure 6.6) (Baskin and Kikby, 1990) and 3-mercaptopyruvate (CAS 2464-23-5) (Way *et al.*, 1985) have also been suggested for use in cyanide poisoning. Some more complex sources of sulphane sulphur have been suggested recently (Baskin *et al.*, 1999).

6.2.6 Summary

Table 6.2 gives recommended antidotal treatment for cyanide poisoning in different locations. Oxygen (100 %) should be given in all suspected cases of cyanide poisoning together with cardiorespiratory support as appropriate. If the diagnosis is unequivocal, and especially if the patient is unconscious, give dicobalt edetate, 600 mg i.v. over 1 min, followed by 300 mg i.v. if recovery does not occur within 1 min. Alternatively, give 10 mL of 3 % sodium nitrite (300 mg) i.v. over 5–20 min, followed by 50 mL 25 % sodium thiosulphate (12.5 g) over 10 min. Amyl nitrite (0.2–0.4 mL) administered via an Ambu bag with 100 % oxygen or one ampoule (0.3 mL) on a cloth inhaled for 30 s in each minute (new ampoule every 3 min, maximum six ampoules) may be used as first aid treatment prior to arrival at a facility where other antidotes are available, but is unlikely to be efficacious alone.

TABLE 6.2
Summary of cyanide antidotes used clinically

Place of use	Antidote
Industry	Amyl nitrite
Ambulance	Amyl nitrite; oxygen (100 %)
A&E and/or ITU	Oxygen (100 %); nitrites or DMAP; dicobalt edetate (Kelocyanor)[a] *or* hydroxocobalamin; sodium thiosulphate

Note
[a]Not to be used unless diagnosis of poisoning with cyanide is certain

CHAPTER 6

6.3 HYDROGEN SULPHIDE POISONING

Hydrogen sulphide is an extremely toxic gas. Fortunately, acute poisoning with this agent is relatively rare. If a victim is found in time then removal from the contaminated atmosphere is usually efficacious in bringing about recovery, and thus clinical experience with antidotal treatment is very limited. Nevertheless, it appears possible to by-pass the toxicity of hydrogen sulphide as well as that of cyanide by giving oxygen. Secondly, sodium nitrite (section 6.2.3.1) has also been advocated in hydrogen sulphide poisoning and in poisoning with other sulphides as sulphide is an even more potent inhibitor of cytochrome oxidase than cyanide (Nicholls, 1975; Smith *et al.*, 1977) and also binds to ferric iron in methaemoglobin. In animal models, sodium nitrite is effective in ameliorating the toxicity of sulphides (Scheler and Kabisch, 1963; Smith, 1969a). However, Beck *et al.* (1981) have suggested that in the presence of oxygen the sulphmethaemoglobin complex is short-lived and leads directly to the oxidation of sulphide by molecular oxygen. Thus, nitrite might only be effective in the first few minutes after hydrogen sulphide exposure.

REFERENCES

Antal J. Experimentelle Untersuchungen zur Therapie der Cyanvergiftungen. *Ungar Arch Med* 1894; 3: 117–28.

Astier A, Baud FJ. Complexation of intracellular cyanide by hydroxocobalamin using a human cellular model. *Hum Exp Toxicol* 1996; 15: 19–25.

Ballantyne B, Marrs TC (eds). *Clinical and Experimental Toxicology of Cyanides*. Bristol: Wright, 1987.

Baskin SI, Kirkby SD. The effect of sodium tetrathionate on cyanide conversion of thiocyanate by enzymatic and non-enzymatic mechanisms. *J Appl Toxicol* 1990; 10: 379–82.

Baskin SI, Nealley EW, Lempka JC. Cyanide toxicity in mice pretreated with diethylamine nitric acid complex. *Hum Exp Toxicol* 1996; 15: 13–18.

Baskin SI, Porter DW, Rockwood GA, Romano JA, Patel HC, Kiser RC, Cook CM, Ternay AL. *In vitro* and *in vivo* comparison of sulfur donors as antidotes to acute cyanide intoxication. *J Appl Toxicol* 1999; 19: 173–83.

Beck JF, Bradbury CM, Connors AJ, Donini JC. Nitrite as an antidote for acute hydrogen sulphide intoxication? *Am Ind Hyg Assoc J* 1981; 42: 805–9.

Benz FW, Nerland DE, Pierce WM, Babiuk C. Acute acrylonitrile toxicity: studies on the mechanism of the antidotal effect of D- and L-cysteine and their *N*-acetyl derivatives in the rat. *Toxicol Appl Pharmacol.* 1990; 102: 142–50.

Bhattacharya R. Therapeutic efficacy of sodium nitrite and 4-dimethylaminophenol or hydroxylamine co-administration against cyanide poisoning in rats. *Hum Exp Toxicol* 1995; 14: 29–33.

Brouard A, Blaisot B, Bismuth C. Hydroxocobalamine in cyanide poisoning. *J Tox Clin Exp* 1987; 7: 155–68.

Bryson DD. Cyanide poisoning [letter]. *Lancet* 1978; i: 92.

Bryson DD. Acute industrial cyanide intoxication and its treatment. In: *Clinical and Experimental Toxicology of Cyanides*. Ballantyne B, Marrs TC (eds). Bristol: John Wright, 1987: 348–58.

Burrows GE, Way JL. Antagonism of cyanide toxicity by phenoxybenzamine [abstract]. *Fed Proc* 1976; 35: 533.

Chen KK, Rose CL. Treatment of acute cyanide poisoning. *J Am Med Assoc* 1956; 162: 1154–5.

Chen KK, Rose CL, Clowes GHA. Methylene blue, nitrites, and sodium thiosulphate against cyanide poisoning. *Proc Soc Exp Biol Med* 1933a; 31: 250–1.

Chen KK, Rose CL, Clowes GHA. Potentiation of antidotal action of sodium tetrathionate and sodium nitrite in cyanide poisoning. *Proc Soc Exp Biol Med* 1933b; 31: 252–3.

Chen KK, Rose CL, Clowes GHA. Amyl nitrite and cyanide poisoning. *J Am Med Assoc* 1933c; 100; 1920–2.

Chen KK, Rose CL, Clowes GHA. Comparative values of several antidotes in cyanide poisoning. *Am J Med Sci* 1934; 188: 767–81.

Cottrell JE, Casthely P, Brodie JD, Patel K, Klein A, Turndorf H. Prevention of nitroprusside-induced cyanide toxicity with hydroxocobalamin. *N Engl J Med* 1978; 298: 809–11.

Crawford R, Campbell DGD, Ross J. Carbon monoxide poisoning in the home: recognition and treatment. *Br Med J* 1990; 301: 977–9.

Crompton M, Palmieri F, Capano M, Quagliariello E. The transport of thiosulphate in rat liver mitochondria. *FEBS Lett* 1974; 46: 247–50.

Demedts P, Wauters A, Franck F, Neels H. Monitoring of cyanocobalamin and hydroxocobalamin during treatment of cyanide intoxication [letter]. *Lancet* 1995; 346: 1706–7.

van Dijk A, Glerum JH, van Heijst ANP, Douze JMC. Clinical evaluation of the cyanide antagonist 4-DMAP in a lethal cyanide poisoning case. *Vet Hum Toxicol* 1987; 29 (Suppl 2): 38–9.

Dodds C, McKnight C. Cyanide toxicity after immersion and the effects of dicobalt edetate. *Br Med J* 1985; 291: 785–6.

Dorr RT. Antidotes to vesicant chemotherapy extravasations. *Blood Rev* 1990; 4: 41–60.

Ducassé JL, Celsis P, Marc-Vergnes JP. Non-comatose patients with acute carbon monoxide poisoning: hyperbaric or normobaric oxygenation? *Undersea Hyperbar Med* 1995; 22: 9–15.

Eckert K-G, Eyer P. Formation and transport of xenobiotic glutathione-S-conjugates in red cells. *Biochem Pharmacol* 1986; 35: 325–9.

Evans CL. Cobalt compounds as antidotes for hydrocyanic acid. *Br J Pharmacol* 1964; 23: 455–75.

Eyer P, Gaber H. Biotransformation of 4-dimethylaminophenol in the dog. *Biochem Pharmacol* 1978; 27: 2215–21.

Eyer P, Kampffmeyer HG. Biotransformation of 4-dimethylaminophenol in the isolated perfused rat liver and in the rat. *Biochem Pharmacol* 1978; 27: 2223–8.

Eyer P, Kiese M. Biotransformation of 4-dimethylaminophenol: reaction with glutathione, and some properties of the reaction products. *Chem Biol Interact* 1976; 14: 165–78.

Eyer P, Lengfelder E. Radical formation during autoxidation of 4-dimethylaminophenol and some properties of the reaction products. *Biochem Pharmacol* 1984; 33: 1005–13.

Eyer P, Kiese M, Lipowsky G, Weger N. Reactions of 4-dimethylaminophenol with hemoglobin and autoxidation of 4-dimethylaminophenol. *Chem Biol Interact* 1974; 8: 41–59.

Eyer P, Hertle H, Kiese M, Klein G. Kinetics of ferrihemoglobin formation by some reducing agents and the role of hydrogen peroxide. *Mol Pharmacol* 1975; 11: 326–34.

Frankenberg L. Enzyme therapy in cyanide poisoning: effect of rhodanese and sulfur compounds. *Arch Toxicol* 1980; 45: 315–23.

Friedberg KD, Grützmacher J, Lendle L. Aquocobalamin (Vitamin 12a) als spezifisches Blausäureantidot. *Arch Int Pharmacodyn* 1965; 154; 327–50.

Frost DV, Lapidus M, Plaut KA, Scherfling E, Fricke HH. Differential stability of various analogs of cobalamin to vitamin C. *Science* 1952; 116: 119–21.

Geiger JC. Cyanide poisoning in San Francisco. *J Am Med Assoc* 1932; 99: 1944–5.

Geiger JC. Methylene blue solutions in potassium cyanide poisoning: report on cases 2 and 3. *J Am Med Assoc* 1933; 101: 269.

Gordh T, Norberg B. Studies on oxygen treatment in connection with experimental hydrocyanic acid poisoning. *Acta Physiol Scand* 1947; 13: 26–34 [abstract in *Excerpta Med* (Sect II) 1948; 1: 429].

Gréhant N. Traitement par l'oxygène, à la pression atmosphérique, de l'homme empoisonné par l'oxyde de carbone. *CR Acad Sci* 1901a; 133: 574–6.

Gréhant N. Nouvelles recherches sur la dissociation de l'hémoglobine oxycarbonée. *CR Acad Sci* 1901b; 133: 951–2.

Hall A, Doutre W, Kulig K, Rumack B, Ludden T. Nitrite/thiosulfate treated acute cyanide poisoning: estimation of some toxicokinetic parameters in an antidote treated patient. *Vet Hum Toxicol* 1987; 29 (Suppl 2): 40–1.

CHAPTER 6

Hambright P. *Anti-cyanide Drugs: Annual Summary Report.* Fort Detrick, MD: US Army Medical Research and Development Command, 1986 (unclassified report).

Hart GB, Strauss MB, Lennon PA, Whitcraft DD. Treatment of smoke inhalation by hyperbaric oxygen. *J Emerg Med* 1985; 3: 211–15.

van Heijst ANP, Douze JMC, van Kesteren RG, van Bergen JEAM, van Dijk A. Therapeutic problems in cyanide poisoning. *Clin Toxicol* 1987; 25: 383–98.

Heubner W. Studien über Methämoglobinbildung: Dritte Mitteilung. *N-S Arch Pathol Pharmacol* 1913; 72: 241–81.

Hewick DS, Butler AR, Glidewell C, McIntosh AS. Sodium nitroprusside: pharmacological aspects of its interaction with hydroxocobalamin and thiosulphate. *J Pharm Pharmacol* 1987; 39: 113–17.

Hillman B, Bardhan KD, Bain JTB. The use of dicobalt edetate (Kelocyanor) in cyanide poisoning. *Postgrad Med J* 1974; 50: 171–4.

Holmes RK, Way JL. Mechanism of cyanide antagonism by sodium nitrate [abstract]. *Pharmacologist* 1982; 24: 182.

Houeto P, Borron SW, Sandouk P, Imbert M, Levillain P, Baud FJ. Pharmacokinetics of hydroxocobalamin in smoke inhalation victims. *J Toxicol Clin Toxicol* 1996; 34: 397–404 [see also correspondence in *J Toxicol Clin Toxicol* 1997; 35: 409–17].

Houeto P, Hoffman JR, Imbert M, Levillain P, Baud FJ. Relation of blood cyanide to plasma cyanocobalamin concentration after a fixed dose of hydroxocobalamin in cyanide poisoning. *Lancet* 1995; 346: 605–8.

Howard RJMW, Blake DR, Pall H, Williams A, Green ID. Allopurinol/N-acetylcysteine for carbon monoxide poisoning [letter]. *Lancet* 1987; ii: 628–9

Hug E. Acción del nitrito de sodio y del hiposulfito de sodio en el tratamiento de la intoxicación provocada por el cianuro de potasio en el conejo. *Rev Soc Argentinians Biol* 1933; 9: 91–7.

Hug E. Supériorité de la combinaison du nitrite de sodium et de l'hyposulfite de sodium pour le traitement de l'intoxication cyanhydrique. *Presse Med* 1934; 42: 594–7.

Isom GE, Johnson JD. Sulphur donors in cyanide intoxication. In: *Clinical and Experimental Toxicology of Cyanides.* Ballantyne B, Marrs TC (eds). Bristol: Wright, 1987: 413–26.

Ivankovich AD, Braverman B, Stephens TS, Shulman M, Heyman HJ. Sodium thiosulphate disposition in humans: relation to sodium nitroprusside toxicity. *Anesthesiology* 1983; 58: 11–17.

Ivankovich AD, Braverman B, Kanuru RP, Heyman HJ, Paulissian R. Cyanide antidotes and methods of their administration in dogs: a comparative study. *Anesthesiology* 1980; 52: 210–16.

Jacobs K. Report on experience with the administration of 4-DMAP in severe prussic acid poisoning. Consequences for medical practice [in German]. *Zentralbl Arbeitsmed* 1984; 34: 274–7.

James J, Warin RP. Sensitivity to cyanocobalamin and hydroxocobalamin. *Br Med J* 1971; 2: 262.

Jansco P, Szinicz L, Eyer P. Biotransformation of 4-dimethylaminophenol in man. *Arch Toxicol* 1981; 47: 39–45.

Johanning RJ, Zaske DE, Tschida SJ, Johnson SV, Hoey LL, Vance-Bryan K. A retrospective study of sodium nitroprusside use and assessment of the potential risk of cyanide poisoning. *Pharmacotherapy* 1995; 15: 773–7.

Keniston RC, Cabellon S, Yarbrough KS. Pyridoxal 5'-phosphate as an antidote for cyanide, spermine, gentamicin, and dopamine toxicity: an *in vivo* rat study. *Toxicol Appl Pharmacol* 1987; 88: 433–41.

Kiese M, Weger N. Formation of ferrihaemoglobin with aminophenols in the human for the treatment of cyanide poisoning. *Eur J Pharmacol* 1969; 7: 97–105.

Klimmek R, Fladerer H, Szinicz L, Weger N, Kiese M. Effects of 4-dimethylaminophenol and Co_2EDTA on circulation, respiration and blood homeostasis in dogs. *Arch Toxicol* 1979; 42: 75–84.

Klimmek R, Krettek C, Szinicz L, Eyer P, Weger N. Effects and biotransformation of 4-dimethylaminophenol in man and dog. *Arch Toxicol* 1983; 53: 275–88.

Krapez JR, Vesey CJ, Adams L, Cole PV. Effects of cyanide antidotes used with sodium nitroprusside infusions: sodium thiosulfate and hydroxocobalamin given prophylactically to dogs. *Br J Anaesth* 1981; 53: 793–804.

Kruszyna H, Kruszyna R, Smith RP. Cyanide and sulfide interact with nitrogenous compounds to influence the relaxation of various smooth muscles. *Proc Soc Exp Biol Med* 1985; 179: 44–9.

Kruszyna R, Kruszyna H, Smith RP. Comparison of hydroxylamine, 4-dimethylaminophenol and nitrite protection against cyanide poisoning in mice. *Arch Toxicol* 1982; 49: 191–202.

Lang K. Die Rhodanbildung im Tierkörper. *Biochem Z* 1933a; 259: 243–56.

Lang K. Die Rhodanbildung im Tierkörper. II. *Biochem Z* 1933b; 263: 262–7.

Lang S. Studien über Entgiftungstherapie. I. Ueber Entgiftung der Blausäure. *N-S Arch Pathol Pharmacol* 1895; 36: 75–99.

Lee-Chiong TL. Smoke inhalation injury: when to suspect and how to treat. *Postgrad Med J* 1999; 105; 55–62.

Leung P, Sylvester DM, Chiou F, Way L, Way JL. Effect of naloxone HCl on cyanide intoxication [abstract]. *Fed Proc* 1984; 43: 545.

Levasseur L, Galliot-Guilley M, Scherrmann JM, Baud FJ. Effects of mode of inhalation of carbon monoxide and of normobaric oxygen administration on carbon monoxide elimination from the blood. *Hum Exp Toxicol* 1996; 15: 898–903.

McKiernan MJ. Emergency treatment of cyanide poisoning [letter]. *Lancet* 1980; ii: 86.

Marques HM, Brown KL, Jacobsen DW. Kinetics and activation parameters of the reaction of cyanide with free aquocobalamin and aquocobalamin bound to a haptocorrin from chicken serum. *J Biol Chem* 1988; 263: 12378–83.

Marrs TC. The choice of cyanide antidotes. In: *Clinical and Experimental Toxicology of Cyanides*. Ballantyne B, Marrs TC (eds). Bristol: Wright, 1987: 383–401.

Marrs TC. Antidotal treatment of acute cyanide poisoning. *Adverse Drug React Acute Pois Rev* 1988; 4: 179–206.

Marrs TC, Swanston DW, Scawin J. Heinz-body anaemia produced by 4-DMAP [abstract]. *Hum Toxicol* 1984; 3: 332.

Mathieu D, Nolf M, Durocher A, Saulnier F, Frimat P, Furon D, Wattel F. Acute carbon monoxide poisoning. Risk of late sequelae and treatment by hyperbaric oxygen. *J Toxicol Clin Toxicol* 1985; 23: 315–24.

Mathieu D, Wattel F, Mathieu-Nolf M, Durak C, Tempe JP, Bouachour G, Sainty JM. Randomized prospective study comparing the effect of HBO versus 12 hours NBO in non-comatose CO poisoned patients: results of the interim analysis [abstract]. *Undersea Hyperb Med* 1996; 23 (Suppl): 7–8

Maynard RL, Waller R. Carbon monoxide. In: *Air Pollution and Health*. Holgate ST, Koren HS, Samet JM, Maynard RL (eds). London: Academic Press, 1999; 749–96.

Meert KL, Heidemann SM, Sarnaik AP. Outcome of children with carbon monoxide poisoning treated with normobaric oxygen. *J Trauma: Injury Infect Crit Care* 1998; 44: 149–54.

Meredith TJ, Jacobsen D, Haines JA, Berger J-C, van Heijst ANP (eds). *Antidotes for Poisoning by Cyanide. IPCS/CEC Evaluation of Antidotes Series*, Volume 2. Cambridge: Cambridge University Press, 1993.

Mushett CW, Kelley KL, Boxer GE, Rickards JC. Antidotal efficacy of vitamin B_{12a} (hydroxocobalamin) in experimental cyanide poisoning. *Proc Soc Exp Biol Med* 1952; 81: 234–7.

Myers RAM, Snyder SK, Emhoff TA. Subacute sequelae of carbon monoxide poisoning. *Ann Emerg Med* 1985; 14: 1163–7.

Nadler JE, Green H, Rosenbaum A. Intravenous injection of methylene blue in man with reference to its toxic symptoms and effect on the electrocardiogram. *Am J Med Sci* 1934: 188: 15–21.

CHAPTER 6 ■

Nagler J, Provoost RA, Parizel G. Hydrogen cyanide poisoning: treatment with cobalt EDTA. *J Occup Med* 1978; 20: 414–16.

Nicholls P. The effect of sulphide on cytochrome aa$_3$. Isosteric and allosteric shifts of the reduced α-peak. *Biochim Biophys Acta* 1975; 396: 24–35.

Norkool DM, Kirkpatrick JN. Treatment of acute carbon monoxide poisoning with hyperbaric oxygen: a review of 115 cases. *Ann Emerg Med* 1985; 14: 1168–71.

Odunuga OO, Adenuga GA. Sodium nitrite alone protects the brain microsomal Ca^{2+}-ATPase against potassium cyanide-induced neurotoxicity in rats. *Biosci Rep* 1997; 17: 543–6.

Pace N, Strajman E, Walker EL. Acceleration of carbon monoxide elimination in man by high pressure oxygen. *Science* 1950; 111: 652–4.

Paulet G. Sur la valeur du nitrite d'amyle dans le traitement de l'intoxication cyanhydrique. *CR Soc Biol* 1954; 148: 1009–14.

Paulet G. *L'intoxication Cyanhydrique et son Traitement*. Paris: Masson, 1960: 62–6.

Paulet G. Nouvelles perspectives dans le traitement de l'intoxication cyanhydrique. *Arch Mal Prof* 1961; 22: 120–7.

Pedigo LG. Antagonism between amyl nitrite and prussic acid. *Trans Med Soc Va* 1888; 19: 124–31.

Perschau RA, Modell JH, Bright RW, Shirley PD. Suspected sodium nitroprusside-induced cyanide intoxication. *Anesth Analg* 1977; 56: 533–7.

Posner MA, Tobey RE, McElroy H. Hydroxocobalamin therapy of cyanide intoxication in guinea-pigs. *Anesthesiology* 1976; 44: 157–60.

Raphael J-C, Elkharrat D, Jars-Guincestre M-C, Chastang C, Chasles V, Vercken J-B, Gajdos P. Trial of normobaric and hyperbaric oxygen for acute carbon monoxide intoxication. *Lancet* 1989; ii: 414–19.

Reenstra WW, Jencks WP. Reactions of cyanide with cobalamins. *J Am Chem Soc* 1979; 101: 5780–91.

Riou B, Baud FJ, Astier A, Barriot P, Lecarpentier Y. In vitro demonstration of the antidotal efficacy of hydroxocobalamin in cyanide poisoning. *J Neurosurg Anesthesiol* 1990; 2: 296–304.

Riou B, Gérard J-L, Drieu La Rochelle C, Bourdon R, Berdeaux A, Giudicelli J-F. Hemodynamic effects of hydroxocobalamin in conscious dogs. *Anesthesiology* 1991; 74: 552–8.

Rump S, Edelwejn Z. Effects of centrophenoxine on electrical activity of the rabbit brain in sodium cyanide intoxication. *Int J Neuropharmacol* 1968; 7: 103–13.

Scheinkestel CD, Bailey M, Myles PS, Jones K, Cooper DJ, Millar IL, Tuxen DV. Hyperbaric or normobaric oxygen for acute carbon monoxide poisoning: a randomised controlled clinical trial. *Med J Aust* 1999; 170: 203–10.

Scheler W, Kabisch R. The antagonistic effect on the acute H$_2$S-intoxication in mice by methaemoglobin-forming agents [in German]. *Acta Biol Med Ger* 1963; 11: 194–9.

Schulz V, Bonn R, Kämmerer H, Kriegel R, Ecker N. Counteraction of cyanide poisoning by thiosulphate when administering sodium nitroprusside as a hypotensive treatment. *Klin Wochenschr* 1979; 57: 905–7.

Schulz V, Gross R, Pasch T, Busse J, Loeschcke G. Cyanide toxity of sodium nitroprusside in therapeutic use with and without sodium thiosulphate. *Klin Wochenschr* 1982; 60: 1393–400.

Schwartz C, Morgan RL, Way LM, Way JL. Antagonism of cyanide intoxication with sodium pyruvate. *Toxicol Appl Pharmacol* 1979; 50: 437–41.

Shea M, Koziol JA, Howell SB. Kinetics of sodium thiosulphate, a cisplatin neutralizer. *Clin Pharmacol Ther* 1984; 35: 419–25.

Smith L, Kruszyna H, Smith RP. The effect of methaemoglobin on the inhibition of cytochrome *c* oxidase by cyanide, sulfide or azide. *Biochem Pharmacol* 1977; 26: 2247–50.

Smith RP. The significance of methemoglobinemia in toxicology. In: *Essays in Toxicology*. Blood FR (ed.). New York: Academic Press, 1969a: 83–113.

Smith RP. Cobalt salts: effects in cyanide and sulfide poisoning and on methemoglobinemia. *Toxicol Appl Pharmacol* 1969b; 15: 505–16.

Smith RP. Some features of the reaction between cobaltinitrite and hemoglobin. *Toxicol Appl Pharmacol* 1970; 17: 634–47.

Sörbo B. The pharmacology and toxicology of inorganic sulfur compounds. In: *Sulfur in Organic and Inorganic Chemistry*, Volume 2. Senning A (ed.). New York: Dekker, 1972: 143–69.

Spenzer JG. On antidotes for hydrocyanic acid. *Cleveland Med Gaz* 1895; 10: 353–8.

Sylvester DM, Hayton WL, Morgan RL, Way JL. Effects of thiosulphate on cyanide pharmacokinetics in dogs. *Toxicol Appl Pharmacol* 1983; 69: 265–71.

Szinicz LL. The nephrotoxicity of aminophenols. Effects of 4-dimethylaminophenol on isolated kidney tubules in rats [in German]. *Fortschr Med* 1984; 47/8: 1206–8.

Takano T, Miyzaki Y, Nashimoto I, Kobayashi K. Effect of hyperbaric oxygen on cyanide intoxication: *in situ* changes in intracellular oxidation reduction. *Undersea Biomed Res* 1980: 7: 191–7.

Terzic M, Milosevic M. Action protectrice de l'éthylène-diamine-tétra-acétate-dicobaltique dans l'intoxication cyanée. *Thérapie* 1963; 18: 55–61.

Thom SR, Taber RL, Mendiguren II, Clark JM, Hardy KR, Fisher AB. Delayed neuropsychologic sequelae after carbon monoxide poisoning: prevention by treatment with hyperbaric oxygen. *Ann Emerg Med* 1995; 25: 474–80.

Vick JA, Froehlich HL. Studies of cyanide poisoning. *Arch Int Pharmacodyn* 1985; 273: 314–22.

Way JL. Cyanide intoxication and its mechanism of antagonism. *Annu Rev Pharmacol Toxicol* 1984; 24: 451–81.

Way JL, Burrows G. Cyanide intoxication: protection with chlorpromazine. *Toxicol Appl Pharmacol* 1976; 36: 93–7.

Way JL, Gibbon SL, Sheehy M. Effect of oxygen on cyanide intoxication. 1. Prophylactic protection. *J Pharmacol Exp Ther* 1966; 153: 381–5.

Way JL, End E, Sheehy MH, de Miranda P, Feitknecht UF, Bachand R, Gibson SL, Burrows GE. Effects of oxygen on cyanide intoxication. IV. Hyperbaric oxygen. *Toxicol Appl Pharmacol* 1972; 22: 415–21.

Way JL, Holmes R, Way JL. Cyanide antagonism with mercaptopyruvate. *Fed Proc* 1985; 44: 718.

Way JL, Leung P, Sylvester DM, Burrows G, Way JL, Tamulinas C. Methaemoglobin formation in the treatment of acute cyanide intoxication. In: *Clinical and Experimental Toxicology of Cyanides*. Ballantyne B, Marrs TC (eds). Bristol: Wright, 1987: 402–12.

Weaver LK. Hyperbaric oxygen in carbon monoxide poisoning: conflicting evidence that it works. *Br Med J* 1999; 319: 1083–4.

Weeke E. [57]Co-Cyanocobalamin in the determination of the glomerular filtration rate. *Scand J Clin Lab Invest* 1968; 21: 139–44.

Werner B, Persson H, Kulling P (eds). Symposium. Carbon monoxide poisoning: mechanism of damage, late sequelae and therapy. *J Toxicol Clin Toxicol* 1985; 23: 247–326.

Westley J. Mammalian detoxification with sulphane sulphur. In: *Ciba Foundation Symposium – Cyanide Compounds in Biology*. Evered D, Harnett S (eds). London: Ciba, 1988: 201–18.

Westley J, Adler H, Westley L, Nishida C. The sulfurtransferases. *Fundam Appl Toxicol* 1983; 3: 377–82.

Wirth W. Zur Behandlung der Blausäurevergiftung. *Zentralblatt J Gewerghyg Unfallverk* 1937; 24: 258–61.

Worm-Petersen J, Poulsen E. Transport of vitamin B_{12} from blood to cerebrospinal fluid. *Biochem Pharmacol* 1961; 8: 323–4.

CHAPTER 6

Antidotes to Chemical Warfare Agents

Contents

7.1 INTRODUCTION

On 22 April 1915, the German army launched a massive chlorine gas cloud attack at Ypres, France. Some 5,000 Allied troops died and a further 15,000 became casualties. Subsequently, both sides strove not only to find new, more effective chemical warfare agents for a range of purposes (Table 7.1) and to devise improved methods of deploying them on the battlefield, but also to develop and mass produce means whereby their own forces could be provided with some protection against chemical attack. In addition, methods of treating casualties were continually scrutinized with the aim of not only minimizing suffering, but also speeding the return of casualties to their units.

An activated charcoal filter was at the heart of the British small box respirator and animal respirators that were introduced in response to the use of chlorine in 1915. With entry of the USA into the war in 1917, it was found that charcoal derived from red cedar or other conifers was a good adsorbent for chlorine and phosgene but provided little protection against chloropicrin. Charcoal from coconuts was more effective – a factory set up in the Philippines had 1,000 tons in stock in early 1919. Charcoal made from other nuts was also an effective adsorbent for a range of compounds. In Germany, denied overseas resources by blockade, it had been found that impregnating softwood with zinc chloride before heating produced an effective adsorbent (Moore, 1987).

Massive preparations for chemical warfare were made before and during World War II. Sulphur mustard was used in quantity by Italy in Ethiopia in 1935–6 and by Japan in China, but the substances available were not released in Europe, except perhaps in anger in very small quantity or by accident (83 people died and some 500 were seriously injured in Bari, Italy, in December 1943 when, during an air raid, the ammunition ship *John Harvey* exploded, releasing large quantities of sulphur mustard into the harbour). This was despite the fact that in Germany a new class of volatile organophosphorus (OP) acetylcholinesterase (AChE) inhibitors were developed (Table 7.1) and some compounds, notably tabun, were produced in large quantity (some 12,000 tons were seized by the Allies in 1945, the human lethal dose being thought to be *c.* 1 mg).

Since 1945 chemical warfare agents have been used sporadically, notably in the Iran–Iraq war in the 1980s, when sulphur mustard and an OP nerve agent, probably tabun, were used extensively. In addition to use in warfare, terrorist actions, such as the release of an OP on the Tokyo subway, and accidental exposure, such as that experienced by at least 23 Baltic fisherman in 1984 resulting from sulphur mustard from shells caught in nets (Aasted *et al.*, 1987) – some 50,000 tons of German chemical warfare munitions were dropped into the Baltic by Allied forces at the end of World War II – provide examples whereby human exposure to chemical warfare agents continues to this day. Finally, mention must also be made of a related class of agents, so-called tear gases or riot control agents, some of which were used in gas attacks in World War I. Later variants (notably CS) continue to be employed at times of civil unrest.

Of course many chemical warfare agents or related compounds are used in industry. Phosgene, for example, is commonly used as a synthetic intermediate, whereas chloropicrin has been used as a soil fumigant. Thus, human exposure from accidental or deliberate release of such compounds is always a possibility. Sulphur mustard has even been used to treat psoriasis. Although prevention of poisoning remains the first line of defence against industrial chemicals and chemical warfare agents alike, such measures may not be always either practicable or totally effective.

TABLE 7.1

Some chemical warfare and riot control agents

Code	Name	Formula
World War I and II chemical agents		
AC (French 4)	Hydrogen cyanide (prussic acid)	HCN
BA	Bromoacetone	CH_3COCH_2Br
BBC	70 % CA/30 % phenylacetonitrile	
BZ	3-Quinuclidinyl benzoate	
CA	Camite (phenylbromoacetonitrile)	$C_6H_5CHBrCN$
CBR	Arsenic trichloride/CG	
CG (D-stoff)	Phosgene	$COCl_2$
CK	Cyanogen chloride	CNCl
CX	Phosgene oxime	Cl_2CNOH
DA (Clark I)	Diphenylchloroarsine	$(C_6H_5)_2AsCl$
DC (CDA; Clark II)	Diphenylcyanoarsine	$(C_6H_5)_2AsCN$
DM	Adamsite (10-chloro-5, 10-dihydrophenarsazine)	
DP	Diphosgene	$ClCOOCCl_3$
ED	Ethyldichloroarsine	$C_2H_5AsCl_2$
H (HD, HS, LOST, BB)	Sulphur mustard (mustard, mustard gas)	$ClCH_2CH_2SCH_2CH_2Cl$
HL	37–50 % H/50–63 % L	
HN-1	Nitrogen mustard	$(ClCH_2CH_2)_2NC_2H_5$
HN-2	Nitrogen mustard	$(ClCH_2CH_2)_2NCH_3$
HN-3	Nitrogen mustard	$(ClCH_2CH_2)_3N$
HT	60 % H/40 % T	
L (M-1)	Lewisite	$ClCH=CHAsCl_2$
MD	Methyldichloroarsine	CH_3AsCl_2
NC	80 % PS/20 % tin(IV) chloride	
PD	Phenyldichloroarsine	$C_6H_5AsCl_2$
PG	75 % PS/25 % CG	
PS	Chloropicrin (Klop)	Cl_3CNO_2
Q	Sesquimustard	$Cl(CH_2)_2S(CH_2)_2S(CH_2)_2Cl$
SA	Arsine	AsH_3
SK (KSK)	Ethyl iodoacetate	$ICH_2COOC_2H_5$
T	Bis[2-(2-chloroethylthio) ethyl]ether	$Cl(CH_2)_2S(CH_2)_2O(CH_2)_2S(CH_2)_2Cl$
VN	Vincennite (50 % AC/30 % arsenic trichloride/16 % tin(IV) chloride/5 % chloroform)	
Z	Disulphur decafluoride	F_5SSF_5

Code	Name	Formula
OP nerve agents		
GA	Tabun (ethyl-*N*,*N*-dimethyl phosphoramidocyanidate)	$(CH_3)_2N-\overset{\overset{\displaystyle O}{\|}}{\underset{\underset{\displaystyle CN}{\|}}{P}}-OCH_2CH_3$
GB	Sarin (isopropylmethyl phosphonofluoridate)	$F-\overset{\overset{\displaystyle CH_3}{\|}}{\underset{\underset{\displaystyle O}{\|}}{P}}-OCH(CH_3)_2$
GD	Soman (pinacolylmethyl phosphonofluoridate)	$H_3C-\overset{\overset{\displaystyle CH_3}{\|}}{\underset{\underset{\displaystyle CH_3}{\|}}{C}}-CH(CH_3)-O-\overset{\overset{\displaystyle O}{\|}}{\underset{\underset{\displaystyle CH_3}{\|}}{P}}-F$
GE	Isopropylethyl phosphonofluoridate	$(CH_3)_2CHO-\overset{\overset{\displaystyle O}{\|}}{\underset{\underset{\displaystyle F}{\|}}{P}}-CH_2CH_3$
GF	Cyclosarin (cyclohexylmethyl phosphonofluoridate)	$\text{cyclohexyl}-O-\overset{\overset{\displaystyle O}{\|}}{\underset{\underset{\displaystyle CH_3}{\|}}{P}}-F$
VE[a]	*O*-Ethyl-*S*-[2-(diethylamino) ethyl]ethyl phosphonothioate	$CH_3CH_2O-\overset{\overset{\displaystyle CH_2CH_3}{\|}}{\underset{\underset{\displaystyle O}{\|}}{P}}-S(CH_2)_2N\overset{CH_2CH_3}{\underset{CH_2CH_3}{}}$
VG[a]	*O*,*O*-Diethyl-*S*-[2-(diethylamino)ethyl] phosphorothioate	$CH_3CH_2O-\overset{\overset{\displaystyle OCH_2CH_3}{\|}}{\underset{\underset{\displaystyle O}{\|}}{P}}-S(CH_2)_2N\overset{CH_2CH_3}{\underset{CH_2CH_3}{}}$
VM[a]	*O*-Ethyl-*S*-[2-(diethylamino) ethyl] methyl phosphonothioate	$CH_3CH_2O-\overset{\overset{\displaystyle CH_3}{\|}}{\underset{\underset{\displaystyle O}{\|}}{P}}-S(CH_2)_2N\overset{CH_2CH_3}{\underset{CH_2CH_3}{}}$
VX[a]	*O*-Ethyl-*S*-[2-(diisopropylamino) ethyl]methyl phosphonothioate	$CH_3CH_2O-\overset{\overset{\displaystyle CH_3}{\|}}{\underset{\underset{\displaystyle O}{\|}}{P}}-S(CH_2)_2N\overset{CH(CH_3)_2}{\underset{CH(CH_3)_2}{}}$
Riot control agents		
CN	2-Chloroacetophenone	
CS	2-Chlorobenzilidene malononitrile	
CR	Dibenz(b,f)-1,4-oxazepine	

Note
a   Sometimes referred to as A or F agents.

Battlefield antidotes to hydrogen cyanide, OP nerve agents, phosgene and sulphur mustard are discussed below. The development of OP nerve agents especially prompted much research into pharmacological protection against these agents as well as antidotal treatment of casualties. However, the treatment of poisoning with OP nerve agents has clearly much in common with the treatment of OP pesticide poisoning (section 5.9). Similarly, the treatment of cyanide poisoning is discussed extensively in section 6.2, while the use of dimercaprol and other sulphydryl-containing compounds to treat poisoning with organoarsenicals is also discussed briefly in section 2.2.

7.2 HYDROGEN CYANIDE

Hydrogen cyanide, used either alone or as a mixture with other poisons (Vincennite, Table 7.1), was not thought particularly effective when used as a chemical warfare agent during World War I, primarily because it is easily dispersed. However, the possibility of future use in chemical warfare remains. Of course, cyanide poisoning may also occur as a result of industrial accident, occupational exposure, deliberate self-poisoning and in a range of other circumstances.

It is important to be realistic about the efficacy of cyanide antidotes, used in the field, against hydrogen cyanide deployed as a chemical warfare agent. Most antidotes to cyanide (section 6.2) have been developed for use in civilian practice, which commonly involves ingestion of cyanide salts such as sodium cyanide. By comparison, hydrogen cyanide is very rapidly absorbed when inhaled. Moreover, blood cyanide concentrations start to fall when hydrogen cyanide exposure ceases and, therefore, if the dose of hydrogen cyanide has not proved fatal, and if there is no further exposure, the casualty will usually recover without antidotal treatment (Marrs *et al.*, 1996). On the other hand, if potentially lethal blood cyanide concentrations have been attained, antidotal treatment would have to be instituted within a minute or two in order to have any chance of success.

For many years it was believed that oxygen had no role in treating cyanide poisoning. It was thought that the blood was fully oxygenated in cyanide poisoning and it was oxygen utilization that was interrupted. However, a number of experimental studies have suggested that this view might be wrong, and nowadays oxygen is recommended as a component of the first-line treatment of cyanide poisoning (section 6.2.2).

A large number of compounds have been studied as antidotes for cyanide, and several have been introduced into clinical practice with varying degrees of success (section 6.2). The antidotal regimes use the principle of enhanced enzymic detoxification (e.g. administration of sodium thiosulphate) and enhanced binding of cyanide to heavy metals, such as cobalt or iron, the latter in the form of endogenous methaemoglobin generated from haemoglobin using, for example, sodium nitrite or 4-dimethyl-aminophenol (DMAP), although nitrites (sodium nitrite, amyl nitrite) may act simply as vasodilators. All the antidotes in clinical use have been shown to be effective in experimental animals. However, the relatively poor clinical results obtained probably reflect the difficulty of treating poisoning of rapid onset that is rarely seen in clinical practice.

With the exception of amyl nitrite and oxygen, all cyanide antidotes have to be administered i.v., generally in large (> 10 mL) volumes. On a battlefield this is not likely to be practicable, as the attendant and the casualty would probably be wearing full chemical/biological protective equipment. At a first aid post it might be possible to administer other cyanide antidotes, but this might well be too late. As a result, the possibility of administering cyanide antidotes such as hydroxylamine hydrochloride, DMAP or sodium nitrite i.m. has been studied (Vick and von Bredow, 1996).

7.2.1 Prophylaxis against cyanide poisoning

Because of the potential difficulties with field treatment of hydrogen cyanide poisoning as discussed above, the possibility of prophylaxis against cyanide poisoning has been studied. Bright (1987) concluded that an orally active drug with a long duration of activity and low toxicity would be required. One group of compounds that has been studied with this application in mind is the aminophenones. These substances are methaemoglobin formers, superficially similar to the aminophenols, but their mechanism of action is rather different. The proximate methaemoglobin former with 4-aminopropiophenone (*para*-aminopropiophenone, PAPP; CAS 70-69-9) is *N*-hydroxyl-aminopropiophenone (Graffe *et al.*, 1964; Marrs *et al.*, 1991). Oxidation of Fe^{2+} to Fe^{3+} in haemoglobin is accompanied by conversion of the hydroxylaminopropiophenone to the nitroso derivative, which is reduced, in the erythrocyte, back to the hydroxy-aminopropiophenone by NADPH, thus setting up a catalytic cycle (Figure 7.1). A methaemoglobinaemia of 12–15 %, generated by PAPP, was effective against the sublethal effects of a dose of about the LD_{50} of hydrogen cyanide. PAPP is thought to show promise as a prophylactic agent because of its long half-life (Bright and Marrs, 1986).

Other compounds have been studied as candidate prophylactic cyanide antidotes, including long-chain aminophenones such as 4-aminooctanoylphenone (Bright, 1987) and 8-aminoquinoline derivatives (Steinhaus *et al.*, 1990). Combined sodium nitrite/hydroxylamine prophylaxis has also been suggested (Bhattacharya *et al.*, 1993).

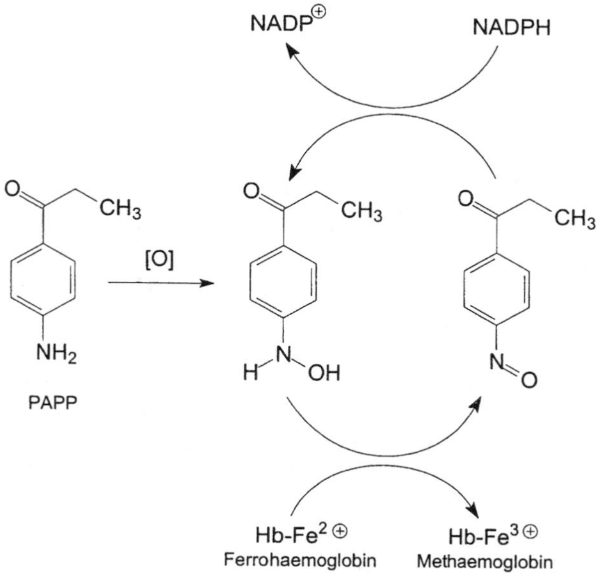

■ CHAPTER 7 ■

Figure 7.1: Suggested mechanism of methaemoglobin production by 4-aminopropiophenone (PAPP)

7.3 ORGANOPHOSPHORUS NERVE AGENTS

The standard treatment for OP nerve agent poisoning, as with OP insecticide poisoning, is combination therapy with atropine, or another anticholinergic drug, and an oxime enzyme reactivator such as pralidoxime or obidoxime (Marrs *et al.*, 1991; Bismuth *et al.*, 1992; Heath and Meredith, 1992). This combination has been evaluated in numerous studies and, in animals, can ensure survival of many multiples of lethal doses of nerve agents. A CNS depressant, such as diazepam, further increases survival in animal studies and has specific effects in humans in the management of convulsions and muscle fasciculations (Sellström, 1992).

7.3.1 Use of atropine

Atropine (section 5.3) is a muscarinic cholinergic antagonist. It has little effect at nicotinic sites such as autonomic ganglia and almost none at the neuromuscular junction. The efficacy of atropine in treating OP poisoning has been studied in a variety of experimental animals, often in combination with other drugs, usually oximes, and also in conjunction with diazepam and pyridostigmine pretreatment. It is often said that these drugs act synergistically, but that is a generalization (Marrs *et al.*, 1996). It is important to institute treatment of OP nerve agent poisoning as soon as possible. The initial dose of atropine should be 2 mg i.v., and this should be repeated at 15-min intervals. Reversal of bradycardia and drying of salivary secretions are the most useful clinical signs for assessing the adequacy of atropinization. In severe OP poisoning, very large doses of atropine may be needed.

Casualties overdosed with atropine may experience hallucinations and delirium, and care is necessary in the use of atropine in hot climates because the drug interferes with sweating. Atropine may also interfere with bladder function.

Atropine eyedrops have proved more useful in OP nerve agent poisoning than in OP pesticide poisoning, presumably because of the route-specific effects of OPs of high vapour pressure, such as miosis and ciliary muscle paralysis; these can be distressing and painful (Nozaki and Aikawa, 1995).

7.3.2 Use of oximes

Oximes (section 5.9.2) hasten the reactivation of the phosphorylated or phosphonylated complex formed when OP nerve agents react with AChE, thereby reactivating the enzyme. There are some national differences in the oxime favoured. Clinicians in France, the UK and the USA all favour the monopyridinium oxime, pralidoxime, although the pralidoxime salts used differ. In France, the methylsulphate is preferred, in the UK the mesilate (methanesulphonate) and in the USA the chloride. The methiodide is also described in some pharmacopoeias. Pralidoxime is a quaternary ammonium compound, and thus fully ionized at all pH values, and therefore pralidoxime bioavailability from formulations using the different salts should be similar. Nevertheless, the product literature reveals disconcerting differences in the doses advocated in terms of pralidoxime itself (Anonymous, 1986, 1987). German clinicians favour obidoxime, a bispyridinium oxime that, unlike pralidoxime, is effective against tabun but which is possibly hepatotoxic (section 5.9.2). The Hagedorn oximes, especially HI-6 and HLö-7 (Table 5.1), are attractive options as they have some activity against nearly all OP nerve agents, including tabun and GF (Worek *et al.*, 1998a,b; Kassa and Cabal, 1999). Indeed, on the basis of animal studies, HLö-7 comes near to being a universal antidote against OPs (section 5.9.2).

The most serious gap in the efficacy of combinations of atropine and oximes is in poisoning by soman, in which case ageing, that is monoalkylation of the phosphonylated AChE complex, renders oximes ineffective. Although ageing of the inhibited enzyme is a potential problem with all OP anticholinesterases if treatment is delayed, ageing with soman occurs with a half-life of a few minutes. Some studies of newer oximes such as HI-6 and HLö-7 (Bismuth *et al.*, 1992; Kassa, 1995; Worek *et al.*, 1997; Kassa and Bajgar, 1998; Worek *et al.*, 1998b) have shown some indication of efficacy in the peripheral nervous system, but the usefulness of these oximes in the field is not well established. There have been several approaches to the problem of the treatment of soman poisoning, including prophylaxis with carbamates such as pyridostigmine or physostigmine (as discussed below), the injection of cholinesterase itself and the use of antibodies to soman and other nerve agents (Inns and Marrs, 1992; Ci *et al.*, 1995; Liao and Rong, 1995). A range of quinuclidinium–imidazolium compounds (Figure 7.2) have also been synthesized and investigated as to their effects on soman poisoning in mice (Simeon-Rudolf *et al.*, 1998). The rationale for this approach was that some ligands bind to the allosteric site adjacent to the catalytic site of AChE (section 5.9.2), thereby providing protection to the catalytic site.

As discussed above, pralidoxime, but not obidoxime, seems to be ineffective in tabun poisoning. The reason for this is not connected to ageing, but may be due to the fact that the nitrogen atom bonded to the phosphorus atom causes the phosphorus in the phosphonylated enzyme to be less prone to nucleophilic attack as a result of electron donation (Bismuth *et al.*, 1992).

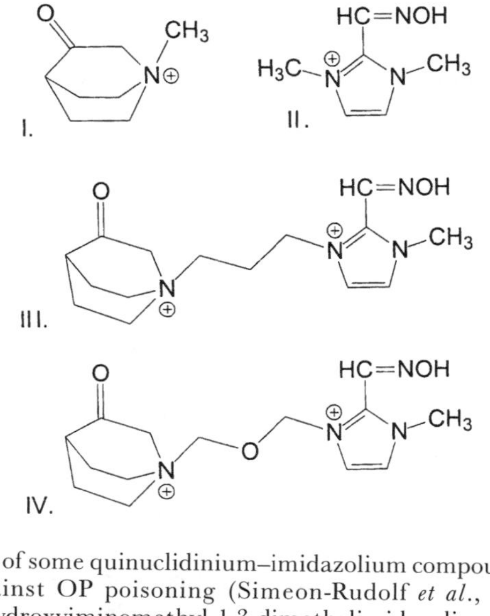

■ CHAPTER 7 ■

Figure 7.2: Structures of some quinuclidinium–imidazolium compounds investigated as possible protective agents against OP poisoning (Simeon-Rudolf *et al.*, 1998). I, 3-Oxo-1-methyl-quinuclidinium; II, 2-hydroxyiminomethyl-1,3-dimethylimidazolium; III, 3-oxo-1-[3-(2-hydroxy-iminomethyl-3-methyl-1-imidazolio)propyl]quinuclidinium; IV, 3-oxo-1-[3-(2-hydroxy-iminomethyl-3-methyl-1-imidazolio)-2-oxapropyl]quinuclidinium

7.3.3 Use of central nervous system depressants

The third component of the standard treatment of OP poisoning, including poisoning with OP nerve agents, is the use of CNS depressants, usually diazepam (Sellström, 1992). Diazepam was introduced primarily on a symptomatic basis to counteract convulsions. It also has a beneficial action on muscle fasciculations. There is evidence that in animals the combination of an oxime, atropine and diazepam is considerably superior to the individual drugs alone against the lethal effects of OP nerve agents (Inns and Leadbeater, 1983).

Other CNS depressants have been suggested for use in treating OP poisoning, including other benzodiazepines (clonazepam, midazolam), barbiturates (phenobarbitone, pentobarbitone) and phenytoin.

7.3.4 Use of enzymes

A number of workers have studied the possible use of AChE or butyrylcholinesterase as treatment for, or prophylaxis against, OP nerve agent poisoning. Reports of recent developments in this area, including the use of modified human enzyme or enzymes from other sources such as bacteria, can be found in Broomfield et al. (1999), Maxwell et al. (1999) and Hoskin et al. (1999).

7.3.5 Prophylaxis

One possible answer to the problem of ageing of soman-inhibited AChE is the use of prophylaxis so that either reactivation takes place before there is time for ageing to occur or inhibition is prevented. The former approach consists of prophylactic treatment with oximes; at one time pralidoxime mesylate tablets were issued to British military forces. More recently, the most widely used approach to the prophylaxis of soman poisoning has been undertaken using the carbamate drugs physostigmine or pyridostigmine (Dunn and Sidell, 1989). In military circles these drugs are called OP pretreatments, as they have no antidotal effect if given after poisoning. These carbamates react with AChE by carbamylating the active site of the enzyme in a manner similar to carbamate pesticides (section 5.9.2). However, the carbamylated enzyme reactivates much more rapidly than the phosphorylated/phosphonylated enzyme, and no reaction takes place analogous to ageing. Moreover, the carbamylated enzyme is unavailable for reaction with the OP. It is necessary to ensure that not too large a proportion of the enzyme is carbamylated: sufficient carbamylation is required to protect against any OP which may be present, but not so much as to interfere with military performance.

The action of pyridostigmine, unlike that of physostigmine, is almost entirely peripheral, but the action of the latter is shorter in duration and it is pyridostigmine that has generally been adopted for military prophylaxis (Keeler et al., 1991). On the battlefield, the dose of pyridostigmine bromide is one tablet (30 mg) 8-hourly. After approximately 24 h the erythrocyte AChE stabilizes at about 20 % inhibited.

A number of animal studies have shown the efficacy of pyridostigmine in protecting against soman poisoning, generally in combination with post-exposure treatment with an anticholinergic drug and an oxime, and often diazepam as well (Gordon et al., 1978; Inns and Leadbeater, 1983; Leadbeater et al., 1985; Anderson et al., 1991). As discussed above, the potential problem that carbamate prophylaxis might inactivate sufficient enzyme to interfere with military performance has been considered. This problem has been addressed in some small animal studies, and has also been the subject of studies in primates and in human volunteers (Marrs *et al.*, 1996). A study in marmosets showed that physostigmine prophylaxis at a dose causing approximately 30 % blood AChE depression did not affect behavioural parameters, EEG and cortical evoked visual response. Moreover, the treatment was effective, in combination with post-poisoning atropine treatment, against the lethal effects of twice the lethal dose of soman (Philippens *et al.*, 2000).

The first use of pyridostigmine bromide tablets on a large scale as OP nerve agent prophylaxis took place during the Gulf War and some adverse effects were recorded. Thus, Sharabi *et al.* (1991) recorded rhinorrhoea, nausea, abdominal pain and frequency of micturition. These effects were mostly mild, occurring some 1.6 h after dosing, and were not associated with AChE depression. Overall, AChE depression of about 20 % was recorded: 18.8 ± 3.5 in the symptomatic group ($n = 9$); 19.3 ± 6.6 in the asymptomatic group ($n = 12$). On the other hand, pyridostigmine bromide has been suggested as a possible cause of the so-called Gulf War syndrome (Pennisi, 1996; Haley *et al.*, 1997a,b; Haley and Kurt 1997; Iowa Persian Gulf Study Group, 1997).

7.4 PHOSGENE

Like sulphur mustard, phosgene (Table 7.1) was developed as a chemical warfare agent during World War I. It was used first by the German army in December 1915. Phosgene was the most effective lethal agent used in the Great War, sulphur mustard the most effective incapacitating agent. These compounds have other similarities: both are alkylating agents, and in neither case is there a specific and effective antidote. Of course, there are also differences: phosgene causes pulmonary oedema due to damage to the gas-exchanging region of the lung and is not a vesicant. Phosgene is the only compound that (i) has been used in chemical warfare and (ii) is produced on a large scale and transported in large quantities in peacetime. The risk of an accident involving many civilian casualties is real (World Health Organization, 1997).

Phosgene weakens the tight junctions between epithelial (type I alveolar) and, perhaps, endothelial cells of the blood–air barrier in the lung. Once the junctions are damaged, the permeability of the barrier to water, electrolytes and colloids is increased, and flooding of the alveoli may follow. Permeability pulmonary oedema (non-cardiogenic pulmonary oedema) is difficult to treat as no means of restoring the normal permeability of the barrier is available. Because of this, therapy has been largely supportive, with rest and supplementary oxygen forming the mainstays (Gilchrist and Matz, 1933). That rest is important was clearly demonstrated during World War I: men exposed to phosgene, but apparently unharmed, collapsed with florid pulmonary oedema when they undertook heavy work (Vedder, 1925). The latent period before adverse effects appear can last for 24 h after exposure.

Recent studies have shown that phosgene damages F-actin filaments in both pulmonary artery endothelial cells and bronchial epithelial cells maintained in culture (Werrlein *et al.*, 1994). This offers an explanation for the increase in barrier permeability that follows exposure. In addition to disruption of F-actin organization within cells, disruption of the basal lamina was also recorded. Interestingly, phosgene caused a phenotypic shift in the cultured airway epithelial cells: the cells developed dendritic

CHAPTER 7

processes and came to resemble the antigen-presenting cells of the normal airway epithelium. Whether this change occurs *in vivo* and, if so, whether it is significant is unknown. These observations link with that of Gurtner *et al.* (1992), who showed that 3',5'-cyclic adenosine monophosphate (cAMP) played a role in maintaining cytoskeletal structure. Raising concentrations of cAMP might then be a rational way of treating poisoning with phosgene.

Sciuto *et al.* (1996a) exposed rabbits to 1500 ppm phosgene. After sacrifice, lungs were removed and perfused. At about 1 h after exposure to phosgene, dibutyryl(DB) cAMP was administered either via a pulmonary artery cannula or directly into the trachea. DBcAMP is known to increase concentrations of cAMP by direct formation of cAMP as a result of intracellular deacylation, and by inhibition of phosphodiesterase (DBcAMP is a more effective inhibitor of phosphodiesterase than theophylline). A significant reduction in both the increase in lung weight (reflecting trans blood–air barrier leakage) and formation of arachidonic acid-derived mediators of inflammation was noted in the group treated with DBcAMP compared with the control group. It was further noted that GSH concentrations were maintained; in fact, the GSH/GSSG ratio was increased 3.6-fold. It was reported that DBcAMP produced these effects when given via the trachea – very much reduced effects were produced following dosing via the vascular perfusate. Perhaps the most remarkable finding of this study was that the proposed therapy worked when given an hour after exposure to phosgene.

Phosgene exposure is believed to lead to free radical generation in lung tissue. This may in turn lead to lipid peroxidation. If free radical formation forms a part of the mechanism by which phosgene damages the lung, then the increase in the GSH/GSSG ratio reported by Sciuto *et al.* (1996a) may form part of the mechanism by which DBcAMP opposes the effects of phosgene. Recent studies have linked free radical formation to activation of the transcription factor NFκB and thence to the upregulation of production of inflammatory mediators (Gilmour *et al.*, 1997). Reduced glutathione is an important antioxidant found in high concentrations in airway lining fluid. If it plays a part in defending against the effects of phosgene then the administration of aerosolized antioxidants might also be useful. Furthermore, Sciuto *et al.* (1995) have shown that NAC given in the same way as DBcAMP in the work described above, i.e. after exposure to phosgene, prevented much of the increase in lung weight and the release of inflammatory mediators seen in control subjects. NAC (section 4.16) is available for inhalational as well as i.v. and oral use in man and thus might be tried as a treatment for phosgene poisoning. Sciuto *et al.* (1996b) have also shown that ibuprofen given after exposure to phosgene in animal models can reduce the toxic effects of phosgene. This work follows that of Kennedy *et al.* (1989, 1990).

The developments described above may represent very important progress in treating phosgene poisoning.

A drug that has been advocated by some (Stavrakis, 1971), but not by others (Diller, 1978, 1980), in the management of phosgene poisoning is hexamethylenetetramine (HMT, hexamine, methenamine, Urotropin; CAS 100-97-0; Figure 7.3). This compound has a long history in the chemical warfare literature. It was discovered in Russia (Prentiss, 1937) that hexamine could 'neutralize' phosgene, and the compound was used in the PH (phenolate–hexamine) anti-gas helmet issued to British troops in 1916. Steroids and aminophylline have also been recommended for use in treating phosgene poisoning. The evidence on the efficacy of steroids is inconclusive: Diller (1978) thought that a case for their use could be made, whereas Bradley and Unger (1982) took the

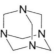

Figure 7.3: Molecular structure of hexamethylenetetramine

opposite view. The similarity of phosgene-induced pulmonary oedema to the adult respiratory distress syndrome (ARDS) has encouraged some clinicians to use steroids in phosgene poisoning. The case for aminophylline, a phosphodiesterase inhibitor, is strengthened by the work on DBcAMP referred to above. Despite this, clinical efficacy remains unproven.

Antibiotics should be used to treat pneumonia that may occur following exposure to phosgene, and prophylactic use immediately on diagnosing phosgene-induced lung damage has been advocated. Support for such an approach was provided by Selgrade *et al.* (1995), who showed in rats that exposure to phosgene leads to impairment of defences against bacterial challenge.

7.5 VESICANTS

7.5.1 Arsenicals

In contrast to other vesicants, such as sulphur mustard, there is effective and specific therapy for poisoning with organic arsenicals. Since World War II, dimercaprol (British anti-lewisite, BAL, 2,3-dimercaptopropanol; section 2.2.4) has been the standard treatment for poisoning by arsenic compounds, including lewisite as well as other organic arsenicals (Table 7.1), and would be used on the battlefield. Dimercaprol is thought to bind to lewisite to form a less toxic compound which can then be excreted (Figure 7.4).

In animals, it has been shown that dimercaprol is able to protect against the effects of lewisite and reverse the enzyme inhibition produced after exposure to the poison. Dimercaprol has to be used parenterally, and in systemic lewisite poisoning has to be given i.m. It was also available as an ointment for use against skin burns, and was used effectively in treating previously intractable dermatitis contracted from exposure to Adamsite (10-chloro-5,10-dihydrophenarsazine, DM – Table 7.1) dust (Longcope *et al.*, 1946). Because it cannot be given by mouth or i.v., dimercaprol is less than ideal as an antidote. Moreover, the dose is limited by the toxicity of the drug, and i.m. injections of dimercaprol (the drug is formulated dissolved in groundnut oil and benzyl benzoate is added as a preservative) are painful (Modell *et al.*, 1946; Sulzberger *et al.*, 1946).

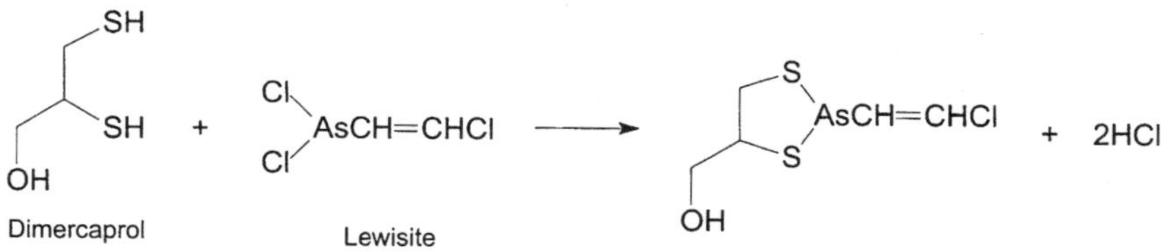

■ CHAPTER 7 ■

Figure 7.4: Proposed reaction of dimercaprol with lewisite

Furthermore, the fact that it cannot be given i.v. means that administration of a loading dose is impractical.

The dosage schedule given below has been recommended for use in severe arsenic poisoning (Parfitt, 1999):

Day 1:	400–800 mg i.m. in divided doses
Days 2–3:	200–400 mg i.m. in divided doses
Days 4–12:	100–200 mg i.m. in divided doses

The range of doses is to allow for variations in the severity of poisoning and in body weight. The UK Ministry of Defence (1972) suggested doses of 2.5 mg/kg 4-hourly for four doses, then 2.5 mg/kg twice daily.

Administration is by deep i.m. injection. The injection site should be varied. The drug may produce unpleasant reactions. Systemic reactions may include headache, feelings of constriction of the chest, increased blood pressure, tachycardia, nausea and vomiting. Conjunctivitis, lachrymation, rhinorrhoea, sweating, anxiety and agitation have also been reported. These effects pass in a few hours. Pain at the injection site may last for up to 24 h. Despite the potential for adverse effects from dimercaprol, Klaassen (1996) has emphasized the need to maintain a high plasma dimercaprol concentration in treating arsenic poisoning so that the rapidly excreted 2:1 complex of dimercaprol–arsenic should predominate over the 1:1 complex.

Dimercaprol can be used topically. Skin contamination should be treated with dimercaprol ointment (see above). This should not be used in conjunction with silver sulfadiazine ointment as dimercaprol will chelate silver (Maynard, 1999). Eye contamination can be treated by dimercaprol (5–10 % w/v in vegetable oil) instilled into the conjunctival sac. As the eye is very rapidly damaged by lewisite, this should be performed as a matter of urgency.

Two water-soluble analogues of dimercaprol, *meso*-2,3-dimercaptosuccinic acid (DMSA) and 2,3-dimercapto-1-propanesulphonate (DMPS), have also been studied in the treatment of poisoning with metal ions (sections 2.2.5 and 2.2.7). These drugs have two major advantages when compared with dimercaprol: they can be given orally and their therapeutic ratios are more favourable (in mice DMSA and DMPS are about 20 and 10 times less toxic, respectively, than dimercaprol – Table 2.5). The disadvantages of dimercaprol largely relate to systemic administration and the water-soluble analogues are unlikely to be better than dimercaprol ointment.

DMSA and DMPS appear to be effective lewisite antidotes in animal studies. Inns *et al.* (1990) have shown that in rabbits poisoned with i.v. lewisite, dimercaprol, DMPS, and DMSA were equieffective antidotes in molar terms, as would be expected, but that the water-soluble analogues could be given at higher doses. Inns and Rice (1993) studied the antidotal efficacy of dimercaprol, DMSA, and DMPS against lewisite applied to the skin of rabbits and concluded that, at equimolar doses (40 µmol/kg), there was little difference between the efficacy of dimercaprol, DMPS and DMSA. However, the low toxicity of DMPS and DMSA enabled their use at higher doses. Protection ratios (LD_{50} with treatment/LD_{50} without treatment) were 13 and 16.9, respectively, for DMPS and DMSA at a dose of 160 µmol/kg i.m.

In addition to effects on LD_{50}, there appeared to be beneficial activity against the hepatocellular damage characteristic of lewisite poisoning. There may be further advantages to using DMSA and DMPS. Aposhian *et al.* (1984) showed that, in the kidneys of mice or in a mouse kidney system *in vitro*, dimercaprol was less effective than DMPA, DMPS or DMSA in reversing arsenite inhibition of the pyruvate dehydrogenase complex. Furthermore, they observed that dimercaprol increased the arsenic content of brains of rabbits poisoned with sodium arsenite (i.e. mobilized the arsenic in a biologically disadvantageous direction), whereas DMPS and DMSA did not. It is, however, possible that the arsenic mobilized was not biologically active.

7.5.2 Sulphur mustard

Sulphur mustard (mustard gas, bis(2-chloroethyl)sulphide, dichlorodiethylsulphide, H, HD) is a highly reactive, lipophilic, alkylating agent (Marrs *et al.*, 1996). Exposure to vapour leads to damage to the upper respiratory tract, eyes and skin. Absorption across these surfaces is followed by damage to rapidly dividing cells throughout the body, the gut epithelium, the lymphatic system and the bone marrow being particularly affected. Damage to the bone marrow leads to the marked leucopenia seen in severely affected casualties (Balali-Mood and Navaeian, 1986). The rapid reaction of the ethylenesulphonium ion formed by internal rearrangement of sulphur mustard (Figure 7.5) with endogenous nucleophilic molecules leading to the formation of covalent bonds suggests that finding effective therapeutic agents will be difficult (Lindsay and Hambrook, 1998).

Employed on a large scale during World War I and in Ethiopia in 1936, sulphur mustard was used again during the Iran–Iraq war in the mid 1980s (Balali-Mood and Navaeian, 1986; Balali-Mood *et al.*, 1986). Sulphur mustard casualties from this conflict were treated in London (Marrs *et al.*, 1996) and in Belgium (Colardyn *et al.*, 1986;

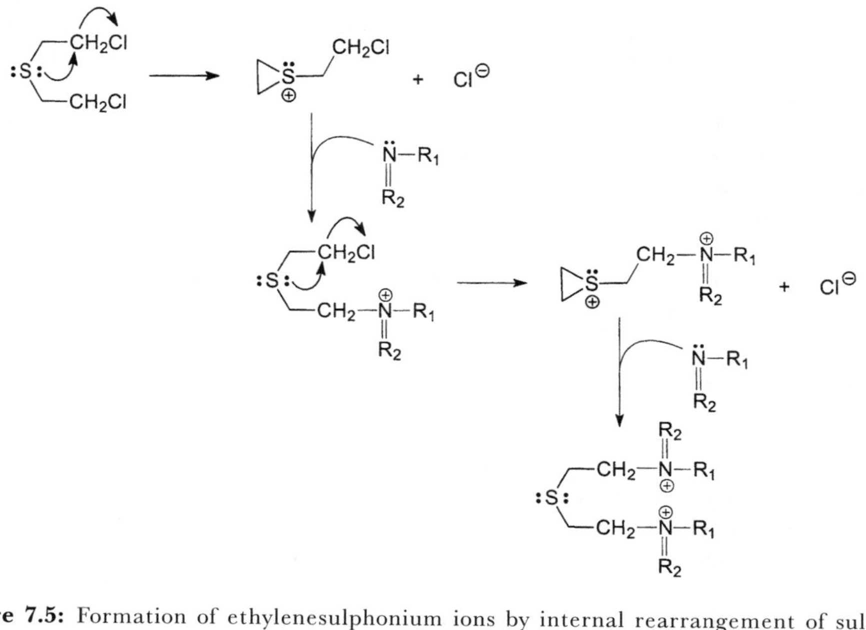

Figure 7.5: Formation of ethylenesulphonium ions by internal rearrangement of sulphur mustard and subsequent reaction with nucleophilic molecules

Willems, 1989). Sulphur mustard has considerable potential as a terrorist weapon: it is comparatively easy to produce and exposure can lead to severe injuries that require prolonged hospital treatment. As far as is known, sulphur mustard, unlike the OP nerve agents, has not been used by terrorist groups.

Research in treating sulphur mustard casualties has been sporadic, depending on the use of the compound in warfare. Research designed to find antidotes to blister-producing compounds, including sulphur mustard and lewisite (section 7.5.1), carried out in the UK during World War II led to the discovery of dimercaprol, but this substance proved ineffective as regards sulphur mustard poisoning (Dixon and Needham, 1946). More recent work has shed much light on the biochemical toxicity of sulphur mustard but has done little to either (i) explain the remarkable blistering property of the compound or (ii) suggest effective antidotes. At present, it seems to be impossible to reverse the binding of sulphur mustard to key intracellular components, though some advances have been made in developing substances with potential as prophylactic compounds. None has yet, to the authors' knowledge, developed to the stage of being issued to troops or civilians likely to be asked to deal with sulphur mustard casualties.

Treatment of lesions produced by mustard gas is dealt with below by the organ system affected. Before treatment is begun, thorough decontamination must be carried out. This is essential both from the patient's standpoint and to ensure that medical and nursing staff are not exposed to vapour emitted from contaminated clothing and skin. Decontamination of casualties should not be undertaken by anyone unprotected against the effects of sulphur mustard present either as a liquid or as a vapour. Thus, gloves (two pairs of standard surgical gloves, changed regularly and disposed of safely) are essential. Protection of the eyes and respiratory tract by a satisfactory respirator is desirable, although civilian attendants may not have immediate access to such equipment. The desirability of working in a well-ventilated area, preferably outdoors, is obvious. Decontamination may be accomplished by thorough washing with soap and water. Fuller's earth has been a standard decontaminant in military circles, but recently dilute bleach has been preferred and is very effective (Morgan-Jones and Hodgetts, 1996). Checking that casualties have been adequately decontaminated before they are moved indoors is desirable, but difficult to achieve unless equipment such as the UK Chemical Agent Monitor is available. It should be noted that the detector can be 'misled' by substances other than chemical warfare agents, including harmless substances, and clinical judgement should be exercised in interpreting positive readings from the detector.

Details of the management of skin and eye damage are given in Marrs et al. (1996), and thus only a brief summary is provided here.

7.5.2.1 Skin lesions

Silver sulfadiazine (silver sulphadiazine, Flamazine) (1 % w/w) cream is useful for preventing infections of damaged areas. Steroid creams such as beclometasone (beclomethasone) dipropionate (Propaderm) have been used and are of value in reducing itching, which may be severe. Damaged skin should be treated in the same way as thermal burns. Management by exposure is probably more effective and less troublesome than treatment by application of wet dressings. Use of the topical antiseptic chloramine T (sodium N-chloro-4-methylbenzenesulphonamide; CAS 127-65-1) may inactivate sulphur mustard (Klimmek et al., 1983; Figure 7.6), but clinical experience in the use of this agent in sulphur mustard exposure is lacking.

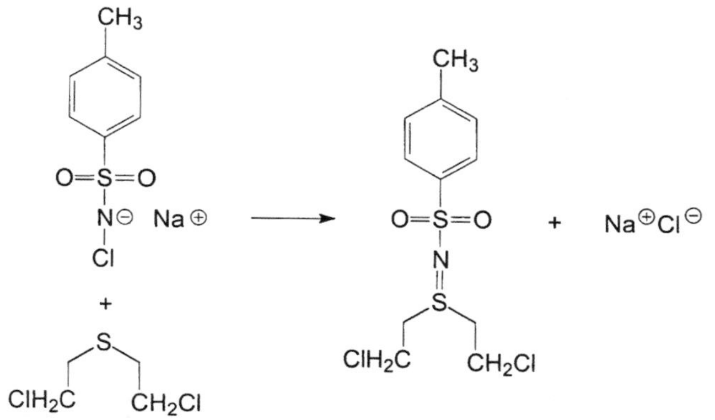

Figure 7.6: Proposed reaction of chloramine T with sulphur mustard (Klimmek *et al.*, 1983)

7.5.2.2 *Effects on the respiratory tract*

Inhalation of sulphur mustard vapour damages the epithelium of the upper respiratory tract. Damage seldom extends to the gas exchange part of the lung though alveoli lying adjacent to small conducting airways may be damaged, presumably by diffusion of the poison through the wall of the airway. The damaged airway epithelium sloughs and is expectorated. Cough may be troublesome and retrosternal pain has been described. Healing is by epithelial regeneration, and experimental work suggests that inhaled steroids may increase the rate of healing (Calvet *et al.*, 1996). It seems likely that epithelial regeneration in the airways depends on secretory cells rather than basal cells. Damage to the epithelium also occurs in asthma, inflammatory mediators being responsible (Barnes, 1994). Studies of patients suffering from asthma support the finding that inhaled steroids can enhance airway epithelial repair (Laitinen *et al.*, 1992).

7.5.2.3 *Effects on the eye*

The urgency with which eye decontamination is required if liquid sulphur mustard has found its way into the eye cannot be stressed too strongly. Nitrogen mustards (less likely to be encountered than sulphur mustard) produce even more severe eye damage. Water or 0.9 % (w/v) sodium chloride should be used, but do not delay while looking for some fluid other than water! The suggested treatment of sulphur mustard-induced eye damage is outlined in Table 7.2.

It will be appreciated that a number of different 'drops' could be used, and an expert ophthalmological opinion is needed as soon as possible. Eye damage from sulphur mustard can lead to long-lasting photophobia and involuntary lachrymation. Years later, keratitis, leading to blindness, may occur in a minority of cases.

7.5.2.4 *Prophylaxis*

Sulphur mustard is a very reactive alkylating agent and forms covalent bonds with nucleophilic moieties. Given this, attempts have been made to develop compounds that would bind avidly to sulphur mustard and to nitrogen mustards and thus prevent these compounds attacking key intracellular components. Thiols have been examined

CHAPTER 7

■ 261

TABLE 7.2
Treatment of sulphur mustard-induced eye damage

1	Saline irrigation
2	Petroleum jelly (Vaseline) on follicular margins to prevent sticking
3	Potassium ascorbate (10 % w/v) and sodium citrate (10 % w/v) drops alternately every 30 min of the waking day – discontinue as soon as a stable epithelial covering has formed
4	Pain relief
	– hyoscine drops (0.25 % w/v) to reduce pain due to spasm of the iris and to prevent sticking of the iris to the lens
	– tetracaine (amethocaine) hydrochloride (0.5 % w/v) drops
5	Chloramphenicol eyedrops to prevent infection
6	Dark glasses to ease photophobia

in detail as candidate drugs, though none has been shown to be effective if given some time *after* exposure (Callaway and Pearce, 1958; Connors *et al.*, 1964; Fasth and Sörbo, 1973; Dorr *et al.*, 1988). In animal models, if the thiol is provided prior to exposure then some protection has been demonstrated both *in vitro* and to a lesser extent *in vivo*. Early work focused on a thiosulphate/citrate mixture. More recently, GSH (Amir *et al.*, 1998), cysteine, *N*-acetylcysteine (NAC) and esters of cysteine (cyclohexyl, cyclopentyl, isopropyl, methyl) have been considered (Wilde and Upshall, 1994; Langford *et al.*, 1996) in addition to diisopropylglutathione ester (Lindsay and Hambrook, 1998). Aryl thiols (2,6-dimethoxybenzenethiol and 2,3,4-trimethoxybenzenethiol) have also been studied (Langford *et al.*, 1996), as has HMT (Lindsay and Hambrook, 1997; Andrew and Lindsay, 1998).

The lipophilicity of esters seems to confer some advantage, probably as a result of more rapid uptake into cells. It is clear that providing a high extracellular concentration of substances likely to bind rapidly and permanently to sulphur mustard might offer some degree of protection: such is the part played by the high concentration of GSH in the lining fluid of the airways and gut (Kosower and Kosower, 1978; Bray and Taylor, 1993; Hiraishi *et al.*, 1994). The role of intracellular GSH is less well understood. It has been shown that 90 % depletion of intracellular GSH in cultured macrophage/monocytes (J774 cell line) by buthionine sulphoxamine (BSO) did not cause cell death (Amir *et al.*, 1998). This is a greater degree of depletion than that caused by a dose of sulphur mustard that would be lethal to the cell. Raising intracellular GSH concentrations prior to exposure to sulphur mustard did confer a measure of protection. Taking this work forward to clinical use presents considerable difficulties. In the civilian setting prophylaxis has no part to play and will not be discussed further.

One approach that has been suggested but not, as far as is known, tried is the use of colony-stimulating factors such as granulocyte–macrophage colony-stimulating factor (GM-CSF) to oppose the effects of sulphur mustard on the bone marrow. The reader is referred to textbooks of haematology for details of these compounds.

In conclusion, the management of sulphur mustard exposure remains symptomatic: no specific and effective antidote is available. The lack of a specific antidote for sulphur mustard poisoning has led to a number of compounds including heparin, atropine, vitamin E and the vitamin B complex being advocated as therapies. No evidence of their clinical efficacy has appeared in the western literature. The work of Anguelov *et al.* (1996) may be consulted for details of studies in rats and rabbits. A modest level of protection was achieved when a complex cocktail of drugs was used in prophylaxis.

REFERENCES

Aasted A, Darre E, Wulf HC. Mustard gas: clinical, toxicological, and mutagenic aspects based on modern experience. *Ann Plas Surg* 1987; 19: 330–3.

Amir A, Chapman S, Gozes Y, Sahar R, Allon N. Protection by extracellular glutathione against sulfur mustard induced toxicity *in vitro*. *Hum Exp Toxicol* 1998; 17: 652–60.

Anderson DR, Harris LW, Lennox WJ, Solana RP. Effects of subacute pretreatment with carbamate together with acute adjunct pretreatment against nerve agent exposure. *Drug Chem Toxicol* 1991; 14: 1–19.

Andrew DJ, Lindsay CD. Protection of human upper respiratory tract cell lines against sulphur mustard toxicity by hexamethylenetetramine (HMT). *Hum Exp Toxicol* 1998; 17: 373–9.

Anguelov A, Belchev L, Angelov G. Experimental sulfur mustard gas poisoning and protective effect of different medicines in rats and rabbits. *Indian Vet J* 1996; 73: 546–51.

Anonymous. *Protopam Chloride Brand of Pralidoxime Chloride*. New York: Ayerst Laboratories, 1986.

Anonymous. *Data Sheet: Contrathion, Pralidoxime, Pralidoxima*. Paris: Laboratoires SERB, 1987.

Aposhian HV, Carter DE, Hoover TD, Hsu C-A, Maiorino RM, Stine E. DMSA, DMPS, and DMPA – as arsenic antidotes. *Fund Appl Toxicol* 1984; 4: S58–70.

Balali-Mood M, Navaeian A. Clinical and paraclinical findings in 233 patients with sulphur mustard poisoning. In: *Proceedings of the 23rd International Meeting of The International Association of Forensic Toxicologists*. Heyndrickx B (ed.). Ghent: The International Association of Forensic Toxicologists, 1986: 464–73.

Balali-Mood M, Farhoodi M, Panjvani FK. Report of three fatal cases of war gas poisoning. In: *Proceedings of the 23rd International Meeting of The International Association of Forensic Toxicologists*. Heyndrickx B (ed.). Ghent: The International Association of Forensic Toxicologists, 1986: 475–82.

Barnes PJ. Cytokines as mediators of chronic asthma. *Am J Respir Crit Care Med* 1994; 150: S42–9.

Bhattacharya R, Jeevaratnam K, Raza SK, Das Gupta S. Protection against cyanide poisoning by the co-administration of sodium nitrite and hydroxylamine in rats. *Hum Exp Toxicol* 1993; 12: 33–6.

Bismuth C, Inns RH, Marrs TC. Efficacy, toxicity and clinical use of oximes in anticholinesterase poisoning. In: *Clinical and Experimental Toxicology of Organophosphates and Carbamates*. Ballantyne B, Marrs TC (eds). Oxford: Butterworth-Heinemann, 1992: 555–77.

Bradley BL, Unger KM. Phosgene inhalation: a case report. *Texas Med* 1982; 78: 51–3.

Bray TM, Taylor CG. Tissue glutathione, nutrition, and oxidative stress. *Can J Physiol Pharmacol* 1993; 71: 746–51.

Bright JE. A prophylaxis for cyanide poisoning. In: *Clinical and Experimental Toxicology of Cyanides*. Ballantyne B, Marrs TC (eds). Bristol: John Wright, 1987: 359–82.

Bright JE, Marrs TC. Kinetics of methaemoglobin production (2). Kinetics of the cyanide antidote p-aminopropiophenone during oral administration. *Hum Toxicol* 1986; 5: 303–7.

Broomfield CA, Lockridge O, Millard CB. Protein engineering of a human enzyme that hydrolyzes V and G nerve agents: design, construction and characterization. *Chem–Biol Interact* 1999; 119–20: 413–18.

Callaway S, Pearce KA. Protection against systemic poisoning by mustard gas, di(2-chloroethyl) sulphide, by sodium thiosulphate and thiocit in the albino rat. *Br J Pharmacol* 1958; 13: 395–8.

Calvet JH, Coste A, Levame M, Harf A, Macquin-Mavier I, Escudier E. Airway epithelial damage induced by sulfur mustard in guinea pigs, effects of glucocortiocoids. *Hum Exp Toxicol* 1996; 15: 964–71.

Ci Y-X, Zhou Y-X, Guo Z-Q, Rong K-T, Chang W-B. Production, characterization and application of monoclonal antibodies against the organophosphorus nerve agent Vx. *Arch Toxicol* 1995; 69: 565–7.

■ CHAPTER 7 ■

Colardyn F, de Keyser K, Vogelaers D, Vandenbogaerde J. The clinics and therapy of victims of war gases. In: *Proceedings of the 23rd International Meeting of The International Association of Forensic Toxicologists*. Heyndrickx B (ed.). Ghent: The International Association of Forensic Toxicologists, 1986: 506–10.

Connors TA, Jeney A, Jones M. Reduction of the toxicity of 'radiomimetic' alkylating agents in rats by thiol pretreatment. III. The mechanism of the protective action of thiosulphate. *Biochem Pharmacol* 1964; 13: 1545–50.

Diller WF. Medical phosgene problems and their possible solution. *J Occup Med* 1978; 20: 189–93.

Diller WF. The methenamine misunderstanding in the therapy of phosgene poisoning. *Arch Toxicol* 1980; 46: 199–206.

Dixon M, Needham DM. Biochemical research on chemical warfare agents. *Nature* 1946; 158: 432–8.

Dorr RT, Soble M, Alberts DS. Efficacy of sodium thiosulfate as a local antidote to mechlorethamine skin toxicity in the mouse. *Cancer Chemother Pharmacol* 1988; 22: 299–302.

Dunn MA, Sidell FR. Progress in medical defense against nerve agents. *J Am Med Assoc* 1989; 262: 649–52.

Fasth A, Sörbo B. Protective effect of thiosulfate and metabolic thiosulfate precursors against toxicity of nitrogen mustard (HN_2). *Biochem Pharmacol* 1973; 22: 1337–51.

Gilchrist HA, Matz PB. The residual effects of warfare gases: the use of phosgene gas, with report of cases. *Med Bull Veterans' Administration* 1933; 10: 1–36.

Gilmour PS, Brown DM, Beswick PH, MacNee W, Rahman I, Donaldson K. Free radical activity of industrial fibers: role of iron in oxidative stress and activation of transcription factors. *Environ Health Perspect* 1997; 105 (Suppl 5): 1313–17.

Gordon JJ, Leadbeater L, Maidment MP. The protection of animals against organophosphate poisoning by pretreatment with a carbamate. *Toxicol Appl Pharmacol* 1978; 43: 207–16.

Graffe W, Kiese M, Rauscher E. The formation *in vivo* of p-hydroxylaminopropiophenone from p-aminopropiophenone and its action *in vivo* and *in vitro*. *N-S Arch Exp Pathol Pharmacol* 1964; 249: 168–75.

Gurtner GH, Scuito AM, Knoblauch A. The role of cAMP in the regulation of pulmonary vascular permeability. In: *Lung Vascular Injury: Molecular and Cellular Response*. Johnson A, Ferro TJ (eds). New York: Dekker, 1992: 99–111.

Haley RW, Kurt TL. Self-reported exposure to neurotoxic chemical combinations in the Gulf War: a cross-sectional epidemiologic study. *J Am Med Assoc* 1997; 277: 231–7.

Haley RW, Kurt TL, Hom J. Is there a Gulf War Syndrome? Searching for syndromes by factor analysis of symptoms. *J Am Med Assoc* 1997a; 227: 215–22.

Haley RW, Hom J, Roland PS, Bryan WW, Van Ness PC, Bonte FJ, Devous MD, Mathews D, Fleckenstein JL, Wians FH, Wolfe GI, Kurt TL. Evaluation of neurologic function in Gulf War veterans: a blinded case–control study. *J Am Med Assoc* 1997b; 277: 223–30.

Heath AJW, Meredith T. Atropine in the management of anticholinesterase poisoning. In: *Clinical and Experimental Toxicology of Organophosphates and Carbamates*. Ballantyne B, Marrs TC (eds). Oxford: Butterworth Heinemann, 1992: 543–54.

Hiraishi H, Terano A, Ota S, Mutoh H, Sugimoto T, Harada T, Razandi M, Ivey KJ. Protection of cultured rat gastric cells against oxidant-induced damage by exogenous glutathione. *Gastroenterology* 1994; 106: 1199–207.

Hoskin FCG, Walker JE, Stote R. Degradation of nerve gases by CLECS and cells: kinetics of heterogenous systems. *Chem–Biol Interact* 1999; 199–20: 439–44.

Inns RH, Leadbeater L. The efficacy of bispyridinium derivatives in the treatment of organophosphate poisoning in the guinea pig. *J Pharm Pharmacol* 1983; 35: 427–33.

Inns RH, Marrs TC. Prophylaxis against anticholinesterase poisoning. In: *Clinical and Experimental Toxicology of Organophosphates and Carbamates*. Ballantyne B, Marrs TC (eds). Oxford: Butterworth Heinemann, 1992: 602–10.

Inns RH, Rice P. Efficacy of dimercapto chelating agents for the treatment of poisoning by percutaneously applied dichloro(2-chlorovinyl)arsine in rabbits. *Hum Exp Toxicol* 1993; 12: 241–6.

Inns RH, Rice P, Bright JE, Marrs TC. Evaluation of the efficacy of dimercapto chelating agents for the treatment of systemic organic arsenic poisoning in rabbits. *Hum Exp Toxicol* 1990; 9: 215–20.

Iowa Persian Gulf Study Group. Self-reported illness and health status among Gulf War veterans: a population-based study. *J Am Med Assoc* 1997; 277: 238–45.

Kassa J. Comparison of the efficacy of two oximes (HI-6 and obidoxime) in soman poisoning in rats. *Toxicology* 1995; 101: 167–74.

Kassa J, Bajgar J. Changes of acetylcholinesterase activity in various parts of brain following nontreated and treated soman poisoning in rats. *Mol Chem Neuropathol* 1998; 33: 175–84.

Kassa J, Cabal J. A comparison of the efficacy of actylcholinesterase reactivators against cyclohexyl methylphosphonofluoridate (GF agent) by *in vitro* and *in vivo* methods. *Pharmacol Toxicol* 1999; 84: 41–5.

Keeler JR, Hurst CG, Dunn MA. Pyridostigmine used as a nerve agent pretreatment under wartime conditions. *J Am Med Assoc* 1991; 266: 693–5.

Kennedy TP, Michael JR, Hoidal JR, Hasty D, Sciuto AM, Hopkins C, Lazar R, Bysani GK, Tolley E, Gurtner GH. Dibutyryl cAMP, aminophylline and β-adrenergic agonists protect against pulmonary edema caused by phosgene. *J Appl Physiol* 1989; 67: 2542–52.

Kennedy TP, Rao NV, Noah W, Michael JR, Jafri MH, Gurtner GH, Hoidal JR. Ibuprofen prevents oxidant lung injury and in vitro lipid peroxidation by chelating iron. *J Clin Invest* 1990; 86: 1565–73.

Klaassen CD. Heavy metals and heavy-metal antagonists. In: *Goodman and Gilman's The Pharmacological Basis of Therapeutics*, 9th edn. Hardman JG, Limbird LE, Molinoff PB, Ruddon RW (eds). New York: McGraw-Hill, 1996: 1649–71.

Klimmek R, Szinick L, Weger N. *Chemische Gifte und Kampfstoffe: Wirkung und Therapie*. Stuttgart: Hippokrates, 1983: 57.

Kosower NS, Kosower EM. The glutathione status of cells. *Int Rev Cytol* 1978; 54: 109–60.

Laitinen LA, Laitinen A, Haahtela T. A comparative study of the effects of an inhaled corticosteroid, budesonide, and a β$_2$-agonist, terbutaline, on airway inflammation in newly diagnosed asthma: a randomised, double blind, parallel-group controlled trial. *J Allergy Clin Immunol* 1992; 90: 32–42.

Langford AM, Hobbs MJ, Upshall DG, Blain PG, Williams FM. The effect of sulphur mustard on glutathione levels in rat lung slices and the influence of treatment with arylthiols and cysteine esters. *Hum Exp Toxicol* 1996; 15: 619–24.

Leadbeater L, Inns RH, Rylands JM. Treatment of poisoning by soman. *Fundam Appl Toxicol* 1985; 5: S225–31.

Liao W-G, Rong K-T. An explanation on the limited efficacy of detoxication against VX toxicity by purified specific antibodies. *Fundam Appl Toxicol* 1995; 27: 90–4.

Lindsay CD, Hambrook JL. Protection of A549 cells against the toxic effects of sulphur mustard by hexamethylenetretamine. *Hum Exp Toxicol* 1997; 16: 106–14.

Lindsay CD, Hambrook JL. Diisopropylglutathione ester protects A549 cells from the cytotoxic effects of sulphur mustard. *Hum Exp Toxicol* 1998; 17: 606–12.

Longcope WT, Luetscher JA, Wintrobe MM, Jäger V. Clinical uses of 2,3-dimercaptopropanol (BAL). VII. The treatment of arsenical dermatitis with preparations of BAL. *J Clin Invest* 1946; 25: 528–33.

Marrs TC, Inns RH, Bright JE, Wood SG. The formation of methaemoglobin by 4-amino-propiophenone (PAPP) and 4-(N-hydroxy)aminopropiophenone. *Hum Exp Toxicol* 1991; 10: 183–8.

Marrs TC, Maynard RL, Sidell FR. *Chemical Warfare Agents. Toxicology and Treatment*. Chichester: Wiley, 1996.

Maxwell DM, Saxena A, Gordon RK, Doctor BP. Improvements in scavenger protection against organophosphorus agents by modification of cholinesterases. *Chem–Biol Interact* 1999; 119–20: 419–28.

Maynard RL. Toxicology of chemical warfare agents. In: *General and Applied Toxicology*, 2nd edn. Ballantyne B, Marrs TC, Syversen T (eds). London: Macmillan, 2000: 2079–109.

Modell W, Gold H, Cattell M. Clinical uses of 2,3-dimercaptopropanol (BAL). IV. Pharmacologic observations on BAL by intramuscular injection in man. *J Clin Invest* 1946; 25: 480–7.

Moore W. *Gas Attack! Chemical Warfare 1915–18 and Afterwards*. London: Cooper, 1987: 168–9.

Morgan-Jones D, Hodgetts T. Sarin. *J Accid Emerg Med* 1996; 13: 431–2.

Nozaki H, Aikawa N. Sarin poisoning in Tokyo subway [letter]. *Lancet* 1995; 345: 1446–7.

Parfitt K. (ed.) *Martindale: The Complete Drug Reference*, 32nd edn. London: Pharmaceutical Press, 1999: 979–80.

Pennisi E. Chemicals behind the Gulf War Syndrome? *Science* 1996; 272: 479–80.

Philippens IHCHM, Vanwersch RAP, Groen B, Olivier B, Bruijnzeel PLB, Melchers BPC. Subchronic physostigmine pretreatment in marmosets: absence of side effects and effectiveness against soman poisoning with negligible postintoxication incapacitation. *Toxicol Sci* 2000; 53: 84–91.

Prentiss AM. *Chemicals in War: A Treatise on Chemical Warfare*. New York: McGraw-Hill, 1937: 536.

Sciuto AM, Strickland PT, Kennedy TP, Gurtner GH. Protective effects of *N*-acetylcysteine treatment after phosgene exposure in rabbits. *Am J Respir Crit Care Med* 1995; 151: 768–72.

Sciuto AM, Strickland PT, Kennedy TP, Guo Y-L, Gurtner GH. Intratracheal administration of DBcAMP attenuates edema formation in phosgene-induced acute lung injury. *J Appl Physiol* 1996a; 80: 149–57.

Sciuto AM, Stotts RR, Hurt HH. Efficacy of ibuprofen and pentoxifylline in the treatment of phosgene-induced acute lung injury. *J Appl Toxicol* 1996b; 16: 381–4.

Selgrade MK, Gilmour MI, Yang YG, Burleson GR, Hatch GE. Pulmonary host defenses and resistance to infection following subchronic exposure to phosgene. *Inhalation Toxicol* 1995; 7: 1257–68.

Sellström Ä. Anticonvulsants in anticholinesterase poisoning. In: *Clinical and Experimental Toxicology of Organophosphates and Carbamates*. Ballantyne B, Marrs TC (eds). Oxford: Butterworth-Heinemann, 1992: 578–86.

Sharabi Y, Danon YL, Berkenstadt H, Almog S, Mimouni-Bloch A, Zisman A, Dani S, Atsmon J. Survey of symptoms following intake of pyridostigmine during the Persian Gulf war. *Isr J Med Sci* 1991; 27: 656–8.

Simeon-Rudolf V, Reiner E, Škrinjarić-Špoljar M, Radić B, Lucić A, Primozić I, Tomić S. Quinuclidinium-imidazolium compounds: synthesis, mode of interaction with acetyl-cholinesterase and effect upon soman intoxicated mice. *Arch Toxicol* 1998; 72: 289–95.

Stavrakis P. The use of hexamethylenetetramine (HMT) in treatment of phosgene poisoning. *Ind Med* 1971; 40: 30–1.

Steinhaus RK, Baskin SI, Clark JH, Kirby SD. Formation of methemoglobin and metmyoglobin using 8-aminoquinoline derivatives or sodium nitrite and subsequent reaction with cyanide. *J Appl Toxicol* 1990; 10: 345–51.

Sulzberger MB, Baer RL, Kanof A. Clinical uses of 2,3-dimercaptopropanol (BAL). III. Studies on the toxicity of BAL on percutaneous and parenteral administration. *J Clin Invest* 1946; 25: 474–9.

UK Ministry of Defence. *Medical Manual of Defence against Chemical Agents. JSP 312*. London: HMSO, 1972: 20.

Vedder EB. *The Medical Aspects of Chemical Warfare*. Baltimore: Williams and Wilkins, 1925: 77–124.

Vick JA, von Bredow JD. Effectiveness of intramuscularly administered cyanide antidotes on methemoglobin formation and survival. *J Appl Toxicol* 1996; 16: 509–16.

Werrlein RJ, Madren-Whalley JS, Kirby SD. Phosgene effects on F-actin organization and concentration in cells cultured from sheep and rat lung. *Cell Biol Toxicol* 1994; 10: 45–58.

Wilde PE, Upshall DG. Cysteine esters protect cultured rodent lung slices from sulphur mustard. *Hum Exp Toxicol* 1994; 13: 743–8.

Willems JL. Clinical management of mustard gas casualties. *Ann Med Militaires Belgicae* 1989; 3 (Suppl): 1–61.

Worek F, Bäcker M, Thiermann H, Szinicz, Mast U, Klimmek R, Eyer P. Reappraisal of indications and limitations of oxime therapy in organophosphate poisoning. *Hum Exp Toxicol* 1997; 16: 466–72.

Worek F, Widmann R, Knopff O, Szinicz L. Reactivating potency of obidoxime, pralidoxime, HI 6 and HLö 7 in human erythrocyte acetylcholinesterase inhibited by highly toxic organophosphorus compounds. *Arch Toxicol* 1998a; 72: 237–43.

Worek F, Eyer P, Szinicz L. Inhibition, reactivation and aging kinetics of cyclohexyl-methylphosphonofluoridate-inhibited human cholinesterases. *Arch Toxicol* 1998b; 72: 580–7.

World Health Organization. *Environmental Health Criteria 193: Phosgene*. Geneva: WHO, 1997.

■ CHAPTER 7 ■

Antidotal Treatment of Paraquat Poisoning

Contents

8.1 INTRODUCTION

Paraquat (1,1'-dimethyl-4,4'-dipyridinium dichloride; methyl viologen) is available in more than 100 countries and is sold in concentrated (up to 20 % w/v) form for professional use and as granules (2.5–8 % w/w) for use in the garden. Occupational poisoning has occurred by dermal absorption when concentrated spray solutions have leaked from backpacks, but in general paraquat is poorly absorbed through intact skin or from the respiratory tract. However, paraquat is sometimes used as a means of suicide by deliberate ingestion and has a high fatality rate. Deaths have also occurred from accidental ingestion of concentrates.

Paraquat is rapidly absorbed from the gastrointestinal tract and may become sequestered in the epithelial alveolar cells in the lung, where it sets up a redox cycle involving molecular oxygen, resulting in the production of superoxide radical anion and depletion of intracellular NADPH (Figure 8.1). Detoxification of superoxide by superoxide dismutase within the cell results in the formation of hydrogen peroxide, and this in turn may cause further NADPH depletion by reaction with GSH catalysed by the selenium-containing enzyme glutathione peroxidase. Reduction of ferric iron to ferrous iron by superoxide and subsequent oxidation to ferric iron by reaction with hydrogen peroxide (Fenton reaction) can result in the production of hydroxyl radicals, which are highly reactive and can cause lipid peroxidation, destruction of cell membranes and ultimately cell death (Figure 8.1).

Clinically, an acute alveolitis develops, causing haemorrhagic pulmonary oedema or adult respiratory distress syndrome. The lethal dose of paraquat for an adult is estimated to be 2–4 g; therefore, ingestion of as little as 10–20 mL of a 20 % (w/v) solution can be fatal. The features of upper gastrointestinal and respiratory tract damage reflect the corrosive nature of the solution swallowed, whereas the systemic features depend more on the amount of paraquat ingested. The development of renal failure compromises the only efficient method of eliminating absorbed paraquat.

Reduction of morbidity and mortality in paraquat poisoning relies at present on methods designed to prevent absorption. These measures include limiting the supply of concentrates, the addition of stenching and emetic agents and adequate labelling/public awareness campaigns. Despite much research into the mechanisms of paraquat poisoning and its potential treatment, only early gastrointestinal decontamination and supportive measures have a therapeutic role (Vale *et al.*, 1987). No clinical evidence as yet supports the use of any antidote in the management of paraquat poisoning.

8.2 INVESTIGATIONS AND PROGNOSIS

The diagnosis of paraquat poisoning is usually made on the basis of a history of ingestion together with the presence of oral injury. A urine spot test should be performed to confirm paraquat exposure: 100 mg sodium dithionite should be added to 10 mL of 1 mol/L sodium hydroxide solution, and 1 mL of this mixture is in turn added to 1 mL urine – an intense royal blue colour (due to the production of paraquat radical cation, Figure 8.1) indicates the presence of paraquat. A negative test within 4–6 h of exposure indicates that not enough paraquat has been absorbed to cause toxicity in the lungs in the ensuing days. Patients who have a positive urine spot test should therefore have a blood sample taken for plasma paraquat measurement. The prognosis for an individual who has ingested paraquat can be predicted from a nomogram that relates plasma

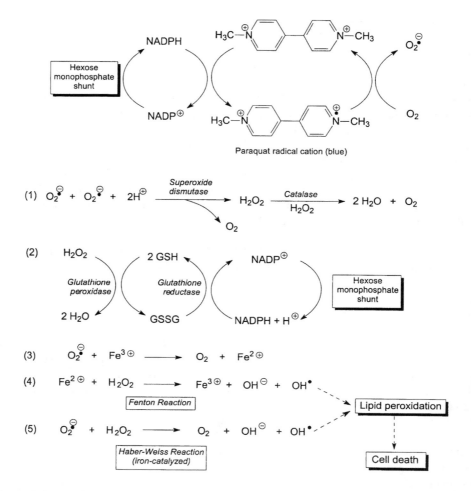

Figure 8.1: Possible mechanisms by which paraquat causes depletion of lung NADPH and cell death [adapted from Smith (1988)]. Formation of superoxide radical anion is followed by (1–5) detoxification of superoxide radical anion and associated reactions

paraquat concentrations up to 24 h after exposure to the probability of survival (Proudfoot *et al.*, 1979).

8.2.1 Supportive care

In vitro and *in vivo* activated charcoal absorbs paraquat and is as effective as fuller's earth (Gaudreault *et al.*, 1985). The administration of adsorbent as soon as possible effectively reduces paraquat absorption from the gastrointestinal tract in animal models (Idid and Lee, 1996), and thus activated charcoal should be given if the patient presents within 1 h of ingestion. Symptomatic measures include use of antiemetics, mouthwashes and analgesics and rigorous rehydration to replace gastrointestinal fluid loss.

As the absorption of paraquat peaks at 2 h post ingestion and sequestration of paraquat into the alveolar epithelial cells occurs within 4 h, any technique designed to increase elimination of absorbed paraquat must be instituted as soon as possible (Honoré et al., 1994). Most elimination methods, such as haemoperfusion and haemodialysis, appear to remove only a very small proportion of absorbed paraquat (Vale et al., 1977). When renal function is conserved, elimination by the kidney is 3–10 times more efficient than haemoperfusion (Proudfoot et al., 1987). It is therefore possible that methods for enhancing elimination may prove ineffective.

Palliative care is the best approach in patients with plasma paraquat concentrations above the 'survival' line (Proudfoot et al., 1979). There is a range of treatment options available for patients whose plasma paraquat concentrations lie below the line, but the efficacy of the majority of options is unproven. Supplemental oxygen is not given unless absolutely necessary because of animal evidence of increased severity of pulmonary damage where the proportion of oxygen in the inspired air (Fio_2) is raised (Rhodes et al., 1976; Fogt and Zilker, 1989). Producing low inspired oxygen concentrations in patients by increasing the proportion of nitrogen in the air is generally unsuccessful as the hypoxaemia produced worsens lung oedema, in turn necessitating increase of the Fio_2 (Fogt and Zilker, 1989). Attempts to reduce the extent of lung inflammation and scarring using radiotherapy are of limited efficacy (Webb et al., 1984; Smith, 1988). Lung transplantation has been used in a few patients (Matthew et al., 1968; Kamholz et al., 1984), but without success.

8.3 ANTIDOTAL TREATMENT

Some potential antidotes have shown promise in experimental studies, partly because they are administered prophylactically or early in the course of poisoning and partly because of interspecies differences. Antidotes that show promise in rodents, such as those containing the magnesium ion, which is thought to have an anti-oxidant role *in vivo*, sadly do not show the same promise in clinical studies. Clinical efficacy data are lacking because of heterogeneity of patient populations, the paucity of controlled trials and numerous confounding variables, and the fact that most patients present after most of the ingested paraquat has been absorbed.

Most efforts to develop an antidote have been directed towards maintaining or enhancing detoxification of the superoxide radical (Table 8.1). These have included administration of superoxide dismutase (Harley et al., 1977; Michelson et al., 1981; Bateman, 1987), vitamin E (Bus et al., 1977; Redetzki and Wood, 1980; Combs and Peterson, 1983), ascorbate (Harley et al., 1977; Schvartsman et al., 1984), selenium (as sodium selenate – Combs and Peterson, 1983), N-acetylcysteine (NAC) (Dawson et al., 1984; Wegener et al., 1988), riboflavin and niacin (Brown et al., 1981; Schvartsman et al., 1984), and methylthioninium chloride (Kelner et al., 1988). None of these has been shown to have a beneficial effect in human poisoning.

The use of the iron chelator deferoxamine (DFO) has been suggested because ferric iron can catalyse the production of hydoxyl radicals from hydrogen peroxide (Figure 8.1). DFO decreases cytotoxicity of paraquat on alveolar cells in mice, and protects mice from lethal doses of paraquat (Kohen and Chevion, 1985; Ogino and Awai, 1988; van der Wal et al., 1990). DFO might act not only by inhibition of paraquat-induced iron-catalysed free radical generation, but also by inhibiting paraquat uptake by alveolar type II epithelial cells (van der Wal et al., 1990). DFO seems to be an interesting therapeutic possibility, but efficacy and optimal dosing regimes have not been evaluated in humans.

TABLE 8.1
Some suggested antidotal treatments for paraquat poisoning [modified from Hall (1998)]

N-Acetylcysteine (sections 2.2.8.1 and 4.16)	Nitric oxide (CAS 10102-43-9)
Ambroxol (surfactant synthesis inducer; CAS 18683-91-5)	Paraquat-specific antibodies
Ascorbate (vitamin C, section 4.13.1)	Putrescine (CAS 110-60-1)
Clofibrate (CAS 637-07-0)	Riboflavin (vitamin B_2; section 4.14)
Colchicine (CAS 64-86-8)	Selenium-containing compounds
Corticosteroids (dexamethasone, CAS 50-02-2; methylprednisolone, CAS 83-43-2)	Spermine (CAS 71-44-3)
Deferoxamine (desferrioxamine, DFO; section 2.3)	Superoxide dismutase (CAS 9054-89-1)
Hypo-oxygenation	Valinomycin (CAS 2001-95-8)
Immunosuppressants (cyclophosphamide; CAS 6055-19-2)	Vitamin E (α-tocopherol; CAS 59-02-9)
Magnesium salts	Xanthine oxidase inhibitors
Methylthioninium chloride (methylene blue; section 4.13.2)	Zinc salts (section 4.18)
Niacin (nicotinic acid, CAS 59-67-6)	

Others have tried to prevent the accumulation of paraquat in alveolar epithelial cells via blockage of the polyamine uptake pathway(s). *In vitro* studies with putrescine and spermine (Figure 8.2), and also with the cyclic antibiotic valinomycin (Figure 8.3), have demonstrated competition for uptake (Smith, 1988; Masek and Richards, 1990; Hoet *et al.*, 1994), but studies *in vivo* have not shown antidotal effect (Bateman, 1987; Dunbar *et al.*, 1988; Pond, 1995).

Recently, antibodies from IgG- and IgM-secreting cell lines have been raised in murine hybridomas and show high selectivity and affinity for paraquat (Bowles *et al.*, 1988; Johnston *et al.*, 1988). Paraquat-specific antibodies inhibit the uptake of paraquat by type II alveolar cells from the rat and reduce toxicity (Wright *et al.*, 1987; Chen *et al.*, 1994). After i.v. injection of 0.1 mg/kg paraquat, the plasma paraquat concentration in rats pretreated with anti-paraquat antibodies was increased and the amount excreted in the urine was significantly decreased compared with controls (Nagao *et al.*, 1989). However, although use of anti-paraquat antibodies succeeded in sequestering paraquat in the plasma compartment, it could not prevent paraquat from accumulating in tissues (Nagao *et al.*, 1989). Such *in vitro* and *in vivo* studies suggest that, as the concentrations of paraquat in the lung are not changed, paraquat antibodies neither prevent paraquat uptake by the lung nor favour its release. More recently a single-chain F_v fragment specific for paraquat has been produced from hybridoma cells secreting a paraquat-specific murine monoclonal antibody (Devlin *et al.*, 1995). It remains to be seen if these paraquat antibodies have different efficacy *in vitro* and *in vivo*.

It has been noted that magnesium and/or potassium restriction enhances paraquat toxicity in rats (Minakata *et al.*, 1998). When activated charcoal and magnesium citrate were administered concomitantly, the survival rate in mice improved significantly, but this may be due to catharsis alone and may not be a direct protective effect (Gaudreault

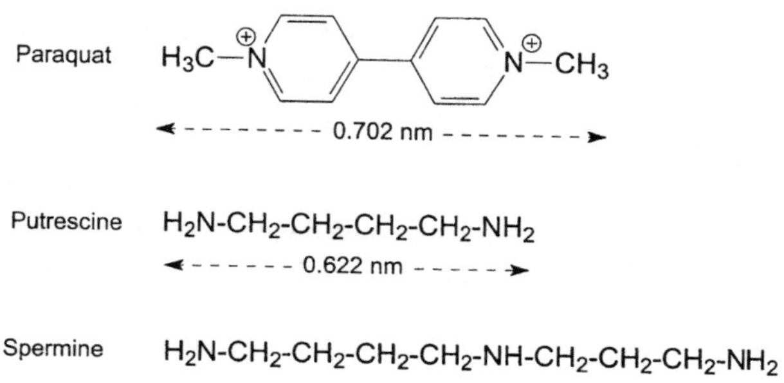

Paraquat $H_3C-\overset{\oplus}{N}$ ... $\overset{\oplus}{N}-CH_3$

◄ - - - - - - - - 0.702 nm - - - - - - - - ►

Putrescine $H_2N-CH_2-CH_2-CH_2-CH_2-NH_2$

◄ - - - - - - 0.622 nm - - - - - ►

Spermine $H_2N-CH_2-CH_2-CH_2-CH_2-NH-CH_2-CH_2-CH_2-NH_2$

Figure 8.2: Molecular formulae of paraquat, putrescine and spermine showing geometric standards of the distance between nitrogen atoms. There is thought to be a paraquat accumulation receptor on the outside of the alveolar epithelial cell membrane containing two negatively charged sites more than 0.5 nm apart (actual distance unknown) [adapted from Smith (1988)]

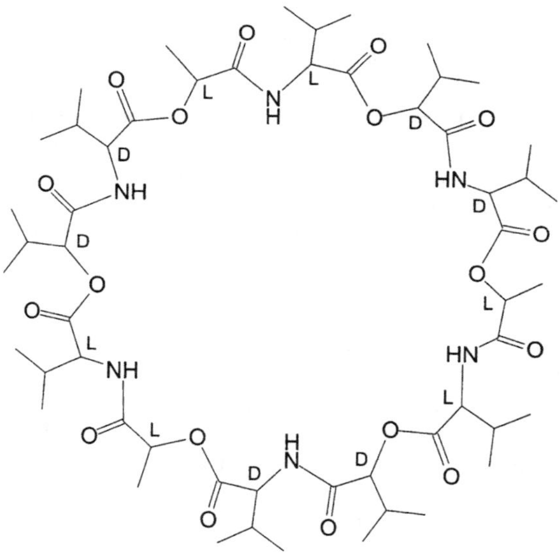

Figure 8.3: Structural formula of valinomycin

et al., 1985). Case reports of the use of magnesium salts in man have appeared (Ochoa Gomez and Gil Paraiso, 1993), but early results from controlled studies are equivocal (M Wilks, personal communication, 2000).

Cyclophosphamide and glucocorticoids alter the polymorphonuclear granulocyte reaction to paraquat and, although high doses of both agents have been used, variable efficacy has been reported (Addo *et al.*, 1984; Nogué *et al.*, 1989; Perriëns *et al.*, 1992; Lin *et al.*, 1996, 1999). Cyclophosphamide (1 g/d, 2 days) and methylprednisolone (1 g/d, 3 days) was given as pulse therapy and reported mortality was 25 % versus 70.6 % (Lin *et al.*, 1996). However, a previous study and a case report of high-dose cyclophosphamide and dexamethasone in paraquat poisoning indicated that treatment with these drugs was ineffective (Nogué *et al.*, 1989; Perriëns *et al.*, 1992).

Inhaled nitric oxide has also been suggested for use in the later stages of poisoning (Köppel *et al.*, 1994; Hall, 1998). One patient treated with fuller's earth, forced diuresis, haemofiltration, NAC, methylprednisolone, cyclophosphamide, vitamin E, colchicine and delayed continuous nitric oxide inhalation survived with return to normal pulmonary function, despite a predicted chance of survival of only 30 % (Eisenman *et al.*, 1998).

REFERENCES

Addo E, Ramdial S, Poon-King T. High dosage cyclophosphamide and dexamethasone treatment of paraquat poisoning with 75 % survival. *West Indian Med J* 1984; 33: 220–6.

Bateman DN. Pharmacological treatments of paraquat poisoning. *Hum Toxicol* 1987; 6: 57–62.

Bowles M, Johnston SC, Schoof DD, Pentel PR, Pond SM. Large scale production and purification of paraquat and desipramine monoclonal antibodies and their Fab fragments. *Int J Immunopharmacol* 1988; 10: 537–45.

Brown OR, Heitkamp M, Song C-S. Niacin reduces paraquat toxicity in rats. *Science* 1981; 212: 1510–2.

Bus JS, Aust SD, Gibson JE. Lipid peroxidation as a proposed mechanism for paraquat toxicity. In: *Biochemical Mechanisms of Paraquat Toxicity*. Autor AP (ed.). New York: Academic Press, 1977: 157–74.

Chen N, Bowles MR, Pond SM. Prevention of paraquat toxicity in suspensions of alveolar type II cells by paraquat-specific antibodies. *Hum Exp Toxicol* 1994; 13: 551–7.

Combs GF, Peterson FJ. Protection against acute paraquat toxicity by dietary selenium in the chick. *J Nutr* 1983; 113: 538–45.

Dawson JR, Norbeck K, Anundi I, Moldéus P. The effectiveness of *N*-acetylcysteine in isolated hepatocytes, against toxicity of paracetamol, acrolein, and paraquat. *Arch Toxicol* 1984; 55: 11–15.

Devlin CM, Bowles MR, Gordon RB, Pond SM. Production of a paraquat-specific murine single chain Fv fragment. *J Biochem* 1995; 118: 480–7.

Dunbar JR, DeLucia AJ, Acuff RV, Ferslew KE. Prolonged intravenous paraquat infusion in the rat. I. Failure of coinfused putrescine to attenuate pulmonary paraquat uptake, paraquat-induced biochemical changes, or lung injury. *Toxicol Appl Pharmacol* 1988; 94: 207–20.

Eisenman A, Armali Z, Raikhlin-Eisenkraft B, Bentur L, Bentur Y, Guralnik L, Enat R. Nitric oxide inhalation for paraquat-induced lung injury. *J Toxicol Clin Toxicol* 1998; 36: 575–84.

Fogt F, Zilker T. Total exclusion from external respiration protects lungs from development of fibrosis after paraquat intoxication. *Hum Toxicol* 1989; 8: 465–74.

Gaudreault P, Friedman PA, Lovejoy FH. Efficacy of activated charcoal and magnesium citrate in the treatment of oral paraquat intoxication. *Ann Emerg Med* 1985; 14: 123–5.

Hall AH. Nitric oxide inhalation for paraquat: surviving both poisoning and therapy? *J Toxicol Clin Toxicol* 1998; 36: 585–6.

Harley JB, Grinspan S, Root RK. Paraquat suicide in a young woman: results of therapy directed against the superoxide radical. *Yale J Biol Med* 1977; 50: 481–8.

Hoet PHM, Lewis CPL, Demedts M, Nemery B. Putrescine and paraquat uptake in human lung slices and isolated type II pneumocytes. *Biochem Pharmacol* 1994; 48: 517–24.

Honoré P, Hantson P, Fauville JP, Peeters A, Mahieu P. Paraquat poisoning: 'state of the art'. *Acta Clin Belg* 1994; 49: 220–8.

Idid SZ, Lee CY. Effects of fuller's earth and activated charcoal on oral absorption of paraquat in rabbits. *Clin Exp Pharmacol Physiol* 1996; 23: 679–81.

Johnston SC, Bowles M, Winzor DJ, Pond SM. Comparison of paraquat-specific murine monoclonal antibodies produced by *in vitro* and *in vivo* immunization. *Fundam Appl Toxicol* 1988; 11: 261–7.

Kamholz S, Veith FJ, Mollenkopf F, Montefusco C, Nehlsen-Cannarella S, Kaleya R, Pinsker K, Tellis V, Soberman R, Sablay L, Matas A, Gliedman M, Goldsmith J, Fell S, Brodman R, Merav A, Shander A, Hollinger I, Nagashima H. Single lung transplantation in paraquat intoxication. *NY State J Med* 1984; 84: 81–3.

Kelner MJ, Bagnell R, Hale B, Alexander NM. Methylene blue competes with paraquat for reduction by flavo-enzymes resulting in decreased superoxide production in the presence of heme proteins. *Arch Biochem Biophys* 1988; 262: 422–6.

Kohen R, Chevion M. Paraquat toxicity is enhanced by iron and reduced by desferrioxamine in laboratory mice. *Biochem Pharmacol* 1985; 34: 1841–3.

Köppel C, von Wissman Ch, Barckow D, Rossaint R, Falke K, Stoltenburg-Didinger G, Schnoy N. Inhaled nitric oxide in advanced paraquat intoxication. *Clin Toxicol* 1994; 32: 205–14.

Lin J-L, Wei M-C, Liu Y-C. Pulse therapy with cyclophosphamide and methylprednisolone in patients with moderate to severe paraquat poisoning: a preliminary report. *Thorax* 1996; 51: 661–3.

Lin J-L, Leu M-L, Liu Y-C, Chen G-H. A prospective clinical trail of pulse therapy with glucocorticoid and cyclophosphamide in moderate to severe paraquat-poisoned patients. *Am J Respir Crit Care Med* 1999; 59: 357–60.

Masek L, Richards RJ. Interactions between paraquat, endogenous lung amines' antioxidants and isolated mouse Clara cells. *Toxicology* 1990; 63: 315–26.

Matthew H, Logan A, Woodruff MFA, Heard B. Paraquat poisoning – lung transplantation. *Br Med J* 1968; 3: 759–63.

Michelson AM, Puget K, Durosay P. Studies of liposomal superoxide dismutase in rats. *Mol Physiol* 1981; 1: 85–96.

Minakata K, Suzuki O, Saito S, Harada N. Dietary Mg and/or K restriction enhances paraquat toxicity in rats. *Arch Toxicol* 1998; 72: 450–3.

Nagao M, Takatori T, Wu B, Terazawa K, Gotouda H, Akabane H. Immunotherapy for the treatment of acute paraquat poisoning. *Hum Toxicol* 1989; 8: 121–3.

Nogué S, Munné P, Campañá E, Bertrán A, Reig R, Rodamilans M. Fracaso de la combinación ciclofosfamida–dexametasona en la intoxicatión por paracuat. *Med Clin (Barc)* 1989; 93: 61–3.

Ochoa Gomez FJ, Gil Paraiso A. Intoxicación letal por paraquat: aportación de un nuevo caso. *An Med Intern (Madrid)* 1993; 10: 349–50.

Ogino T, Awai M. Lipid peroxidation and tissue injury by ferric citrate in paraquat-intoxicated mice. *Biochim Biophys Acta* 1988; 958: 388–95.

Perriëns JH, Benimadho S, Lie Kiauw I, Wisse J, Chee H. High-dose cyclophosphamide and dexamethasone in paraquat poisoning: a prospective study. *Hum Exp Toxicol* 1992; 11: 129–34.

Pond SM. Treatment of paraquat poisoning. In: *Paraquat Poisoning. Mechanism, Prevention, Treatment*. Bismuth C, Hall AH (eds). New York: Dekker, 1995, 325–34.

Proudfoot AT, Stewart MS, Levitt T, Widdop B. Paraquat poisoning: significance of plasma paraquat concentrations. *Lancet* 1979; ii: 330–2.

Proudfoot AT, Prescott LF, Jarvie DR. Haemodialysis for paraquat poisoning. *Hum Toxicol* 1987; 6: 69–74.

Redetzki HM, Wood CD. Vitamin E and paraquat poisoning [abstract]. *Vet Hum Toxicol* 1980; 22: 668.

Rhodes ML, Zavala DC, Brown D. Hypoxic protection in paraquat poisoning. *Lab Invest* 1976; 35: 496–500.

Schvartsman S, Zyngier S, Schvartsman C. Ascorbic acid and riboflavin in the treatment of acute intoxication by paraquat. *Vet Hum Toxicol* 1984; 26: 473–5.

Smith LL. The toxicity of paraquat. *Adv Drug React Ac Pois Rev* 1988; 1: 1–17.

Vale JA, Crome P, Volans GN, Widdop B, Goulding R. The treatment of paraquat poisoning using oral sorbents and charcoal haemoperfusion. *Acta Pharmacol Toxicol* 1977; 41: 109–17.

CHAPTER 8

Vale JA, Meredith TJ, Buckley BM. Paraquat poisoning: clinical features and immediate general management. *Hum Toxicol* 1987; 6: 41–7.

van der Wal NAA, van Oirschot JFLM, van Dijk A, Verhoef J, van Asbeck BS. Mechanism of protection of alveolar type II cells against paraquat-induced cytotoxicity by deferoxamine. *Biochem Pharmacol* 1990; 39: 1665–71.

Webb DB, Williams MV, Davies BH, James KW. Resolution after radiotherapy of severe pulmonary damage due to paraquat poisoning. *Br Med J* 1984; 288: 1259–60.

Wegener T, Sandhagen B, Chan KW, Saldeen T. N-acetylcysteine in paraquat toxicity: toxicological and histological evaluation in rats. *Ups J Med Sci* 1988; 93: 81–9.

Wright AF, Green TP, Robson RT, Niewola Z, Wyatt I, Smith LL. Specific polyclonal and monoclonal antibody prevents paraquat accumulation into rat lung slices. *Biochem Pharmacol* 1987; 36: 1325–31.

Antidote Interference in Toxicological Analyses

Contents

9.1 INTRODUCTION

Toxicological analyses will often be performed before antidotal treatment is initiated, either to establish the diagnosis or to confirm the severity of exposure (Table 9.1). Clearly, normal precautions in sample collection, transport and storage apply, as in other situations (Flanagan, 1995). Transfusion, for example, will invalidate blood or plasma drug or poison assays until equilibrium between blood and tissue drug or poison concentrations has been re-established. Infusion of large amounts of fluid could also unduly influence sample integrity if the sample were to be collected too close to the infusion site.

If an antidote is administered before sample collection for toxicological analysis the possible effect on either the analytical procedure to be used, or on the interpretation of the results obtained, needs to be considered. Some known or potential problem areas are discussed below.

It is possible that antidote administration will interfere in certain clinical chemistry tests. For example, the cyanide antidote hydroxocobalamin (section 6.2.4.2) is thought to interfere in a number of measurements (Curry et al., 1994; Gourlain et al., 1994) and N-acetylcysteine interferes in chloride ion assay performed using a silver/silver chloride

TABLE 9.1

Emergency toxicological analyses that may influence antidotal treatment

Treatment	Poison	Plasma concentration associated with serious toxicity
1. Protective therapy		
N-Acetylcysteine or methionine	Paracetamol	200 mg/L at 4 h, 30 mg/L at 16 h[a]
Ethanol or fomepizole	Ethylene glycol	0.5 g/L
	Methanol	0.5 g/L
2. Chelation therapy		
Deferoxamine	Aluminium	50–250 μg/L (serum)
	Iron	5 mg/L (serum, children)
		8 mg/L (serum, adults)
Edetate[b] or DMSA[c]	Antimony	200 μg/L (whole blood)
	Cadmium	20 μg/L (whole blood)
	Lead	600 μg/L (whole blood)
DMSA[c] or DMPS[d]	Arsenic	50 μg/L (whole blood)[e]
	Bismuth	100 μg/L (whole blood)
	Mercury	50 μg/L (whole blood)
3. Active elimination therapy		
Prussian Blue[f]	Thallium	50 μg/L (whole blood)

Notes

[a] 100 mg/L at 4 h, 15 mg/L at 16 h for 'high-risk' patients (e.g. those treated with anticonvulsants or rifamipicin, alcoholics, AIDS patients; see Figure 4.22).
[b] Calcium disodium edetate.
[c] *meso*-Dimercaptosuccinic acid.
[d] Dimercaptopropane sulphonate.
[e] Recent ingestion of fish or shellfish renders total arsenic measurements uninterpretable.
[f] Potassium ferrihexacyanoferrate.

electrode (Bishell *et al.*, 1994). However, detailed consideration of this topic is outside the scope of the present work.

9.2 *N*-ACETYLCYSTEINE

N-Acetylcysteine can interfere in some enzyme-based plasma paracetamol assays by reducing colour formation, leading to underestimation of the paracetamol concentration (Tarpey and Leonard, 1997; Mayer and Salpeter, 1998; Tyhach, 1999). The magnitude of the interference reported in the GDS Technology AR1000 paracetamol assay kit, for example, was much greater at plasma NAC concentrations of 1 g/L (some 30 % reduction at a paracetamol concentration of 150 mg/L) than at lower NAC concentrations (Mayer and Salpeter, 1998), but this NAC concentration is similar to those attained at the start of the i.v. NAC dosage schedule used in the UK (section 4.16.1.4). Accidental NAC overdosage of up to 3.6 times in the initial infusion bag has been reported (Ferner *et al.*, 1999), hence it would seem possible that NAC concentrations of 3–4 g/L could be attained in exceptional circumstances. Clearly, if the plasma paracetamol concentration in individual patients is measured on a sample obtained before NAC infusion is commenced then this potential problem is obviated, but it would seem prudent to test methods for this problem before accepting them for clinical use, especially if manipulation of the specified test conditions is undertaken to adapt the methods to particular instruments. There are also anecdotal reports of false positives due to the presence of bilirubin or haemolysis in the GDS method.

9.3 α_1-ACID GLYCOPROTEIN

Administration of exogenous α_1-acid glycoprotein (AAG) could give rise to raised plasma concentrations of protein-bound analyte (basic drugs and/or metabolites). Thus interpretation of analytical results obtained using methods that measure total (free + protein-bound) drug will be rendered difficult to interpret as regards correlation with the clinical condition of the patient, and procedures such as *in vitro* equilibrium dialysis or ultrafiltration would be required in order to measure non-protein-bound ('free') drug.

9.4 ANTIDIGOXIN F_{ab} ANTIBODY FRAGMENTS

As in the case of α_1-acid glycoprotein above, equilibrium dialysis or ultrafiltration is required to measure free, pharmacologically active digoxin after the administration of F_{ab} antibody fragments using conventional immunoassays (Gibb *et al.*, 1983; Hursting *et al.*, 1987). Digestion of the F_{ab} antibody fragment–digoxin complex using a proteolytic enzyme is also required before measurement of 'total' digoxin as the affinity of the F_{ab} fragment for digoxin may well be similar to or greater than the affinity of the antibody used in the immunoasay. Using these techniques, it has been shown that plasma free digoxin falls to almost zero a few minutes after F_{ab} administration, whereas the total digoxin rises rapidly to values some 20- to 40-fold above pretreatment values. Plasma digoxin measurements using conventional methodology are not reliable for 1–2 weeks post treatment (Antman *et al.*, 1990).

Similar considerations would, of course, apply if immunoassays were to be used to measure other potential analytes (Chapter 3) after antivenin/whole antibody or F_{ab}

antibody fragment administration. If chromatographic or other conventional analytical methods were to be used, then again the 'total' plasma drug concentration should bear little relation to the clinical condition of the patient assuming the treatment had been successful in mobilizing poison from tissues into plasma.

9.5 CHELATING AND OTHER AGENTS USED TO TREAT POISONING WITH TOXIC METALS

Guidance on interpretation of analytical toxicology results and mass/amount concentration conversion factors for some metals and trace elements is given in Appendix 4. As with AAG above, administration of a chelating agent should enhance blood or plasma 'total' metal ion concentration, thus rendering any measurement of total metal ion of limited value as regards assessing the severity of exposure or the efficacy of treatment. Urinary excretion of total metal ion, however, can still be used as a means of assessing efficacy and also the need for treatment to be continued. Moreover, as many chelating agents have short plasma half-lives, blood or plasma metal ion assays can be used quite quickly after a course of chelation therapy to assess efficacy and the need for further treatment. Note that administration of oral Prussian Blue (section 2.4.1) does not invalidate whole-blood or urinary thallium assays as the antidote is not absorbed to any notable extent.

9.6 CHOLINESTERASE INHIBITORS AND CHOLINESTERASE REACTIVATORS

Prior administration of cholinesterase inhibitors such as pyridostigmine may compromise subsequent plasma or red cell cholinesterase assay if this is required to help assess the severity of poisoning with an OP compound.

Administration of cholinesterase reactivators such as pralidoxime will often reverse inhibition of plasma cholinesterase and red cell (acetyl)cholinesterase, and this effect will, of course, be reflected in any measurements of these parameters performed once the antidote has been given. However, the results may not reflect inhibition of cholinesterase in central compartments and thus must be interpreted in the light of the clinical condition of the patient.

9.7 CYANIDE ANTIDOTES

Most methods used to measure blood cyanide rely on liberation of hydrogen cyanide from an acidified sample. Use of amyl nitrite and sodium nitrite aims to generate methaemoglobin and thus to increase chelation of cyanide ion in erythrocytes. Administration of dicobalt edetate or hydroxocobalamin also aims to chelate cyanide ion in blood. Thus, both procedures aim to enhance blood total cyanide, making conventional cyanide assay procedures difficult to interpret as regards the severity of exposure and the progress of treatment. A further complication in cyanide measurement is that cyanide is unstable in blood and thus special precautions are needed in the storage and transport of samples if even pretreatment samples are not to be analysed immediately (Flanagan, 1995).

Note also that commonly used methods for measuring methaemoglobin measure

CHAPTER 9

cyanmethaemoglobin as haemoglobin. This will give a falsely optimistic impression of the fraction of haemoglobin that is available to carry oxygen (section 6.2.3).

9.8 FLUMAZENIL

It is possible that commercially available immunoassays designed to detect benzodiazepines and their metabolites in plasma and urine will also detect flumazenil. However, Doem and Unger (1988) and Martens *et al.* (1990) did not observe any such interference after patients had been given up to 5 mg flumazenil. Flumazenil does not appear to have been tested for cross-reactivity in the following currently available benzodiazepine immunoassays: Emit II Plus (Dade Behring), CEDIA (Microgenics) and DRI (Microgenics). Note that interference tests in commercial benzodiazepine and other drugs of abuse immunoassays are usually performed using pure compounds and so the possibility that metabolites will show greater cross-reactivity than parent compounds must always be borne in mind, even if the parent compound shows little or no cross-reactivity.

9.9 OPIOID ANTAGONISTS

As with benzodiazepine immunoassays, there is the possibility that commercially available urine opiate immunoassays will also detect opioid antagonists. Again, interference tests in commercial opiate drugs of abuse immunoassays are usually performed using pure compounds and so the possibility that metabolites will show greater cross-reactivity than parent compounds must always be borne in mind. Table 9.2 gives opioid antagonist cross-reactivity data in some opiate immunoassays that are currently available.

TABLE 9.2

Cross-reactivity data in some opiate immunoassays

	Emit II Plus (Dade Behring)[a]	CEDIA (Microgenics)[b]	DRI (Microgenics)
Diprenorphine	No information	No information	No information
Nalorphine	90 mg/L (positive reaction above)	Positive reaction at 500 mg/L	No information
Nalmefene	20 mg/L	No information	No information
Naloxone	150 mg/L	Positive reaction at 500 mg/L	No reaction at 100 mg/L
Naltrexone	1,000 mg/L	Positive reaction at 500 mg/L	No reaction at 1 g/L

Notes
a   No cross-reactivity up to the concentration cited; not tested above this limit except where stated.
b   Concentrations in samples likely to be much lower than 500 mg/L.

9.10 OXYGEN

Carboxyhaemoglobin (COHb) begins to dissociate once the patient begins to breathe uncontaminated air. Administration of 100 % oxygen at atmospheric pressure accelerates this process; hyperbaric oxygen acts even more quickly. It is thus important that a blood sample for COHb measurement is obtained as soon as possible after CO exposure if the measurement is to be of any value in helping assess the severity of poisoning. A further complication in COHb measurement is that carbon monoxide is unstable in blood, and thus special precautions are needed in sample storage and transport if the analysis is not to be performed immediately (Flanagan, 1995).

9.11 SODIUM BICARBONATE

Administration of an adequate dose of sodium bicarbonate will promote diffusion of strongly acidic drugs such as salicylates and chlorophenoxy herbicides from tissues into plasma if poisoning is serious, and especially if an acidosis was present before bicarbonate administration (Flanagan et al., 1990; Wax and Hoffman, 1991). Plasma drug/poison concentrations in samples drawn after bicarbonate administration may thus bear little relation to the clinical condition of the patient.

REFERENCES

Antman EM, Wenger TL, Butler VP, Haber E, Smith TW. Treatment of 150 cases of life-threatening digitalis intoxication with digoxin-specific Fab antibody fragments: final report of a multicenter study. *Circulation* 1990; 81: 1744–52.

Bishell GP, Lewis H, Rooke RA, Davies HR. Interference by Parvolex with chloride estimation by the Ag/AgCl method. *Ann Clin Biochem* 1994; 31: 181–3.

Curry SC, Connor DA, Raschke RA. Effect of the cyanide antidote hydroxocobalamin on commonly ordered serum chemistry studies. *Ann Emerg Med* 1994; 24: 65–7.

Doem A, Unger P-F. Possible interference of flumazenil on benzodiazepine measurement in blood and urine [letter]. *Am J Emerg Med* 1988; 6: 683.

Ferner RE, Hutchings A, Anton C, Almond S, Jones A, Routledge PA. The origin of errors in dosage: acetylcysteine as a paradigm [abstract]. *Br J Clin Pharmacol* 1999; 47: 581P.

Flanagan RJ. The poisoned patient: the role of the laboratory. *Br J Biomed Sci* 1995; 52: 202–13.

Flanagan RJ, Meredith TJ, Ruprah M, Onyon LJ, Liddle A. Alkaline diuresis for acute poisoning with chlorophenoxy herbicides and ioxynil. *Lancet* 1990; 335: 454–8.

Gibb I, Adams PC. Digoxin assay modifications to eliminate interference following immunotherapy for toxicity [abstract]. *Ann Biol Clin* 1985; 43: 696.

Gourlain H, Caliez C, Laforge M, Buneaux F, Levillain P. Study of the mechanisms involved in hydroxocobalamin interference with determination of some biochemical parameters. *Ann Biol Clin* 1994; 52: 121–4.

Hursting MJ, Raisys VA, Opheim KE, Bell JL, Trobaugh GB, Smith TW. Determination of free digoxin concentrations in serum for monitoring Fab treatment of digoxin overdose. *Clin Chem* 1987; 33: 1652–5.

Martens F, Koppel C, Ibe K, Wagemann A, Tenczer J. Clinical experience with the benzodiazepine antagonist flumazenil in suspected benzodiazepine or ethanol poisoning. *J Toxicol Clin Toxicol* 1990; 28: 341–56.

Mayer M, Salpeter L. More on interference of N-acetylcysteine in measurement of acetaminophen [letter]. *Clin Chem* 1998; 44: 892–3.

Tarpey A, Leonard MB. N-Acetylcysteine interference in commonly used enzymic paracetamol methods [abstract]. *Proc ACB National Meeting* 1997: 67–8

Tyhach RJ. More on interference of N-acetylcysteine in measurement of acetaminophen [letter]. *Clin Chem* 1999; 45: 584–5.

Wax PM, Hoffman RS. Sodium bicarbonate. In: *Contemporary Management in Critical Care*. Volume 1 (Part 3): *Critical Care Toxicology*. Hoffman RS, Goldfrank LR (eds). New York: Churchill Livingstone, 1991: 81–108.

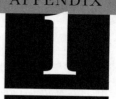
Which Antidote for Which Poison?

See Appendix 2 and individual sections for details of dose and administration.

Poison	Antidote (suggested route of administration)
β-Agonists (e.g. salbutamol)	β-Blockers (i.v.) – avoid in asthmatic patients
Aluminium	Deferoxamine (i.v.)
Amanita phalloides and some other *Amanita* species	Benzylpenicillin (i.v.)
Antiarrhythmic agents	Sodium bicarbonate (i.v.)
Arsenic	Dimercaprol (i.m.), D-penicillamine (oral), DMSA (oral)
Barium	Magnesium sulphate (oral)
Benzodiazepines	Flumazenil (i.v.) – seldom used in practice
β-Blockers (e.g. propranolol)	Glucagon (i.v.), adrenaline (i.v.), isoprenaline (i.v.)
Calcium channel blockers	Calcium chloride or calcium gluconate (i.v.); [glucagon (i.v.)]
Carbamate insecticides	Atropine (i.v.)
Carbon monoxide	Oxygen (high-flow, tight-fitting face-mask); [hyperbaric oxygen]
Carbon tetrachloride	N-Acetylcysteine (i.v.)
Chloroquine	Diazepam (i.v.); adrenaline (i.v.)
Colchicine	Colchicine-specific F_{ab} antibody fragments (i.v.)
Copper salts	D-Penicillamine (oral)
Cyanide	Hydroxocobalamin (i.v.), sodium thiosulphate (i.v.), dicobalt edetate (i.v.); oxygen (high-flow, tight-fitting face mask); amyl nitrite (inhaled as a first aid measure)
Digoxin (and some other cardiac glycosides)	Digoxin-specific F_{ab} antibody fragments (i.v.)
Ethylene glycol	Ethanol (oral or i.v.); fomepizole (i.v.)
Gold	Dimercaprol (i.m.)
Gyrometria mushroom	Pyridoxine (vitamin B_6) (oral or i.m.)
Heparin	Protamine sulphate (i.v.)
Hydrofluoric acid burns	Calcium gluconate gel (topical or s.c.)
Insulin, oral hypoglycaemics	D-Glucose (i.v.); glucagon (i.v.)
Iron salts (e.g. ferrous sulphate)	Deferoxamine (i.v., rarely i.m.)
Isoniazid	Pyridoxine (vitamin B_6) (oral or i.m.)
Lead	Calcium disodium edetate (i.v.); DMSA (oral); DMPS (i.v.); D-penicillamine (oral – rarely used)
Mercury	Dimercaprol (i.m.); D-penicillamine (oral); DMSA (oral); DMPS (i.v.)
Methaemoglobin-forming agents (chlorates, nitrites, etc.)	Methylthioninium chloride (methylene blue) (i.v.)
Methanol	Ethanol (oral or i.v.); fomepizole (i.v.)
Methotrexate	Folinic acid (i.v.)
Opioids (e.g. methadone, morphine)	Naloxone (i.v. or i.m); diprenorphine (i.v., veterinary practice)
Organophosphorus compounds	Atropine (i.v.); pralidoxome (i.v.)
Paracetamol	N-Acetylcysteine (oral or i.v.); D,L-methionine (oral)
Thallium	Prussian Blue (Berlin Blue) (oral)
Theophylline	β-Blockers (i.v.)
Thyroxine	β-Blockers (oral)
Warfarin and superwarfarins	Phytomenadione (i.v.); fresh-frozen plasma (i.v.)

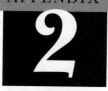

Dosage and Dosage Form of Some Commonly Used Antidotes

The following information is adapted, with permission, from *Poisons Quarterly* 2000; 1(4) (Suppl). For further details of doses of antidotes used in the UK consult TOXBASE (http://www.spib.axl.co.uk/), the UK National Poisons Information Service (0870 600 6266), or the British National Formulary (41st edn, London: British Medical Association and Royal Pharmaceutical Society of Great Britain, March 2001).

A cyanide antidote kit containing amyl nitrite ampoules and dicobalt edetate for injection is available from Cuxson Gerrard (Warley, West Midlands, UK).

N-ACETYLCYSTEINE

Presentation/supply	Injection: 2 g in 10-mL ampoule (200 mg/mL) (Parvolex, Evans)
Principal indication	Paracetamol poisoning (section 4.16.1)
Dose (adult and child)	Initial infusion of 150 mg/kg in 0.2 L 5 % (w/v) D-glucose i.v. over 15 min, then 50 mg/kg in 0.5 L 5 % (w/v) D-glucose over 4 h, then 100 mg/kg in 1 L 5 % (w/v) D-glucose over 16 h
Comments	*N*-Acetylcysteine is stable in 0.9 % (w/v) sodium chloride for 24 h. NAC is most effective if given up to 10 h post ingestion, but may be used up to 36 h or more post ingestion. The volume of infusion fluid used in children should take into account age and weight.

ACTIVATED CHARCOAL

Presentation/supply	Powder: 25-g and 50-g bottles (Carbomix, Penn); granules: 5-g sachets (Medicoal, Torbet); suspension: 50 g (Actidose-Aqua, Cambridge), 25 g and 50 g (Liqui-Char, Oxford)
Indication	Potentially serious ingestion of many poisons (section 1.4.4.1)
Dose	Ten times amount of drug ingested if known, otherwise
Adult	50–100 g immediately and for certain drugs continue with 50 g 4-hourly until charcoal is seen in stools and/or clinical improvement is observed
Child	1 g/kg immediately and for certain drugs continue 4-hourly until charcoal appears in stools or clinical improvement is observed. Charcoal can be given via a nasogastric tube if the child is unable to swallow the material
Comments	Concurrent administration of a laxative such as sorbitol or lactulose may be useful, especially if doses of charcoal are repeated

AMYL NITRITE

Presentation/supply	Vittrella: 0.3 mL (Norton)
Indication	Cyanide poisoning (section 6.2.3.1)
Dose (adult)	0.2–0.4 mL via Ambu bag *or* one vittrella on a cloth inhaled for 30 s every min, new vittrella every 3 min (maximum six vittrellae)

ANTIDIGOXIN ANTIBODY FRAGMENTS

Presentation/supply   Injection: 38 mg fragments/vial (Digibind, GlaxoWellcome)
Principal indication   Digoxin poisoning (section 3.2.1)
Dose (adult and child)   Related to plasma digoxin concentration before antidote administration or amount ingested – see package insert or Figure 3.2

ATROPINE (SULPHATE)

Presentation/supply   Injection: 600 µg in 1-mL ampoule (600 µg/mL); 2 mg in 1-mL ampoule (2 mg/mL) (both Martindale Pharmaceuticals)
Indication (1)   OP or carbamate insecticide poisoning (section 5.3) and OP nerve agent poisoning (section 7.3.1)
Dose
  Adult   1–2 mg i.v. every 10 min until atropinization achieved (dry mouth, pulse > 100 beats/min)
  Child   0.05 mg/kg i.v. every 10 min until atropinization achieved
Comment   Large quantities may be needed over several days
Indication (2)   Pretreatment before gastric decontamination in β-blocker overdose
Dose
  Adult   600 µg s.c. or i.v. (section 5.3)
  Child   30 µg/kg s.c. or i.v. (maximum 600 µg)

BENZATROPINE (MESILATE)

Presentation/supply   Injection: 2 mg in 2-mL ampoule (1 mg/mL) (Cogentin, MSD)
Indication   Dystonic reaction caused by antipsychotic drugs or metoclopramide (section 5.4)
Dose
  Adult   1–2 mg i.m. or i.v., repeated if necessary
  Child   *Not recommended for use in children under 3 years of age, but the following doses have been used in all age groups*: 20 µg/kg i.m. or i.v over 1–2 min, repeated after 15 min if necessary

CALCIUM DISODIUM EDETATE

Presentation/supply   Injection: 1 g in 5-mL ampoule (200 mg/mL) (Ledclair, Sinclair)
Indication   Poisoning with metals, especially lead (section 2.2.2)
Dose (adult and child)   30–40 mg/kg i.v. infusion in 5 % (w/v) D-glucose or 0.9 % (w/v) sodium chloride twice daily for up to 5 days, repeated if necessary after 48 h for a maximum of further 5 days

CALCIUM GLUCONATE

Presentation/supply   Gel: 2.5 % (w/v) in 25-g tube; injection: 10 % (w/v) solution in 10-mL (100 mg/mL) ampoules (both H-F Antidote, Industrial Pharmaceutical Services)

Indication (1)	Hydrofluoric acid skin burns (section 4.3)
Dose (adult and child)	Rub gel into affected area for at least 30 min. If pain persists, inject 10 % solution under site of injury – multiple small volume (0.5 mL) injections are best; aim for intradermal site
Indication (2)	Poisoning with calcium channel blockers (section 4.3)
Dose (adult and child)	10 % solution i.v. 0.2–0.5 mL/kg up to 10 mL over 5–10 min, repeated in 10–15 min if necessary

DANTROLENE (SODIUM)

Presentation/supply	Injection: 20-mg vials (Dantrium Intravenous, Procter and Gamble)
Indications	Severe hyperthermia caused by MAOIs, MDMA, cocaine, amphetamine; neuroleptic malignant syndrome; malignant hyperthermia (section 5.10)
Dose (adult and child)	1 mg/kg by rapid i.v. injection, repeated as required (cumulative maximum 10 mg/kg)

DEFEROXAMINE (MESILATE)

Presentation/supply	Injection: 500-mg and 2-g vials (Desferal, Ciba)
Principal indication	Iron poisoning (section 2.3)
Dose (adult and child)	Up to 15 mg/kg each hour i.v. by slow infusion in 5 % (w/v) D-glucose or 0.9 % (w/v) sodium chloride (normal maximum 80 mg/kg in 24 h)
Comment	Larger doses have been used in serious cases

DICOBALT EDETATE

Presentation/supply	Injection: 300 mg in 20-mL ampoule (15 mg/mL) (Cambridge Laboratories)
Indication	Cyanide poisoning (section 6.2.4.1)
Dose (adult)	300 mg i.v. over 1 min followed by a further 300-mg i.v. if response does not occur within 1 min
Comment	To reduce the toxicity of dicobalt edetate follow the injection immediately with 50 mL i.v. infusion of 50 % (w/v) D-glucose

DIMERCAPROL

Presentation/supply	Injection: 100 mg in 2-mL ampoule (50 mg/mL) in arachis oil (Boots)
Indications	Poisoning with mercury, lead, arsenic (section 2.2.4)
Dose (adult and child)	2.5–3 mg/kg i.m. 4-hourly for 2 days, 2–4 times on day 3, then once or twice daily for 10 days or until recovery

ETHANOL

Presentation/supply   Injection: 5-mL ampoule dehydrated alcohol BP, approximately 4 g ethanol (Macarthy Medical)

Principal indications   Poisoning with ethylene glycol or methanol (section 4.2.1)

Dose (adult and child) 1 g/kg (oral or i.v.), followed by i.v. infusion in 5 % (w/v) D-glucose or 0.9 % (w/v) sodium chloride to achieve ethanol plasma concentration of 1–1.5 g/L (see Table 4.1)

Comment   Ethanol can be added to peritoneal dialysis fluid at a concentration of 1–2 g/L of dialysate

EUROPEAN VIPER VENOM ANTIVENIN (ZAGREB)

Presentation/supply   Injection: one dose (10-mL) ampoule (Farillon; should be available in all UK health regions and is held by UK NPIS)

Indication   Adder *(Vipera berus)* bite (section 3.1.3.5)

Dose (adult and child) One ampoule diluted in 2–3 volumes of 0.9 % (w/v) sodium chloride by slow i.v. injection (over 10–15 min) or i.v. infusion. May be repeated after 1–2 h if no clinical improvement

FOMEPIZOLE

Presentation/supply   Injection: 1.5 mg in 1.5-mL vial (1 g/mL) (Antizol, Cambridge Laboratories)

Principal indications   Poisoning with ethylene glycol or methanol (section 4.2.2)

Dose

  Adult   Loading dose: 15 mg/kg, then 10 mg/kg 12-hourly (four doses), then 15 mg/kg 12-hourly until plasma ethylene glycol or methanol concentration below 0.2 g/L (all doses given by slow i.v. infusion over 30 min)

  Child   Not established but commonly assumed to be same as adult dose; discuss with Poisons Information Service

FOLINATE (CALCIUM) (LEUCOVORIN)

Presentation/supply   Injection: 3 mg in 1-mL and 30 mg in 10-mL ampoules (3 mg/mL calcium folinate); tablets: 15 mg calcium folinate

Indication (1)   Methotrexate rescue (section 4.7)

Dose (adult and child) Oral or i.v. 6-hourly until blood methotrexate concentration below 23 μg/L (50 nmol/L):

  (a) Calcium folinate dose equal to the methotrexate dose if known, or

  (b) 100 mg/m^2 body surface area if methotrexate dose not known

Indication (2)   Poisoning with methanol or formic acid (section 4.7)

Dose (adult and child) 1 mg/kg i.v. or orally, 6-hourly

FLUMAZENIL

Presentation/supply	Injection: 500 µg in 5-mL ampoule (100 µg/mL) (Anexate, Roche)
Indication	Reversal of benzodiazepine sedation in anaesthetic, intensive care and diagnostic procedures – *not licensed or recommended for use in benzodiazepine self-poisoning* (section 5.13)
Dose (suggested for benzodiazepine overdose)	
Adult	Initially 200 µg i.v. over 30 s. If minimal response within 60 s, further 300 µg over 30 s. Further doses of 500 µg over 30 s, at 1-min intervals to total dose of 3 mg. If still no response flumazenil is unlikely to reverse CNS/respiratory depression
Child	Not recommended, but if aged over 4 years 10 µg/kg i.v. for not more than two doses

GLUCAGON

Presentation/supply	Injection: 1-mg vial (10-mg vials discontinued)
Indication	Poisoning with β-adrenoreceptor blocking drugs (section 5.15)
Dose	
Adult	10-mg i.v. bolus repeated as required, or 1–10 mg/h i.v. infusion in either 5 % (w/v) D-glucose or 0.9 % (w/v) sodium chloride, depending on response
Child	*Not recommended in children, but the following dose has been used:* Up to 50 µg/kg hourly i.v. or initial bolus of 50–150 µg/kg over 1 min
Comment	Do not use diluents containing phenol

ISOPRENALINE (HYDROCHLORIDE)

Presentation/supply	Injection: 2 mg in 2-mL ampoule (1 mg/mL) (Saventrine IV, Pharmax)
Indication	Hypotension or low cardiac output due to cardiotoxic drugs such as β-adrenoreceptor blocking drugs and calcium channel blockers if no response to calcium gluconate (section 5.17)
Dose	
Adult	5–50 µg/min i.v. infusion in either 5 % (w/v) D-glucose or 0.9 % (w/v) sodium chloride
Child	0.02 µg/kg each min by i.v. infusion (maximum 0.5 µg/kg each min)
Comment	Huge doses may be needed in adults as response is variable – 10 times the therapeutic dose has been used

KLEAN-PREP®

Presentation/supply	Powder: four sachets to be dissolved in 4 L purified water (Norgine)

Indication	Gut decontamination for substances not bound by activated charcoal such as iron and (especially) slow-release preparations such as those containing lithium salts
Dose	
Adult	2 L/h by mouth until rectal effluent resembles irrigating fluid (usually 2–6 h)
Child > 10 kg	0.5 L/h, given as above
Comment	Discuss use beyond 12–16 h with Poisons Information Service

METHIONINE

Presentation/supply	Tablets: 250 mg (Evans)
Indication	Paracetamol poisoning (section 4.16.1)
Dose	
Adult and child > 6 years	2.5 g initially followed by three doses (2.5 g) 4-hourly
Child < 6 years	1 g initially followed by three doses (1 g) 4-hourly
Comment	Most effective up to 8 h post ingestion; thereafter use NAC

METHYLTHIONINIUM CHLORIDE (METHYLENE BLUE)

Presentation/supply	Injection: 50 mg in 5-mL ampoule (10 mg/mL, 1 % w/v) (David Bull Laboratories)
Indication	Methaemoglobinaemia (section 4.13.2)
Dose (adult and child)	1–2 mg/kg i.v. over 5 min

NALOXONE (HYDROCHLORIDE)

Presentation/supply	Injection: 40 µg in 2-mL ampoule (20 µg/mL) and 400 µg in 1-mL ampoule (400 µg/mL) (Narcan, Du Pont)
Indication	Poisoning with opioids (section 5.19.2)
Dose	
Adult	Initial bolus 400 µg i.v. repeated every 2–3 min to maximum bolus dose of 2 mg (total maximum dose 10 mg). Repeat as required to maintain response
Child	10 µg/kg i.v. repeated every 2–3 min. Up to 100 µg/kg has been used. Repeat as necessary.
Comment	May also be given as an infusion in either 5 % (w/v) D-glucose or 0.9 % (w/v) sodium chloride
Warning	**The plasma half-life of many opioids is long and that of naloxone short, and thus a continuous infusion is often required after an initial bolus dose has been given**

PENICILLAMINE

Presentation/supply	Tablets: 50, 125, 200 mg
Indication	Poisoning with lead, copper, arsenic (section 2.2.6)

Dose
  Adult   1–2 g/d in divided doses
  Child   20 mg/kg daily in divided doses (100 mg/kg daily has been used for arsenic poisoning; maximum dose 1 g daily, 5 days)

PHENTOLAMINE (MESILATE)

Presentation/supply   Injection: 10 mg in 1-mL ampoule (10 mg/mL) (Rogitine, Novartis)

Indication   Severe hypertension caused by amphetamines, MAOIs, clonidine (section 5.1)

Dose
  Adult   Infusion of 0.2–2 mg/min i.v. in either 5 % (w/v) D-glucose or 0.9 % (w/v) sodium chloride – in some cases 5 mg/min may be given initially
  Child   Infusion of 20–100 µg/kg loading dose, then 250–1,000 µg/kg daily (approximately 10–40 µg/kg hourly)

PHYTOMENADIONE (VITAMIN K$_1$)

Presentation/supply   Injection: 2 mg in 0.2-mL ampoule and 10 mg in 1-mL ampoule (both 10 mg/mL) (Konakion MM Paediatric and Konakion MM, Roche)

Indication   Poisoning with coumarin anticoagulants (section 4.10)
Dose (adult and child)   Dependent on severity of poisoning and INR

PRALIDOXIME (MESILATE)

Presentation/supply   Injection: 1 g in 5-mL ampoule (200 mg/mL, 20 % w/v) (manufactured for the UK Department of Health and available in the UK through the NPIS and regional centres)

Indication   OP insecticide and OP nerve agent poisoning (sections 5.9 and 7.3.2)

Dose (adult and child)   30 mg/kg i.v. over 5–10 min, repeated 4- to 6-hourly if necessary.
Comment   May be given as i.v. infusion in either 5 % (w/v) D-glucose or 0.9 % (w/v) sodium chloride at 8 mg/kg hourly after two bolus injections of 30 mg/kg have been given 4 h apart

PROCYCLIDINE (HYDROCHLORIDE)

Presentation/supply   Injection: 10 mg in 2-mL ampoule (5 mg/mL) (Kemadrin, GlaxoWellcome)

Indications   Dystonic reactions caused by antipsychotics and metoclopramide (section 5.21)

Dose
  Adult   5–10 mg i.m. repeated if necessary after 20 min; maximum 20 mg/d, *or* 5 mg i.v. (usually effective within 5 min, but 10 mg or more may be needed, and 30 min may be required for effect)

Child	*Not recommend in children but the following dose has been used:*
	Single dose i.v. (over at least 2 min) or i.m.
	  < 2 years: 0.5–2 mg
	  2–10 years: 2–5 mg
	  > 10 years: 5–10 mg
	Repeat if necessary after 20 min

PRUSSIAN BLUE (BERLIN BLUE SOLUBLE, POTASSIUM FERRIC HEXACYANOFERRATE)

Presentation/supply	Powder: 25-g bottle (Sigma Aldrich, Poole – available through UK NPIS)
Indication	Thallium poisoning (section 2.4.1)
Dose (adult and child)	250 mg/kg daily by mouth in divided doses (fine-bore nasogastric tube)

PYRIDOXINE (HYDROCHLORIDE)

Presentation/supply	Injection: 1 g in 10-mL ampoule (100 mg/mL, 10 % w/v) (Martindale Pharmaceuticals)
Indication	Poisoning with isoniazid, *Gyrometria* species (section 4.12)
Dose	
Adult	1 g for each gram of isoniazid ingested (maximum 10 g – give up to 5 g if history uncertain) by slow i.v. infusion in 5 % (w/v) D-glucose at approximately 500 mg/min. Larger doses have been used but there is a risk of neuropathy
Child	70 mg/kg by slow i.v. infusion to a maximum of 5 g as above
Comment	Pyridoxine not compatible with alkaline solutions; no information on compatibility with 0.9 % (w/v) sodium chloride

SNAKE VENOM ANTIVENIN (SNAKES NOT INDIGENOUS IN UK)

Presentation/supply	Numerous antivenins to non-indigenous snakes held by UK NPIS and by the Pharmacy, Fazakerley Hospital, Liverpool (telephone in UK: 0151 529 5980)
Indication	Bites from snakes not indigenous to the UK (section 3.1)
Dose (adult and child)	As per package insert or TOXBASE (http://www.spib.axl.co.uk/)

SODIUM BICARBONATE

Presentation/supply	Infusion: variety of sterile solutions available
Indication (1)	Poisoning with salicylates, chlorophenoxy herbicides (section 4.15)

Dose
  Adult   1 L 1.26 % (w/v) (iso-osmotic with serum) + 40 mmol potassium ion i.v. over 4 h *and/or* 50-mL boluses of 8.4 % (w/v) solution i.v. (if i.v. administration impossible 3 g orally 4-hourly)

  Child   1 mL/kg 8.4 % (w/v) (= 1 mmol/kg) + 20 mmol potassium ion in 0.5 L 5 % (w/v) D-glucose [or 0.9 % (w/v) sodium chloride] infused i.v. at 2–3 mL/kg hourly

Indication (2)   Poisoning with tricyclic antidepressants, class 1a and 1c antiarrhythmics (section 4.15)

Dose (adult and child) 1–2 mmol/kg [1–2 mL/kg 8.4 % (w/v)] i.v. over 15 min

SODIUM 2,3-DIMERCAPTOPROPANESULPHONATE (DMPS)

Presentation/supply   Capsules: 100 mg; injection: 250 mg in 5-mL ampoule (50 mg/mL) (Dimaval, Heyl, Berlin – available through UK NPIS)

Indication   Poisoning with metals especially mercury, arsenic, bismuth, copper (section 2.2.7)

Dose (adult)   Chronic poisoning: 100 mg orally three times daily
Acute poisoning: 250 mg i.v. every 3–4 h initially, reducing thereafter

SODIUM NITRITE

Presentation/supply   Injection: 300 mg in 10-mL ampoule (30 mg/mL, 3 % w/v) (available as special order from Martindale, Penn or hospital manufacturing unit)

Indication   Cyanide poisoning (section 6.2.3.1)

Dose
  Adult   10 mL of 3 % (w/v) solution (i.e. 300 mg) i.v. over 5–20 min followed by sodium thiosulphate

  Child   0.33 mL/kg of 3 % (w/v) solution (approximately 10 mg/kg) given as for adults

SODIUM NITROPRUSSIDE

Presentation/supply   Injection: 50 mg in 5-mL ampoule (10 mg/mL)

Indication   Severe hypertension due to ergotamine, amphetamine, MAOIs (section 5.24)

Dose (adult and child) Initially 0.3 µg/kg each min by i.v. infusion in either 5 % (w/v) D-glucose or 0.9 % (w/v) sodium chloride, increased until desired response (usual dose 0.5–0.6 µg/kg each min)

Comment   In ergotamine poisoning may be needed for 12–36 h or more

SODIUM THIOSULPHATE

Presentation/supply	Injection: 10 g in 20-mL ampoule (500 mg/mL, 50 % w/v) (available as special order from Martindale, Penn or hospital manufacturing unit)
Indication	Cyanide poisoning (section 6.2.5)
Dose	
Adult	25 mL of 50 % (w/v) solution (i.e. 12.5 g) i.v. over 10 min
Child	0.825 mL/kg of 50 % (w/v) solution (i.e. 412.5 mg/kg) (maximum 25 mL over 10 min)

SUCCIMER (*MESO*-2,3-DIMERCAPTOSUCCINIC ACID, DMSA)

Presentation/supply	Capsules: 100 mg (Chemet, McNeil); 300 mg (Guy's Hospital Pharmacy), both available through UK NPIS
Indication	Lead poisoning (section 2.2.5)
Dose (adult and child)	30 mg/kg daily, 5 days then 20 mg/kg daily, 14 days

Decision Trees to Aid Treatment of Paracetamol Poisoning

The decision trees that follow are based, with permission, on those of Dargan *et al.* (2001) and assume the availability of *N*-acetylcysteine for i.v. use. Although aimed primarily at the treatment of adults, the trees are valid for use in pregnant women and children. It should be emphasized that when patients are discharged they should receive written instructions to return if they develop vomiting or abdominal pain. Particular caution is advised in dealing with children who may have ingested multiple doses of paracetamol, and thus in whom an accurate assessment of the dose has not been possible.

(a) Management of a patient after a single acute ingestion of paracetamol.
(b) Management of a patient after ingestion of more than one potentially toxic dose of paracetamol in the preceding 4–48 h.

REFERENCE

Dargan PI, Wallace CI, Jones AL. Acetaminophen (paracetamol) overdose: an evidence based flowchart to guide management. *Emerg Med J* 2001 (in press).

Appendix 3a. Decision tree: single dose

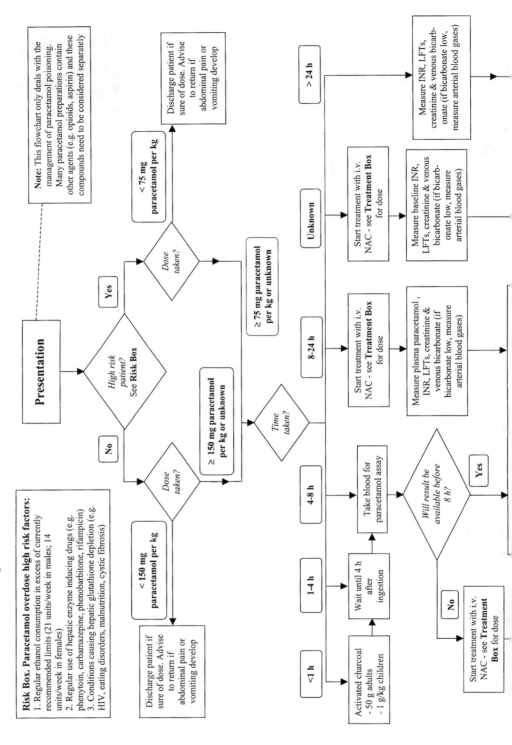

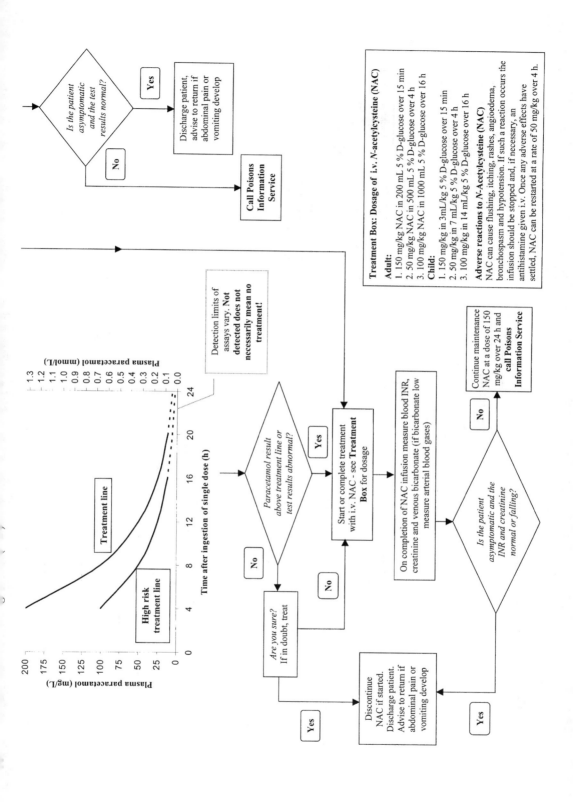

Appendix 3b. Decision tree: multiple doses in last 4-48 h

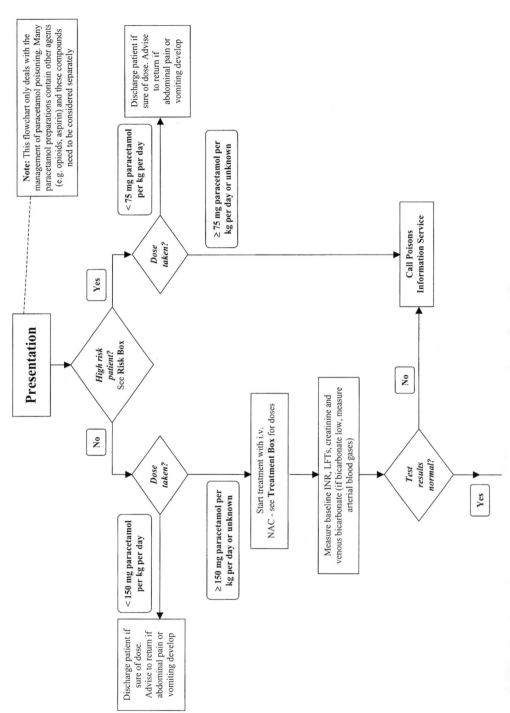

Risk Box. Paracetamol overdose high risk factors:
1. Regular ethanol consumption in excess of currently recommended limits (21 units/week in males; 14 units/week in females)
2. Regular use of hepatic enzyme inducing drugs (e.g. phenytoin, carbamazepine, phenobarbitone, rifampicin)
3. Conditions causing hepatic GSH depletion (e.g. HIV, eating disorders, malnutrition, cystic fibrosis)

Treatment Box: Dosage of i.v. *N*-Acetylcysteine (NAC)

Adult:
1. 150 mg/kg NAC in 200 mL 5 % D-glucose over 15 min
2. 50 mg/kg NAC in 500 mL 5 % D-glucose over 4 h
3. 100 mg/kg NAC in 1000 mL 5 % D-glucose over 16 h

Child:
1. 150 mg/kg in 3mL/kg 5 % D-glucose over 15 min
2. 50 mg/kg in 7 mL/kg 5 % D-glucose over 4 h
3. 100 mg/kg in 14 mL/kg 5 % D-glucose over 16 h

Adverse Reactions to *N*-Acetylcysteine (NAC)
NAC can cause flushing, itching, rashes, angioedema, bronchospasm and hypotension. If such a reaction occurs the infusion should be stopped and, if necessary, an antihistamine given i.v. Once any adverse effects have settled, NAC can be restarted at a rate of 50 mg/kg over 4 h.

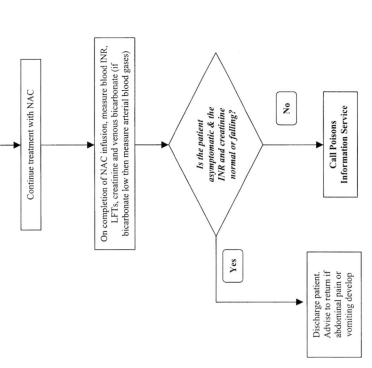

Continue treatment with NAC

On completion of NAC infusion, measure blood INR, LFTs, creatinine and venous bicarbonate (if bicarbonate low then measure arterial blood gases)

Is the patient asymptomatic & the INR and creatinine normal or falling?

Yes

No

Discharge patient. Advise to return if abdominal pain or vomiting develop

Call Poisons Information Service

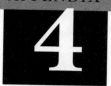
Guide to the Interpretation of Analytical Toxicology Results and Mass/Amount Concentration Conversion Factors for Some Metals and Trace Elements

Appendix 4. Interpretation of analytical results: metals/trace elements

Analyte	'Therapeutic' or 'normal' plasma concentration (less than)	Plasma concentration associated with serious toxicity	Relative atomic formula or mass	Mass/amount conversion	Amount/mass conversion
Aluminium[a]	15 µg/L	60 µg/L	27.0	µg/L × 0.037 = µmol/L	µmol/L × 27.0 = µg/L
(urine)	200 µg/L[b]				
Antimony (whole blood)	10 µg/L	200 µg/L	121.8	µg/L × 8.20 = nmol/L	nmol/L × 0.122 = µg/L
(urine)	1.2 µg/L	20 µg/L			
Arsenic (total)[a,c]	10 µg/L	50 µg/L	74.9	µg/L × 13.35 = nmol/L	nmol/L × 0.075 = µg/L
(total, whole blood)	10 µg/L	50 µg/L			
(total, urine)	10 µg/L	200 µg/L			
Barium	1 µg/L	[Not known]	137.3	µg/L × 7.28 = nmol/L	nmol/L × 0.137 = µg/L
(urine)	5 µg/L				
Beryllium	0.3 µg/L	[Not known]	9.01	µg/L × 110.9 = nmol/L	nmol/L × 0.009 = µg/L
(urine)	1 µg/L				
Bismuth (whole blood)[a]	10 µg/L (dietary)	100 µg/L	209.0	µg/L × 4.78 = nmol/L	nmol/L × 0.209 = µg/L
Cadmium (whole blood)[a]	5 µg/L	20 µg/L	112.4	µg/L × 8.90 = nmol/L	nmol/L × 0.112 = µg/L
(urine)	5 µg/L	20 µg/L			
Chromium	0.35 µg/L	[Not known][d]	52.0	µg/L × 19.2 = nmol/L	nmol/L × 0.052 = µg/L
(urine)	0.25 µg/L				
Cobalt	0.4 µg/L	[Not known]	58.9	µg/L × 17.0 = nmol/L	nmol/L × 0.060 = µg/L
(urine)	1 µg/L				
Copper (total)[e]	0.6–1.6 mg/L	5 mg/L (not Wilson's disease)	63.6	mg/L × 15.7 = µmol/L	µmol/L × 0.064 = mg/L
(urine)	60 mg/L	100 mg/L (Wilson's disease)			
Gold	0.0001 mg/L (dietary)	10 mg/L	197.0	mg/L × 5.08 = µmol/L	µmol/L × 0.197 = mg/L
(total, serum)	3 mg/L (therapy)				
(total, urine)	2 mg/L (therapy)				
Iron (serum)[a,c]	0.5–1.8 mg/L	5 mg/L (children)	55.8	mg/L × 17.92 = µmol/L	µmol/L × 0.056 = mg/L
		8 mg/L (adults)			
Lead (whole blood)	100 µg/L	600 µg/L	207.2	µg/L × 0.00483 = µmol/L	µmol/L × 207.2 = µg/L
Magnesium[f]	10–32 mg/L	95 mg/L	24.3	mg/L × 0.041 = mmol/L	mmol/L × 24.3 = mg/L

Analyte	Reference range	Action level		μg/L → nmol/L	nmol/L → μg/L
Manganese (whole blood)	0.5–1.5 μg/L	[Not known]	54.9	μg/L × 18.2 = nmol/L	nmol/L × 0.055 = μg/L
	4–12 μg/L				
Mercury (whole blood)[a]	10 μg/L	50 μg/L	200.6	μg/L × 4.99 = nmol/L	nmol/L × 0.201 = μg/L
(urine)	10 μg/L	100 μg/L			
Molybdenum	5 μg/L	[Not known]	95.9	μg/L × 10.4 = nmol/L	nmol/L × 0.096 = μg/L
Nickel	1.3 μg/L	[Not known]	58.7	μg/L × 17.0 = nmol/L	nmol/L × 0.059 = μg/L
(urine)	6 μg/L				
Selenium[e]	45–120 μg/L	400 μg/L	79.0	μg/L × 12.66 = nmol/L	nmol/L × 0.079 = μg/L
(urine)	30 μg/L				
	100 μg/L (occupational exposure)				
Silver (whole blood)	0.3 μg/L	[Not known]	107.9	μg/L × 9.27 = nmol/L	nmol/L × 0.108 = μg/L
(urine)	0.8 μg/L				
Strontium (serum)	30 μg/L	[Not known]	87.6	μg/L × 11.4 = nmol/L	nmol/L × 0.088 = μg/L
(urine)	300 μg/L				
Thallium (whole blood)[a]	2 μg/L	50 μg/L	204.4	μg/L × 4.89 = nmol/L	nmol/L × 0.204 = μg/L
(urine)	2 μg/L	200 μg/L			
Tungsten	35 μg/L	[Not known]	183.8	μg/L × 5.44 = nmol/L	nmol/L × 0.184 = μg/L
Vanadium	50 μg/L	[Not known]	50.9	μg/L × 19.6 = nmol/L	nmol/L × 0.051 = μg/L
(urine)	1 μg/L				
Zinc[e]	0.7–1.6 mg/L	5 mg/L	65.4	mg/L × 15.3 = μmol/L	μmol/L × 0.065 = mg/L
(urine)	0.3–0.6 mg/L				

Notes

a See also Table 9.1.

b Deutsche Forschungsgemeinschaft suggested 'action level' 1996.

c Recent ingestion of fish or shellfish renders total arsenic measurements uninterpretable.

d Toxicity of chromium dependent on oxidation state.

e True normal range – deficiency more common problem than poisoning, except in Wilson's disease when serious copper poisoning can occur at relatively low plasma copper concentrations because of ceruloplasmin deficiency.

Index

Note: page numbers in **bold** indicate tables; page numbers in *italic* indicate figures